# FACING the COSTS of LONG-TERM CARE

AN EBRI-ERF POLICY STUDY

By Robert B. Friedland

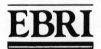

**EMPLOYEE BENEFIT RESEARCH INSTITUTE**

© 1990 Employee Benefit Research Institute
Education and Research Fund
2121 K Street, NW, Suite 600
Washington, DC 20037-2121
(202) 659-0670

**Library of Congress Cataloging-in-Publication Data**

Friedland, Robert Bruce
  Facing the costs of long-term care / by Robert B. Friedland

  p. cm.—(An EBRI-ERF policy study)
  Includes bibliographical references.
  ISBN 0–86643–056–3
  1. Long-term care of the sick—United States—Finance. 2. Aged—Long-term care—United States. 3. Insurance, Long-term care—United States. I. Title. II. Series.
RAA997.F75 1990                                                                89-23681
338.4'33621'60973—dc20                                                              CIP

Printed in the United States of America.

# Table of Contents

PART ONE
DEFINING LONG-TERM CARE

PART TWO
FINANCING LONG-TERM CARE

PART THREE
OPTIONS FOR REFORM

# List of Tables

# List of Charts

# Executive Summary

Restructuring the current financing, organization, and delivery of long-term care is one of the more serious challenges facing our society. Every day millions of Americans face the prospect of impoverishment and endure a physical and emotional struggle to provide or obtain assistance with basic needs. Millions more are at risk of needing help and not finding it or of not having the income and savings to afford that care for as long as the assistance is needed. While insurance is available for medical care and most other financial catastrophes—theft, fires, death during working years—there is a lack of widespread private or public insurance against the costs of long-term care.

The term *long-term care* encompasses the organization, delivery, and financing of a broad range of services and assistance to people with limited ability to function independently on a daily basis over a relatively long period. Assistance may be needed to eat or bathe, change clothes, use the toilet, get out of bed, or move about. Taking medications, managing money, or preparing meals may be impossible. This sort of assistance could be provided in a wide range of settings that includes not only the home but also day care centers, hospitals, clinics, and nursing homes.

Long-term care consists primarily of people caring for others. The technology associated with this care is much less sophisticated than that associated with acute health care. Chair and bed lifts, walkers, electronic monitoring devices, bathroom hand-rails, ramps, and similar devices can make a difference in the lives of those who need assistance. Most long-term care is provided by family and friends, neighbors, and volunteers. But the care and assistance that could be used to supplement and support informal care, or care that is necessary when there is no one else, is not always available.

Our current system of financing and delivering long-term care is fragmented and confusing. It does not encourage the identification and coordination of appropriate services. Efforts to coordinate this care in any systematic and efficient fashion are hampered by the somewhat contradictory effects of existing public programs that finance long-term care, which tend to encourage the use of nursing homes rather than to support strategies to keep people living independently at home.

The financial impoverishment required before a person can receive assistance from the state through the Medicaid program and the interest of federal regulators in minimizing expenditures have produced a system guided by eligibility rules that try to weed out the dishonest and reimbursement rules designed to minimize expenditures, rather than a system guided by the principles of good health care. Both Medicaid and Medicare finance relatively skilled care, discouraging the development of other kinds of services needed to help people remain independent.

Over the next century, the proportion of people at greatest risk of needing long-term care, relative to the proportion of people who can provide physical and financial assistance, will be much larger than it is now. Over the next 23 years—before the baby boom generation begins to enter the ranks of the elderly—the number of persons aged 65 or over is projected to increase 1.7 percent per year, while the population aged 85 or over is projected to increase at more than twice that rate, or 4.1 percent per year. By the time the entire baby boom generation has reached at least age 65 (in the year 2030), the elderly population will have increased by 141 percent, to more than 64.5 million people.

The number of elderly persons is increasing, and they are living longer. Thus, unless there is a substantial improvement in disease prevention or in curing chronic disabilities, a growing number of people are likely to be functionally dependent on others. More people will learn firsthand about our system of delivering and financing long-term care. The demand for long-term care assistance and for public policy change will increase, forcing real economic resources and political inquiry into the long-term care arena.

With or without change in the current organization and delivery of long-term care, the cost of this care is bound to increase. Whether resources will be allocated efficiently and fairly will depend in part on the timing and the nature of the public policy response. This response will be challenged by the demographic shift from a younger to an older America, which will affect employers, employees, and retirees. The shift in the population's age distribution will also have important implications for the financing of Social Security, Medicare, and Medicaid and will create a political imperative for change in the financing of long-term care. Moreover, because the shift is imminent, the window of opportunity for developing long-term care public policy options may never again be as wide open as it is today.

## The Risk and Consequences of Needing Long-Term Care

Medicine and technology have substantially reduced the risk of death from most acute infections. Death is now more likely to occur after medical conditions that may persist for years. This puts everyone at risk of needing assistance to perform essential daily activities or long-term care. Both the prevalence and consequently the risk of nonfatal strokes, heart disease, crippling arthritis, and degenerative brain disease increase with age, but people well under the age of 65 experience motor vehicle accidents; drug overdoses; illness such as multiple sclerosis, muscular dystrophy, and cerebral palsy; severe genetic abnormalities; and other health disorders.

Not everyone who needs long-term care is over the age of 65. In 1984, among people in the community reporting a need for assistance from others to function on a daily basis, less than one-half were elderly. Three quarters were aged 45 or over, but 12 percent were under age 15. Most nursing home residents are very old, but in 1985 nearly 12 percent were under age 65.

Fortunately, most people will never need extensive or expensive assistance. A rough estimate of the lifetime risk of entering a nursing home for a person aged 65 is 30 percent to 40 percent. More of us will be family members faced with the awesome responsibility of caring for a spouse, parent, or relative who needs long-term care. While not everyone will experience this situation, the costs can be staggering for those who do. Individuals who enter a nursing facility for longer than three months are likely never to return home.

While the risk of needing long-term care is relatively moderate, the costs are not. Nursing home costs exceed $25,000 a year, and those of home care for a similar level of assistance can be even greater. Saving for this contingency is very risky, since both the likelihood of needing care and the expected cost of that care are uncertain at best. Pooling the financial risk through insurance would be more efficient—yet insurance has only begun to be available. Many of the same factors that have inhibited the demand for insurance have plagued the development of an insurance market.

## Current Long-Term Care Financing

An estimated $56 billion, or more than 11 percent of all U.S. health care expenditures, was spent on long-term care in 1987. Most long-term care is paid directly by the people who receive assistance, their families, and public programs—particularly Medicaid. Medicare and private insurance were not major sources of financing for this care. Medicare's fundamental purpose is to cover acute and ambulatory care and recuperative care following an acute episode. With the exception of hospice arrangements, all nursing home and home health care covered by Medicare requires that the patient need skilled care. Medicaid does not require that the care be skilled or for recuperative purposes, and therefore covers most of the nursing home care that is publicly financed and a portion of the community-based programs. In 1987, slightly less than one-half (49.3 percent) of all nursing home care was paid directly by nursing home residents and their families; 43.8 percent was paid by Medicaid; 3.7 by federal, state, and local programs (other than Medicaid or Medicare); 1.5 percent by Medicare; 1 percent by private insurance; and 0.7 percent through philanthropic sources.

The lack of affordable private insurance alternatives to Medicaid for financing long-term care has encouraged the elderly to seek ways to become eligible for Medicaid. Paradoxically, the Medicaid program may make it even more difficult for private insurers to market coverage for catastrophic chronic care costs. Misconceptions about the coverage now provided by private health insurance plans, Medicare, and Medicaid and the failure to recognize the risk of high health care costs associated with aging may cause many people to minimize the probability of their needing long-term care and to assume that the financing will be available if it is needed. Some question this, arguing that surveys have found that few elderly are aware of Medicaid coverage.

Medicaid's preeminence in the financing of long-term care has influenced the form of available long-term care services and the way in which these services are delivered. For example, the program's limited coverage of home- or community-based services encourages the provision of care in nursing homes. Medicaid reimbursement policy, which prohibits states from paying nursing homes more than they charge privately paying residents, encourages a two-class system of care. Not all facilities accept Medicaid recipients, and those that do tend to prefer privately paying patients. Facilities that accept Medicaid patients have waiting lists for admission, while those that accept only privately paying patients are more likely to have beds readily available. Furthermore, since patients' assets must be exhausted before they become eligible for coverage, this loss of financial independence may mean that they are more likely to remain institutionalized until they die.

In recent years the private sector has responded to the growing number of elderly persons and to the increasing demand for long-term care and related services. There has been a surge in private insurance options, in particular long-term care insurance and continuing care communities. Over the past five years, private insurer interest in marketing coverage for long-term care has grown substantially. Most major insurers are now either marketing or testing a long-term care product. Whereas 5 or 6 years ago there were only about 12 companies selling long-term care insurance, today more than 100 companies sell this product, covering an estimated 1.3 million people. There are also demonstration projects that integrate insurance and the delivery of long-term care. One such approach—in the form of four social health maintenance organizations (S/HMOs)—extends the HMO model of acute care case management and prepaid financing to long-term care. In addition, a variety of local and federal demonstration programs enable individuals to access their home equity through reverse mortgages or sale leasebacks without leaving their home.

As insurers have learned more about the use of long-term care among policyholders, and as the market for long-term care has changed, insurance products have continued to evolve. Products released today are very different from those offered just a few years ago. Newer policies no longer include many of the restrictions that were imposed on the first products, such as requiring a prior hospitalization before nursing homes are covered or a prior stay in a skilled nursing facility before home health care is covered. In addition, these policies are more likely to have lifetime benefits, rather than benefits that are limited to three or four years, and to provide the opportunity to increase benefits as nursing home costs increase.

Perhaps even more remarkable is the fact that employers have become interested in sponsoring long-term care insurance for employees and their families. Prior to 1987 there were no employer-sponsored policies. By September 1989 at least 35 employers were in the process of offering access to long-term care insurance. An employee's spouse, parents, and parents-in-law are usually eligible to apply for a policy. Employment-based group products have several advantages over individually marketed policies. Because of lower marketing costs, efficiencies in administration, and a reduced likelihood of adverse selection (i.e., the purchase of insurance mainly by those who know in advance that they will be filing a claim), group-marketed long-term care insurance policies are 20 percent to 30 percent less expensive than individually marketed policies. Employees also save by having their employer conduct the search for the best policy. As employers explicitly recognize the importance of long-term care insurance, employees are likely to become aware of the value of this protection, creating even further market expansion.

## The Potential for Private Long-Term Care Insurance

Except for long-term care, insurance is widely held for most of life's contingencies. The feasibility of private long-term care insurance is central to the public policy debate over financing long-term care. The failure of the private market to sell insurance to a large and diverse segment of the population is an important argument for a policy of mandated private insurance, publicly provided insurance, or public financing of long-term care.

The emergence and design of long-term care insurance policies have been influenced by a variety of related factors. Weak market demand, with relatively little tax and regulatory influence, has left policy design to insurers without much input from consumers and legislators. Without strong signals from consumers and adequate data, insurers have found themselves struggling to find marketable products that do not jeopardize their companies' financial health.

Convincing consumers of the financial risk of long-term care has been the most fundamental barrier to the development of long-term care insurance. Public policy can go a long way toward encouraging the demand side and shaping the supply side of the long-term care market. The tax code can be used to call attention to the importance of long-term care insurance. If consumer demand and competition among insurers do not ensure that all policies provide adequate benefits, public policy can intervene by establishing minimum standards with respect to the benefits and the terms under which policies can be sold, using tax incentives or through direct regulation. Public policy can also protect consumers from the consequences of insurer insolvency by establishing financial standards, requiring specific levels of reinsurance, or establishing a public reinsurance program.

Public assistance, to assist the expansion of the private long-term care insurance market, must recognize three policy issues. First, there is no guarantee that the insurance benefit will be sufficient to guarantee access to needed care 20 to 40 years after a policy is purchased. Second, there is no guarantee that an insurer or a policy will still exist when benefits are needed. And third, there seems to be no easy way to ensure a policy's portability or to exchange the prefunded portion of one policy for another.

## The Importance of Long-Term Care to Employers

A public-private partnership exists for most aspects of economic security—again with the exception of long-term care—with employers playing a significant role. Employers provide 65 percent of the

U.S. population with access to group health insurance. Ninety percent of full-time workers in medium-sized and large establishments had employer-provided health insurance in 1988; 45 percent of these employees had coverage that continued after retirement. Among all of the full-time employees, 80 percent had a pension plan.

Like employer-provided health insurance, employer-sponsored long-term care insurance has the potential to increase the share of privately financed long-term care. Several factors have inhibited the development of long-term care insurance as an employee benefit, however. First, it is unlikely that long-term care can be added to employee compensation without modifying the current benefit structure. Second, employers are not likely to offer to pay for new benefits when there is so much uncertainty about the costs and liabilities. Third, long-term care is not offered the same preferential tax treatment as other nonwage employee benefits.

A dollar in compensation used to purchase a qualified, tax-exempt employee benefit is worth more than a dollar to the employee because it is not included in his or her taxable income. Because it is unclear how long-term care insurance would be treated in the tax code, a dollar used by the employer to purchase long-term care insurance may have to be reported by the employee as a dollar of taxable income. Employee contributions toward the premium would not necessarily count as tax-deductible medical expenses. In addition, benefits received when a claim is filed may have to be included as taxable income.

A growing proportion of the labor force consists of working mothers, which has resulted in a continuing preoccupation with day care arrangements for dependents. However, for a growing number and proportion of workers the dependents are chronically ill parents or spouses rather than children. Employers are likely to come under increased pressure to accommodate these concerns. As members of the baby boom generation advance to senior positions in their firms while providing long-term care at home, employers are more likely to consider the actual and potential needs of their employees as caregivers. A growing share of employees may be willing to see their compensation restructured to include some form of long-term care insurance or elder care benefits. As more employers begin to recognize the importance of long-term care, they may become willing to restructure their employee compensation packages to include the purchase of long-term care insurance. Failure to make this adjustment, however, is likely to intensify pressure on the government to establish or expand public programs or to mandate that employers provide this sort of assistance.

# Altering the Public-Private Partnership

Long-term care is currently funded through a combination of public and private financing. While the public and private dollars may be approximately equal, the distribution of the financing burden is not. Most private expenditures for long-term care are paid directly by those who receive the care. On the other hand, most public expenditures for financing long-term care are derived from general revenues. The public policy discussion generally focuses on two aspects of this financing: the issues stemming from the fairness of the patient-based private financing arrangement and the rising cost of publicly financed long-term health care. Despite this dichotomy of concerns, most public action has focused on limiting public program expenditures at the expense of those who need long-term care.

Over the last 10 years, public debate over long-term care financing has shifted away from issues concerning the delivery of care to the question of who should pay. The debate has also shifted toward a private-sector solution because of a heightened awareness of the emerging long-term care cost burden, the acceptance of increasingly tight fiscal constraints, and overall improvements in the elderly's financial position.

The case for using public policy to encourage private financing options for long-term care is based on the argument that the private market can distribute resources and satisfy diverse needs more efficiently. The private market, it is asserted, has been slow to emerge due to inhibiting market barriers. This has led to a call for public intervention to assist in removing these barriers. Government activities that could assist in market development include conducting an educational campaign to encourage demand for long-term care insurance, clarifying or altering tax laws or other laws governing the market, developing a reinsurance program for private insurance, or collecting data to assist in the pricing and development of a private market.

Private insurance is not likely to be affordable or available to many members of the current elderly population. Consequently, it remains to be seen how quickly this market will expand. The best hope for the expansion of the private market for future elderly persons lies in the growing availability of employment-based long-term care insurance. While there is great potential for this market, it must be kept in mind that many workers are still without basic health insurance. More than 80 percent of the uninsured in 1986 were employees or the dependents of full-time workers.

The case for expanding public financing of long-term care through a social insurance or Medicare-like approach is made on the grounds that social insurance can provide universal coverage to all who qualify and the costs can be shared by all taxpayers, based on individual ability to pay, through income taxes, or by workers, through payroll taxes. Administrative economies can be easily realized, and any cost problems associated with adverse selection can be avoided if the program is widely accepted or is mandatory. A universal entitlement program could lessen the differences in access to and quality of care between private paying patients and Medicaid recipients. Unlike private insurance, a social insurance approach could be used to meet other objectives, such as redistributing income, and it could be financed in a variety of ways, including a pay-as-you-go basis.

Regardless of the public policy response, the number of elderly persons will increase in relation to the number of nonelderly and more families will learn firsthand about the current state of the delivery and financing of long-term care. As more people need long-term care, its financial consequences are expected to increase. As more workers, taxpayers, and voters learn about long-term care financing and delivery, the pressure for change is certain to grow. As employers respond to employees who are also caregivers, employers will also learn more and may decide to seek ways to assist future retirees with the financing. The challenge will be to find ways to develop a delivery system that meets the needs of all dependent people and their families and that can make the most effective use of the resources available in each community.

# Foreword

The United States is experiencing a profound demographic shift in the age distribution of its population. The elderly—in particular, persons aged 85 or over—are the fastest growing age group. The aging of our nation's population means that more people are likely to need assistance with simple—but necessary—daily activities that most of us take for granted. In fact, the need for this assistance—known as long-term care—is not unique to the elderly.

Robert B. Friedland, senior research associate at the Employee Benefit Research Institute (EBRI) and the author of this study, estimates that long-term care cost the United States $56 billion in 1987. While government programs—primarily Medicaid, the welfare program for the poor—pay nearly one-half of the cost of care that is purchased, the elderly and their families finance the other half directly from their income and assets. As more people become functionally dependent, the nation's bill for long-term care will increase, raising concern about how escalating costs may affect access to care.

The issue of *who* should pay for long-term care is underscored when the number of persons who are neither willing nor able to pay is considered. In a July 1989 nationwide poll conducted for EBRI by the Gallup Organization, more than one-half of the individuals surveyed said that they would not be willing or able to pay $100 per month— in either insurance premiums or taxes—for access to long-term care; 65 percent of these said that they would not be willing or able to pay $50 a month. The question of who should pay for care has emerged as a major public policy issue, as witnessed by the unrelenting pressure placed upon Congress by many elderly persons to repeal the Medicare Catastrophic Coverage Act of 1988 (MCCA)—which would have required Medicare beneficiaries themselves, primarily those with higher incomes, to finance expanded benefits for all participants. On November 22, 1989, Congress voted to repeal MCCA, with many members who supported repeal calling for a newly expanded program in 1990. We have retained all discussion of the now-repealed act in the belief that repeal will focus renewed attention on long-term care, and that it is important to understand what MCCA *would* and *would not* have done with respect to long-term care.

As a result of these personal and financial challenges, long-term care is becoming a concern of employers as well as public-policy makers. Employers and their employees participate in the financing of long-term care primarily through taxes that support the

Medicaid program. Employers realize that many employees—primarily women, who make up an increasingly large share of the labor force—bear much of the responsibility of caring for an elderly relative in addition to working; some of them are still raising their children. What are the implications for an employer when an employee is physically, emotionally, and perhaps financially stretched thin?

A small but increasing number of employers have responded by making long-term care insurance available to employees and their family members. But the market for private long-term care insurance is still developing, and its growth as an employment-based benefit may be impeded by the cost of insurance and by uncertainty about the income tax status of both the premiums paid on an employee's behalf and the benefits received from such a policy.

With the publication of *Facing the Costs of Long-Term Care*, EBRI continues its longstanding commitment to the timely, thorough, and accurate analysis of public policy employee benefit issues. This study is a valuable resource for experts in the field as well as for anyone seeking to understand the many issues related to long-term care. Friedland examines the nation's changing demographics and the implications for employers, public programs, and current and future employees and retirees; the factors that contribute to the risk of needing long-term care and financial assistance; and the organization, delivery, and financing of long-term care and the restructuring that may be necessary to meet future demands. He analyzes the current long-term care insurance market, including its potential for growth and the prospects for coverage through employers and group arrangements, and concludes with an exploration of how the public and private sectors may work together to ensure that long-term care is both accessible and affordable to the increasing numbers of Americans at risk.

Funding for this study was provided by the sponsors of EBRI and by grants to the EBRI Education and Research Fund from the Atlantic Richfield Foundation, the Southwestern Bell Foundation, the Travelers Foundation, and the American Association of Retired Persons.

The views expressed in this book are solely those of the author and should not be ascribed to those whose assistance is acknowledged or to the officers, trustees, members, or other sponsors of EBRI, its Education and Research Fund, or their staffs.

DALLAS L. SALISBURY
President
Employee Benefit Research Institute
January 1990

# Preface

*Though much is taken, much abides; and though*
*We are not now that strength which in days*
*Moved earth and heaven, that which we are we are;*
*One equal temper of heroic hearts,*
*Made weak by time and fate, but strong in will*
*To strive, to seek, to find, and not to yield.*

—Alfred, Lord Tennyson, *Ulysses*

The Board of Trustees of the Employee Benefit Research Institute (EBRI) showed considerable foresight in 1986 when they directed the Institute to initiate this study. At that time private long-term care insurance was virtually nonexistent. Insurers were skeptical at best, and employers were not even considered a potential source of organizing the financing of long-term care. Since that time, the question of how to organize, deliver, and pay for long-term care has received considerable attention. Today, all large insurers are actively marketing long-term care insurance policies on a nationwide basis. Perhaps as many as 35 employers are in the process of organizing access to long-term care insurance for their employees, their employees' spouses, and even the parents and in-laws of their employees.

The move to expand Medicare coverage, which culminated in the Medicare Catastrophic Coverage Act of 1988, fell short of covering what most elderly fear the most—the need for long-term care. The expansion, however, contained a fundamental change in the way Medicare was to be financed. The additional Medicare benefits were to be financed by the elderly and to be apportioned, in part, by their ability to pay. In conjunction with a basic misunderstanding of both the new benefits and the additional premiums, a coalition of the elderly expressed their displeasure with this fundamental change in Medicare financing. The size of the wake following this legislation caught many by surprise; but one year after its passage, Congress found itself embroiled in a fight over whether to repeal or substantially change the law. Some have suggested that this legislative episode will discourage Congress from considering expanding Medicare to include long-term care. The political lesson, however, may be that expanded benefits must be financed by everyone and that the benefits must be apparent to the potential beneficiaries.

I am deeply indebted to the many people who assisted in the development and production of this book. It could not have been written without the help of Charles Betley, who provided primary research assistance by checking the accuracy and providing invaluable comments and suggestions for every aspect of this study. Assistance was also provided by Elizabeth Owen, who helped to check facts, prepare tables and charts, and compile the bibliography. The research was supported by computer programming provided by Kevin Ward and Jeannette Lee. Jennifer Davis and Wendy Schick also assisted with data analysis and presentation. Diane Stamm significantly improved the clarity of the text with her thorough editing; Deborah Holmes, Stephanie Poe, and Bonnie Newton provided a final editorial review and facilitated the book's production. Mary Catherine Calvert carefully corrected each draft throughout the editing process, and Christine Dolan made everything more accessible by preparing the subject index. Of course, any errors that remain are mine.

Grants from the Atlantic Richfield Foundation, the Southwestern Bell Foundation, the American Association of Retired Persons, and the Travelers Foundation helped to make this study possible. I would like to extend special thanks to the members of the EBRI Work Group on Financing Long-Term Care and the EBRI Research Committee (listed at the end of this preface) for their encouragement, expert guidance, and comments on various drafts. Special mention should be made of the assistance of Bruce Boyd, Kim Bellard, Paul Jackson, Nancy Wanet, Craig Campbell, William Henkel, and Joseph Hollander. Furthermore, the comments of Susan Van Gelder, Emily Andrews, Nancy Saltford, Jack Kittredge, Rick Brandon, and Tom McGuire also helped to significantly improve the final manuscript.

I would also like to thank my colleagues at the Pepper Commission (the U.S. Bipartisan Commission on Comprehensive Health Care) for the opportunity to test and discuss these issues in a very serious way as we prepared staff papers and briefing materials for the Commissioners. Finally, I wish to thank my wife, Melissa, for her patience and her assistance, especially in understanding the medical care needs associated with long-term care.

This book is dedicated to all those who have experienced the anguish and frustration of caring for a loved one who is dependent on others. May our children face a more rational and humane system for delivering long-term care.

ROBERT B. FRIEDLAND, PH. D.
January 1990

# EBRI Work Group on Financing Long-Term Care

John Morgan
The Union Labor Life
   Insurance Company

Al Morgen
Howard Johnson &
   Company

Warren Moser
United Health Care

Gino A. Nalli
The Wyatt Company

Allan C. Northcutt
Southwestern Bell
   Corporation

Robert Paul
Martin E. Segal
   Company

Will Poole
National Rural
   Electric Cooperative
   Association

Melvyn Rodrigues
Atlantic Richfield
   Company

Rich Sanes
Godwins Inc.

Gail P. Schaeffer
John Hancock Mutual
   Life Insurance
   Company

Russell F. Schuck
IBM Corporation

Robert Schumacher
Abbott Laboratories

Frank Sena
CIGNA

Stephanie Sottile
Blue Cross and Blue
   Shield Association

Nancy Wanet
Aetna Life & Casualty

James F. Weil
Metropolitan Life
   Insurance Company

Thomas Woodruff
Mutual of America Life
   Insurance Company

Martin H. Zuckerman
Manufacturers
   Hanover Trust
   Company

# About the Author

Robert B. Friedland, Ph.D., is a senior research associate at the Employee Benefit Research Institute (EBRI), where he conducts and directs public policy research related to private health insurance and public health care financing. Since May 1989, he has served as staff economist for the U.S. Bipartisan Commission on Comprehensive Health Care (the Pepper Commission), helping to develop the commission's report and recommendations on access to health care and long-term care, which is expected to be released in March 1990.

Prior to joining EBRI in 1985, Friedland was senior economist for Maryland's Medical Care Programs, Department of Health and Mental Hygiene; assistant professor of economics in the School of Business and Economics at Towson State University; and a fellow at the National Institute on Aging. He has written and lectured extensively on private and public health insurance coverage, health care costs, and employee and retiree health and welfare benefit plans. Friedland received his Ph.D. in economics from the George Washington University in 1983.

# PART ONE
# DEFINING LONG-TERM CARE

# I. Background and Issues

## Introduction

The term *long-term care* encompasses the organization, delivery, and financing of a broad range of services and assistance to people who are severely limited in their ability to function independently on a daily basis over a relatively long period of time.[1] Functional dependency can result from either physical or mental limitations and is defined in terms of the inability to perform essential activities of daily living (ADLs), such as eating, bathing, dressing, using the toilet, getting into or out of bed, and moving about the house, or activities necessary to remain independent, known as instrumental activities of daily living (IADLs), such as shopping, cooking, doing laundry, managing household finances, and housekeeping.

Long-term care services and technologies can be provided in a wide range of settings. Most care is provided informally by family, friends, neighbors, and volunteers. Care is also provided formally at home through home health care agencies or other community-based services, at adult day care centers, by individuals hired on an independent basis, and through institutions such as nursing homes. Home health care services and adult day care centers can be based in hospitals, clinics, hospices, or nursing homes. Services required by those who need long-term care include skilled nursing care, such as changing catheters or administering medications; physical and occupational therapy; personal care services, such as assistance with bathing, dressing, walking, eating, and using the toilet; counseling; case management or coordination; homemaker services, such as light housekeeping, meal preparation, and shopping; supervision; monitoring; and transportation.

The current system of financing and delivering long-term care is fragmented and confusing. It does not encourage the identification and coordination of appropriate services. Each source of financing has its own complicated and often confusing rules for eligibility and may cover different types of long-term care. Consequently, because the health care system is so fragmented, it is difficult for families to

---

[1]There is no accepted definition of "a relatively long period of time." The 1982 and 1984 National Long-Term Care Surveys defined chronically disabled elderly as those whose limitations had persisted or were expected to persist for at least 90 days.

coordinate the type of care they need. It is difficult for an individual to have all of his or her needs met in one setting, and providers have little incentive to coordinate delivery of services with each other. This fragmentation hinders efficient and cost-effective care.

Until recently, there were few long-term care insurance options that spread financial risk. These products and others (including life care communities and social health maintenance organizations) have been marketed primarily to older people because they are most likely to need long-term care. Most older Americans had not anticipated saving for this insurance and, as a result, the premiums are likely to be higher than many can afford. Even fewer are able to pay for long-term care itself. Most elderly people and their families have little choice but to hope that they do not fall victim to a chronic disability.[2]

While most long-term care is provided informally by family and friends, not all care is provided this way. Care that is purchased is usually paid for directly by patients and their families. The cost of nursing home care, which averaged $22,000 a year in 1985, varies considerably and in some areas may exceed $50,000 a year. In 1987, nursing home residents or their families paid 49 percent of the cost of this care. Medicaid, which provides health care to specific groups of the very poor, is the chief public financer of nursing home care, paying for nearly 44 percent of all such care in 1985. Medicare financed less than 2 percent, and private insurance paid for about 1 percent (chart I.1).

Long-term care expenditures for home- and community-based services are most likely to be paid directly by users. About one-half of home health care expenditures, but very few of the other community-based services, were financed through public programs in 1988. About one-half of all long-term care expenditures for nursing home and home- and community-based care were financed through public programs, mostly Medicaid, while the remainder were paid primarily by those in need of assistance and their families.[3]

This bifurcation of expenditures has engendered contradictory and sometimes perverse incentives. The financial impoverishment required before a nursing home resident can apply for Medicaid assistance encourages people to protect their assets by transferring money or property prior to their illness, or by divorcing, under false pretenses,

---

[2]Throughout this book the term *elderly* refers to people aged 65 or over. It should be noted that the term encompasses a diverse population born over a 35-year period. Similarly, the term *baby boom* will refer to people born between 1945 and 1964, a period of 19 years.

[3]Details on these expenditures are included in chapter IV.

4

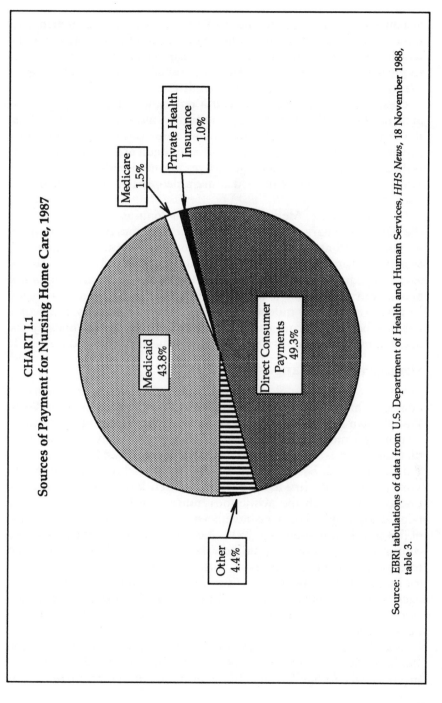

**CHART I.1**

**Sources of Payment for Nursing Home Care, 1987**

Medicare
1.5%

Private Health
Insurance
1.0%

Medicaid
43.8%

Direct Consumer
Payments
49.3%

Other
4.4%

Source: EBRI tabulations of data from U.S. Department of Health and Human Services, *HHS News*, 18 November 1988, table 3.

a spouse who is in a nursing home. Federal regulators seem primarily interested in thwarting and minimizing expenditures. State regulators have similar interests, but they also try to shift as many state services as possible into their Medicaid program to get federal participation while minimizing state expenditures.

These incentives have produced a delivery system guided not by principles of health care but by eligibility rules that try to weed out the dishonest and by reimbursement rules designed to minimize expenditures. In addition, Medicaid and Medicare finance relatively skilled care. This bias has discouraged development of the kinds of long-term care services needed to help people live independently at home.

The dominance of Medicaid in financing long-term care encourages the delivery of care in nursing homes despite individual and family preferences to avoid such care. Most elderly people do not receive assistance from Medicaid until after they have entered a nursing home and have exhausted their savings. Once their resources are gone, some people may not be able to afford to leave the facility because they are no longer financially independent. To compound matters, the people likely to be on Medicaid usually have little or no say in choosing the particular nursing facility that is likely to become their home.

## Demographic Changes

America is growing older, owing in large part to three concurrent demographic trends. First, large groups of people born prior to World War II have reached age 65. Second, advances in sanitation, public health, and medical technology and changes in individual lifestyle, diet, and exercise have led to substantial increases in life expectancy. Third, there has been, except for the two decades following World War II, a steady decline in the proportion of children in the population. Consequently, both the absolute number and the percentage of the population aged 65 or over have been increasing and the percentage of the population under age 16 has been decreasing. At the turn of the century, 4 percent of the total population, or 3.1 million people aged 65 or older, were counted in the census; by 1980 more than 11 percent (or 25.5 million) were counted (Zopf, 1986). The number of Americans aged 65 or over is now estimated to exceed 29.8 million and to represent more than 12 percent of the total population (Bureau of the Census, 1988d).

Since before the turn of the century, people have been living longer. Between 1900 and 1985, life expectancy at birth increased by 28 years (from age 47 to age 75) and life expectancy at age 65 increased by nearly 5 years (age 77 to age 82) (chart I.2). In 1900, median age at death was 55.2 years for men and 58.2 years for women. In 1985, median age at death was 74.7 years for men and 82.4 years for women. For men aged 65 in 1985, life expectancy since 1900 has increased 3.2 years, and for women, 7 years. By the year 2025, it is estimated that life expectancy for 65-year-olds will be approximately 20 years.

Since the turn of the 19th century, with the exception of the period from 1945 to 1957, fertility rates (the number of children born to each woman) have been declining. The general fertility rate declined by one-half between 1800 and 1910, and then fell again by one-half between 1910 and 1980 (Fuchs, 1983). Live births per 1,000 women aged 15 to 44 were approximately 130 in 1900, 117.9 by 1920, and 79.9 by 1940.[4] In 1986, the fertility rate was 64.9 (National Center for Health Statistics, 1987a). From 1945 to 1957, fertility rates increased dramatically, peaking at 122.9 in 1957, but this was still lower than the rates prior to 1900. By 1964, however, fertility rates had returned to the level implied by the trend prior to 1945. The "boom" of children born between 1945 and 1964 added 76 million people to the population—the equivalent of the entire U.S. population in 1900 (Pifer, 1986).

Chart I.3 shows estimates of *total* fertility rates from 1940 to 1985. Total fertility rates estimate how many children a woman is likely to have by the end of her reproductive cycle. Slight upward movements in the total fertility rate since 1972 probably reflect the decision of families to delay having children, but these increases are not likely to affect the declining birth rate.[5] In 1970, total fertility was 2.5 births

---

[4]Live births per 1,000 women aged 15–44 are used to calculate fertility rates rather than births per 1,000 people, or the crude birth rate, to account for changes in the number of women of childbearing age as a proportion of the population (Bureau of the Census, 1975, p. 49, series B5-10).

[5]Whether fertility rates will continue to decline is a matter of some controversy. Most experts believe that fertility rates will not increase substantially. Butz et al. (1982) suggest that when fewer women are in the labor force, the relationship between fertility rates and family income is cyclical. That is, when family income is rising, fertility rates are likely to increase, and when family income declines, fertility rates are likely to fall. In contrast, when more women are in the labor market, the relationship between family income and fertility is no longer simple and is probably counter-cyclical. As family income rises, fertility rates may not increase because the forgone income due to childbearing (and rearing) is greater. If family income is falling, fertility rates could rise, since the cost of forgone income has fallen.

This relatively simple view fits the data quite well (Butz et al., 1982). The economic recessions of 1954 and 1957, a time when relatively few women were in the labor force, were accompanied by declines in fertility rates. However, the prolonged expansion of the 1960s occurred during a time when more women were entering the labor market, and while family income increased fertility rates declined. At the time of the 1970 recession, a substantial number of women were already in the labor market, and

per 1,000 women; by 1983, it was 27 percent lower at 1.81 births per 1,000 women. In 1984, the rate per 1,000 women edged up slightly, and by 1985 it reached 1.84 (chart I.3).

The baby boomers, born between 1945 and 1964, were between the ages of 25 and 44 in 1988 and represent approximately 33 percent of the entire U.S. population (Bureau of the Census, 1988d). This group has already left its mark as its members passed through school, entered the labor market, purchased their first homes, and started to raise families. This has had a relatively dramatic effect on the educational system, the labor market, capital formation, the housing market, and the market for all other goods and services. Parents of baby boomers are now approaching ages at which they are at greatest risk for needing long-term care, which is likely to affect the expectations of this generation. When the baby boom group begins to retire, unless changing expectations alter the delivery of long-term care, the capacity of the system, along with the retirement income and health care systems, will be tested, much as the educational system and the labor market have been.[6]

However, the process will be gradual, for the baby boom generation is likely to retire over a 25-year period, beginning in the year 2004. In

---

fertility rates increased with the decline in family income. During the 1974 and 1982 recessions, family income declined and the fertility rate increased, but only slightly.

Despite this cyclical pattern, however, Easterlin suggests that the fertility rate is likely to increase over time. He hypothesizes that fertility is dependent on family income relative to financial aspirations and expectations—meeting or exceeding aspirations tends to increase fertility (Fuchs, 1983). If incomes do not support aspirations, couples will perceive themselves as badly off (regardless of their actual standing) and have fewer children. Aspirations, he argues, are based on the incomes of each family's parents.

The expansion following World War II and the stagflation of the 1970s suggests this theory can explain the baby boom and the baby bust phenomena; but the theory does not lend itself to rigorous statistical testing owing to the difficulties of expressing aspirations quantitatively. Nevertheless, Easterlin predicts that when the children born during the 1960s and 1970s reach adulthood, there will be another baby boom. This boom will not be as big as the first one, however, and should occur sometime between 1990 and the year 2000.

In two of their three sets of projections, the Social Security Administration actuaries assume that fertility rates will generally increase over the 75-year projection period. From an estimated 1.87 in 1987, total fertility is assumed to increase in 1988 to 1.88 under the "optimistic" alternative I assumptions and to 1.87 under the "intermediate" alternatives II-A and II-B assumptions (*Annual Report*, 1988b). Under the "pessimistic" alternative III assumptions total fertility is expected to decline to 1.86 in 1988. The pessimistic assumptions assume that total fertility will continue to decline, reaching 1.60 in the year 2020. Under the intermediate assumptions it continues to rise, reaching 1.90 in the year 2020, while under the optimistic assumptions it will reach 2.20.

[6]For more discussion of this phenomenon, see, for example, Russell, 1982; Fullerton, 1985; and "The Big Chill (Revisited)," 1985.

8

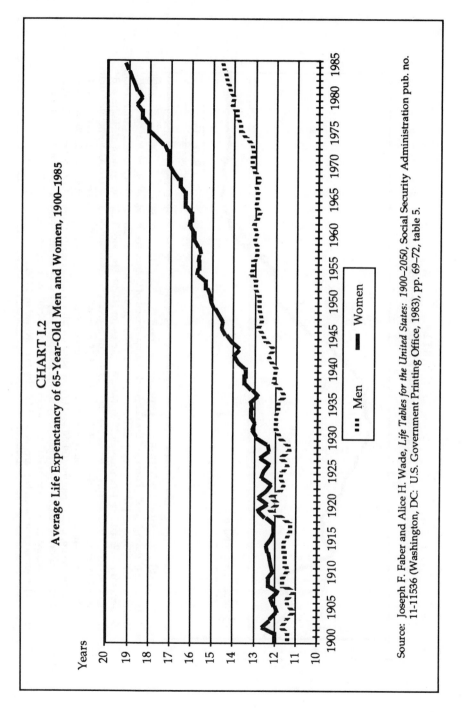

**CHART I.2**

**Average Life Expenctancy of 65-Year-Old Men and Women, 1900–1985**

Years

Men

Women

Source: Joseph F. Faber and Alice H. Wade, *Life Tables for the United States: 1900–2050*, Social Security Administration pub. no. 11-11536 (Washington, DC: U.S. Government Printing Office, 1983), pp. 69–72, table 5.

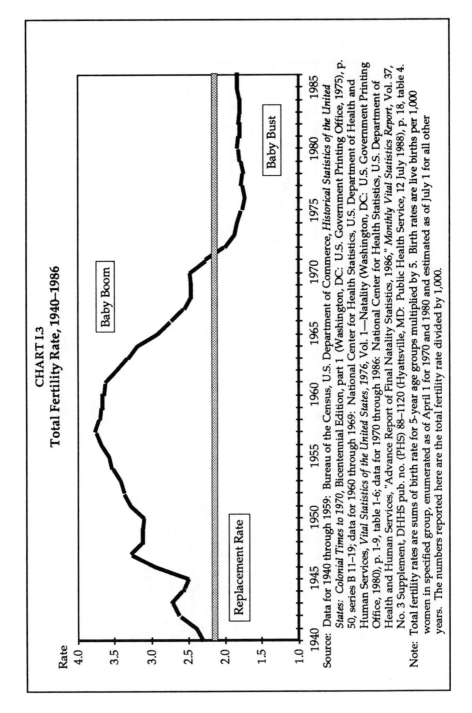

**CHART I.3**
**Total Fertility Rate, 1940–1986**

Baby Boom

Baby Bust

Replacement Rate

Rate
4.0
3.5
3.0
2.5
2.0
1.5
1.0

1940   1945   1950   1955   1960   1965   1970   1975   1980   1985

Source:   Data for 1940 through 1959:  Bureau of the Census, U.S. Department of Commerce, *Historical Statistics of the United States: Colonial Times to 1970*, Bicentennial Edition, part 1 (Washington, DC:  U.S. Government Printing Office, 1975), p. 50, series B 11–19; data for 1960 through 1969:  National Center for Health Statistics, U.S. Department of Health and Human Services, *Vital Statistics of the United States, 1976*, Vol. 1—Natality (Washington, DC:  U.S. Government Printing Office, 1980), p. 1-9, table 1-6; data for 1970 through 1986: National Center for Health Statistics, U.S. Department of Health and Human Services, "Advance Report of Final Natality Statistics, 1986," *Monthly Vital Statistics Report*, Vol. 37, No. 3 Supplement, DHHS pub. no. (PHS) 88–1120 (Hyattsville, MD:  Public Health Service, 12 July 1988). p. 18, table 4.

Note:   Total fertility rates are sums of birth rate for 5-year age groups multiplied by 5.  Birth rates are live births per 1,000 women in specified group, enumerated as of April 1 for 1970 and 1980 and estimated as of July 1 for all other years.  The numbers reported here are the total fertility rate divided by 1,000.

the year 2022, only one-half of the baby boomers will be aged 65 or over, but none will be more than 77 years old. By the year 2030, however, all baby boomers will be aged 65 or over, and some will be as old as 85. However, the percentage of the population aged 65 or over is already increasing, while the percentage of the population under age 16 is decreasing.

Just before the oldest baby boomers reach age 65, the elderly population is expected to approach 14 percent of the total U.S. population. The Census Bureau projects that in the year 2020, when less than one-half of the baby boomers are likely to be aged 65 or older, the elderly will have nearly doubled their current size and will represent nearly 18 percent of the population. In the year 2030, when almost all of the baby boomers will have reached age 65, there will be 120 percent more elderly people than there are today—or almost 65 million, representing 22 percent of the population.

Declining fertility rates since the baby boom have produced smaller population cohorts: the "baby bust" generation—the relatively small number of babies born since 1960—and the "birth dearth" generation of children born since 1972 (Wattenberg, 1987). Since 1972, total fertility rates have been lower than that necessary to maintain a "steady state" population. Many thought that the baby bust would be short-lived due to a tendency toward delayed childbearing, but so far the expected boom from this delay has not materialized. By 1972, total fertility rates had declined to below the replacement rate. Since then, total fertility rates have been less than the replacement rate (2.11 per 1,000 women).

## The Growing Elderly Population: Creating a Political Imperative

The elderly, and especially those aged 85 or over, are the fastest growing age group in the United States (table I.1). They represent a large political constituency as well as a large component of the long-term care market, and much of the political importance of long-term care stems from their growing number. Over the next 23 years—before the baby boom generation begins to enter the ranks of the elderly—the number of persons aged 65 or older is projected to increase 1.7 percent per year, while the population aged 85 or older is projected to increase at more than twice that rate, 4.1 percent per year. By the time the entire baby boom generation has reached at least age 65 (in the year 2030), the elderly population will have increased by 141 percent to more than 64.5 million people. By the year 2050, when all of the baby boomers will have reached age 85, the number of people

## TABLE I.1
## Older Americans in the Total Population, Actual and Projected, 1900–2080

| Year | Aged 65 or over | | Aged 85 or over | | Total |
| | Number (in thousands) | Percentage of total population | Number (in thousands) | Percentage of total population | Population (in thousands) |
|---|---|---|---|---|---|
| 1900 | 3,084 | 4.0% | 123 | 0.2% | 76,303 |
| 1910 | 3,950 | 4.3 | 167 | 0.2 | 91,972 |
| 1920 | 4,933 | 4.7 | 210 | 0.2 | 105,711 |
| 1930 | 6,634 | 5.4 | 272 | 0.2 | 122,775 |
| 1940 | 9,019 | 6.8 | 365 | 0.3 | 131,669 |
| 1950 | 12,270 | 8.1 | 577 | 0.4 | 150,967 |
| 1960 | 16,675 | 9.2 | 940 | 0.5 | 180,671 |
| 1970 | 20,107 | 9.8 | 1,430 | 0.7 | 205,053 |
| 1980 | 25,704 | 11.3 | 2,269 | 1.0 | 227,758 |
| 1985 | 28,540 | 11.9 | 2,695 | 1.1 | 239,279 |
| 1987 | 29,835 | 12.2 | 2,867 | 1.2 | 243,913 |
| 1990 | 31,559 | 12.6 | 3,254 | 1.3 | 250,410 |
| 2000 | 34,882 | 13.0 | 4,622 | 1.7 | 268,267 |
| 2010 | 39,362 | 13.9 | 6,115 | 2.2 | 282,574 |
| 2020 | 52,067 | 17.7 | 6,651 | 2.3 | 294,364 |
| 2030 | 65,604 | 21.8 | 8,129 | 2.7 | 300,629 |
| 2040 | 68,109 | 22.6 | 12,251 | 4.1 | 301,807 |
| 2050 | 68,532 | 22.9 | 15,287 | 5.1 | 299,848 |
| 2080 | 71,631 | 24.5 | 16,966 | 5.8 | 292,235 |

Source: Special Committee on Aging, Senate, U.S. Congress, *Aging America: Trends and Projections*, 1987–88 ed. (Washington, DC: U.S. Department of Health and Human Services, 1988), p. 12, table 1–2; and Bureau of the Census, U.S. Department of Commerce, "Projections of the Population of the United States, by Age, Sex, and Race: 1988 to 2080," *Current Population Reports*, Population Estimates and Projections, Series P-25, no. 1018 (Washington, DC: U.S. Government Printing Office, 1989), p. 7, table F.

aged 85 or older is expected to represent 5.2 percent of the entire population and 24 percent of the elderly.

Whatever problems exist in the current financing and delivery of long-term care are likely to be exacerbated by the shifting age structure of the U.S. population. Furthermore, as the age structure shifts, so will the opportunities to change the system. In part this is seen in the changing composition of ratios of potential dependents. Over the next 65 years, the proportion of people of primary working age (those aged 18 to 64) to children under age 18 and adults over age 65 will increase gradually as the last of the baby boomers enter their prime working years (chart I.4). The ratio of potential dependents to the working age population will decline from 0.62 to 1 in 1985 to 0.58 to 1 in the year 2010—a level similar to that of the decade prior to 1945. As the baby boom generation begins to retire, this ratio increases rapidly, reaching 0.75 to 1 in the year 2035, when more than 21 percent of the U.S. population is expected to be aged 65 or older and 5 percent is expected to be aged 85 or older.

Although referred to as a "dependency ratio," the ratio actually exaggerates the extent of dependency across generations. It does not adjust for employment among "dependents"; the lifetime accumulation of assets, including vested pensions, held by individuals aged 65 or older; healthy people aged 65 or older or sick people younger than age 65; or the trend toward earlier retirement.

In the 80 years depicted in chart I.4, total dependency is not projected to be as high as it was in 1960. Even when the entire baby boom is aged 65 or over (in the year 2030), the dependency ratio will match the 1955 level. The significant difference, however, is that instead of children the dependents will be retirees. Most retirees and their spouses are very independent; only a few will be as dependent as children. To the extent that society would prefer that the cost of long-term care or long-term care insurance be prefunded over an individual's working years, the time to initiate that process to finance long-term care for the baby boom generation is now. The window of opportunity to initiate prefunding to assist the potentially largest group of retirees in U.S. history will diminish with each passing year (Chollet, forthcoming, a).

Estimates by Social Security actuaries of the ratio of Social Security covered workers to beneficiaries is also expected to continue to decline sharply. Since 1960, the number of workers paying into the system relative to beneficiaries declined 1.5 percent per year (chart I.5). Using the intermediate, or II-B, assumptions, between 1987 and the year 2010 the ratio of covered workers to beneficiaries is projected to decline

13

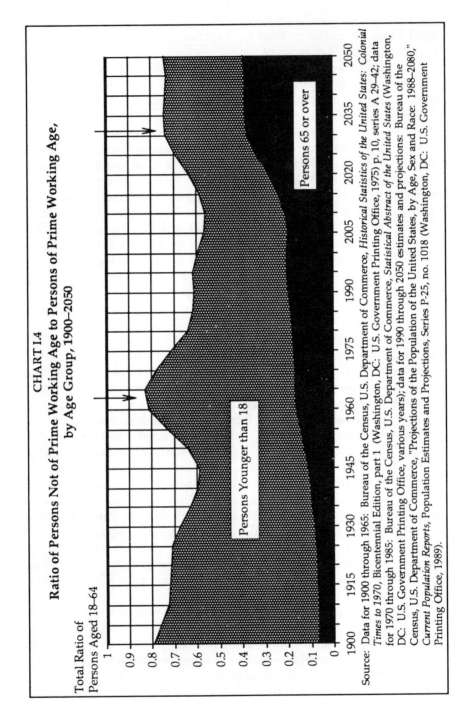

**CHART I.4**

**Ratio of Persons Not of Prime Working Age to Persons of Prime Working Age, by Age Group, 1900–2050**

Total Ratio of Persons Aged 18–64

Persons Younger than 18

Persons 65 or over

Source: Data for 1900 through 1965: Bureau of the Census, U.S. Department of Commerce, *Historical Statistics of the United States: Colonial Times to 1970*, Bicentennial Edition, part 1 (Washington, DC: U.S. Government Printing Office, 1975) p. 10, series A 29–42; data for 1970 through 1985: Bureau of the Census, U.S. Department of Commerce, *Statistical Abstract of the United States* (Washington, DC: U.S. Government Printing Office, various years); data for 1990 through 2050 estimates and projections: Bureau of the Census, U.S. Department of Commerce, "Projections of the Population of the United States, by Age, Sex and Race: 1988–2080," *Current Population Reports*, Population Estimates and Projections, Series P-25, no. 1018 (Washington, DC: U.S. Government Printing Office, 1989).

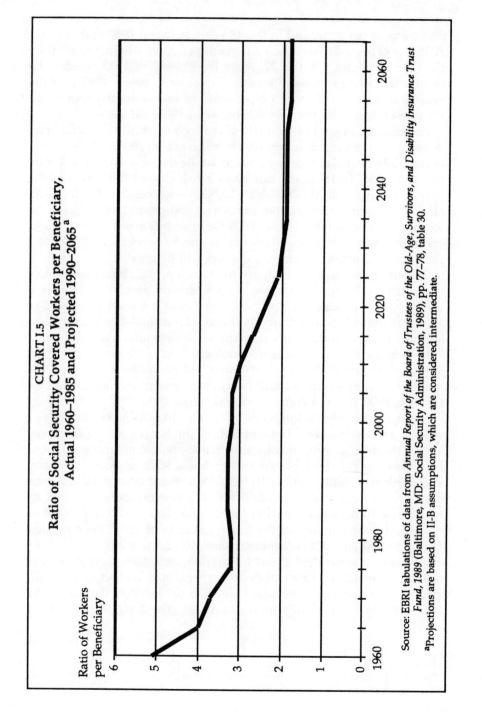

CHART I.5

**Ratio of Social Security Covered Workers per Beneficiary,
Actual 1960–1985 and Projected 1990–2065 [a]**

Ratio of Workers
per Beneficiary

Source: EBRI tabulations of data from *Annual Report of the Board of Trustees of the Old-Age, Survivors, and Disability Insurance Trust Fund, 1989* (Baltimore, MD: Social Security Administration, 1989), pp. 77–78, table 30.

[a]Projections are based on II-B assumptions, which are considered intermediate.

15

0.54 percent per year, and in the 48 years between 1987 and the year 2035 it is expected to decline 1.2 percent per year—slightly more than the rate of decline in the 27 years from 1960 to 1987. Under the pessimistic assumptions, the rate of decline between 1987 and the year 2035 is expected to be 1.6 percent per year—slightly more than the rate of decline in the 27 years between 1960 and 1987.

The relative impact of the ratio of covered workers to beneficiaries depends on worker productivity. The ratio of covered workers to beneficiaries is estimated to be between 1.6 in the year 2030 and 1.9 by the year 2035. In 1960, the ratio was 5.1. If those 1.6 workers in the year 2030 can produce as much as the 5.1 workers did in 1960, holding all else constant, the relative burden of the payroll taxes on those workers will be roughly the same. If the production of those 1.6 workers in the year 2030 is less than that of the 5.1 workers in 1960, then the relative burden on future taxpayers will be greater.

Output per worker, or productivity, for all private business activity in the United States has increased 65.5 percent since 1960. That is, a worker today produces 65 percent more than a worker produced in 1960. Since 1982, productivity has been increasing—but at a decreasing rate. Future productivity is unknown. It depends on many factors, including savings rates and technological advancement. The *1988 Economic Report of the President* (Council of Economic Advisers, 1988) assumes that productivity will continue to rise at an increasing rate through 1990 and at a constant rate through 1993.

Shifts in the population from fewer children to more elderly per worker are expected to have profound public policy implications. Unless the average retirement age increases, public programs financed by active workers on a pay-as-you-go basis, such as Social Security and Medicare, will continually require greater contributions from active employees.[7] Since the mid-1960s, however, there has been an increasing trend toward earlier retirement. In 1960, 26.8 percent of the elderly participated in the labor force; as of 1985, their participation had fallen 14.4 percentage points to 12.4 percent.

We know a great deal about future demographics. Only dramatic changes in mortality rate trends (life expectancy) or changes in immigration can alter the anticipated shifts in the age distribution of the United States. Net immigration can reverse the demographic effects

---

[7]This includes unfunded postretirement medical plans maintained by public and private employers.

of a prolonged decline in the fertility rate.[8] A net migration of 1 million persons a year could compensate for fertility rates below replacement levels, but most observers feel that net immigration is not likely to be this large (Wattenberg, 1987). The World Bank and the United Nations estimate total annual immigration at 435,000 people. Census Bureau estimates of emigration and legal and illegal immigration suggest that prior to the passage of the Immigration and Reform Control Act of 1986, annual net immigration averaged less than 500,000 people.[9]

Longer life expectancies and the maturing of the baby boom generation will increasingly influence the marketplace and the legislative process. Indications of the growing political force and the market potential of the elderly have been seen in such disparate settings as public policy debates over Social Security and Medicare and in the growth in importance of goods and services for older people. The political, economic, and social changes now occurring with the growth of the elderly population may be even greater when the baby boom generation approaches retirement age.

### Retiring Earlier and Living Longer

Retirement is thought of as an event, a process, a role, and a phase of life (Palmore et al., 1985). Undeniably, successive cohorts of workers—men, in particular—are retiring earlier (chart I.6). This is evident both in data on labor force participation and in data on initial recipiency of Social Security. Labor force participation of men aged 55 to 64 in 1987 was more than 21 percentage points lower than the labor force participation of this same age group 30 years earlier. In 1957, 87.6 percent of all men aged 55 to 64 were in the labor force. This rate dropped to 66.5 in 1987. For men aged 65 or older, labor force participation was 16 percent in 1988, compared with 23 percent in 1960 (Bureau of Labor Statistics, 1989).

Labor force participation has also declined for women but not as dramatically. Women who have been in the labor market for a relatively long time may be retiring earlier. However, many women may be reentering or entering the labor market relatively later than men

---

[8]Immigration policy can also have an important effect on the availability of long-term care because new immigrants often work as nursing aides and assistants in nursing homes and for community-based long-term care services.

[9]Over the last seven years, legal immigration has been averaging 551,000 people per year (Wattenberg, 1987). The Census Bureau estimates that immigration has averaged 160,00 people per year and that the number of annual illegal immigrants ranges from 100,000 to 300,000 (Butz et al., 1982).

17

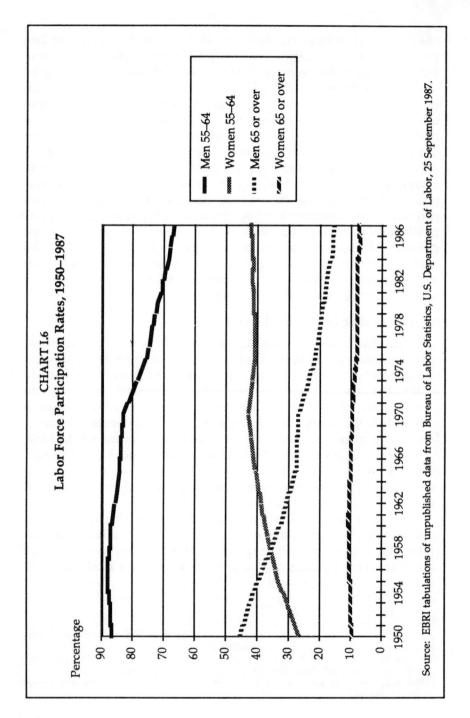

CHART I.6
Labor Force Participation Rates, 1950–1987

Percentage

Men 55–64
Women 55–64
Men 65 or over
Women 65 or over

1950  1954  1958  1962  1966  1970  1974  1978  1982  1986

Source: EBRI tabulations of unpublished data from Bureau of Labor Statistics, U.S. Department of Labor, 25 September 1987.

18

(U.S. General Accounting Office, 1986b). Consequently, the labor force participation rate for women aged 50 to 64 has been increasing since 1960, although at relatively slower rates, while for those aged 65 or older, labor force participation has been declining very slightly. The labor force participation among women aged 65 or older fell from 10.5 percent in 1960 to 7.3 percent in 1987.

Another indication of the trend toward earlier retirement is the average age of acceptance of Social Security benefits. In 1955, the average age of initial benefit acceptance among men was 68.4 years (Andrews, 1986). In 1966, it fell to 66 years of age, and from 1970 to 1986, the average age of initial Social Security benefit recipiency declined from 64.4 to 63.7 (Social Security Administration, 1987). This represents an increasingly large number of retirees. In 1970, 256,000 men, or 27.2 percent of males receiving Social Security benefits, initiated receipt of benefits before age 65. By 1982, the number had increased to 419,000, or 44.5 percent of men who were new beneficiaries. It should be noted that Social Security benefits cannot be collected prior to age 62, and that not all individuals collecting benefits have ceased working.

Many interrelated factors account for the decline in labor force participation at older ages. Factors that have been evaluated include health status (Bazzoli, 1985; Anderson and Burkhauser, 1985; Sickles and Taubman, 1986), the relative importance of self-employment (Fuchs, 1983; Sickles and Taubman, 1986), increases in real wages (which may increase preferences for more leisure), the growth of older workers competing for relatively fewer openings at the top of organizational ladders (Fuchs, 1983), and the growth in Social Security benefits and early retirement provisions in pension plans. In particular, the decline in labor force participation, particularly among men aged 62 to 64 during the late 1970s, parallels the advances in Social Security benefits during this period and the acceleration of early retirement provisions by employers. Between 1973 and 1983, the rate of employer-provided pension receipt increased more than 71 percent. In 1973, 5.4 million individuals aged 50 or over were pension recipients (11.4 percent of the population aged 50 or over). Ten years later, 11.5 million, or 19.5 percent of the population aged 50 or over, were pension recipients (U.S. General Accounting Office, 1986b). Studies suggest that health status and retirement income are the most important factors affecting retirement decisions. Poor health is likely to lead to retirement, but older workers in good health respond to economic incentives to retire. Simulated studies have shown that moderate disincentives, such as increasing the normal age of retirement, are

19

unlikely to lead to substantial changes in retirement decisions (Andrews, 1989; Mitchell and Fields, 1982; Burkhauser and Quinn, 1983; Diamond and Hausman, 1984; Burtless, 1986).

The tendency toward earlier retirement, in conjunction with declines in mortality and fertility rates, has altered the significance of retirement for the individual and society. Retirement affects tax revenues, the cost of the Social Security and Railroad Retirement programs, Medicare, Medicaid, and employer-provided retirement programs. From 1900 to 1986, the life expectancy of a man aged 65 increased 28 percent and that of a woman aged 65 increased 53 percent. On average, current workers can expect to spend more than 16 years in retirement—a period that must be supported by 36 to 42 years of work.[10] A man retiring at age 60 can expect to live at least 18.0 years in retirement. A woman retiring at age 60 can expect to live at least 23 more years. If a man is alive at age 77, he can expect to be retired an additional 8.2 years, for a total of 25 years, based on less than 39 years of employment. If a woman lives to age 83, she can expect to live another 7.3 years, so that she will be retired for more than 30 years, based on 39 years of work (or less if she left the labor force to raise children) (Bureau of the Census, 1986c; Faber and Wade, 1983).

It is difficult to predict whether the tendency to retire earlier will change. Some contend that, given the change in Social Security's normal retirement age from 65 to 67 by the year 2027, the average age of retirement will increase. Simulations suggest that the change will have very little impact (Andrews, 1989). However, if employers also begin to raise normal retirement ages or provide incentives to delay retirement, then the average age of retirement is more likely to increase. But poor health, other sources of retirement income, and individual preferences for retirement could govern the decision to retire earlier.

## The Impact of Demographic Shifts on Public Programs

Retirement has a two-pronged impact on public programs. A decline in labor force participation results in lower federal and state tax revenues and potentially results in an increase in public program

---

[10]Based on data from the National Center for Health Statistics (1988c). This calculation assumes that the individual begins work at age 21, retires at age 65, and lives the average life expectancy of 65-year-olds.

expenditures.[11] The U.S. General Accounting Office (GAO) estimates that the average additional federal income and Social Security tax revenues for each retired person who might have returned to work in 1983 would have been about $4,700 for those under age 62 and $3,800 for those aged 62 to 64. GAO estimates that if between 10 percent and 25 percent of retired pension recipients had returned to work (without replacing other workers), federal revenues in 1983 would have increased by $550 million, to $1.4 billion (U.S. General Accounting Office, 1986b).

Social Security, Medicare, and Medicaid are publicly financed programs that are very important sources of retirement income for the elderly. Workers who qualify (i.e., those who paid FICA taxes during enough quarters of employment) can obtain retirement income from Social Security at age 65 or at an actuarially reduced rate after age 62. Medicare, for which all recipients of Social Security are eligible at age 65, provides protection against the high cost of acute and ambulatory health care. Medicaid, which is a means-tested health care program for specific categories of poor people, pays the health care expenses of those whose Social Security income is so low as to trigger eligibility for Supplementary Security Income (SSI) programs and for people aged 65 or older whose health care costs exceed their income.

Medicare consists of two parts. Part A pays for acute health care expenditures (hospital care and skilled nursing care) and is an entitlement program for Social Security recipients aged 65 or older, anyone receiving Social Security disability payments for two years, and anyone with end-stage renal disease (ESRD). Part B is an optional program that pays for ambulatory physician services. Like Social Security, Part A of Medicare is financed by payroll taxes on essentially a pay-as-you-go basis. That is, current workers finance current benefits. One-quarter of Medicare Part B is financed through premiums paid by beneficiaries who choose to participate in the program, and the remainder is financed through general revenues. About 37.9 million people receive Social Security, and 31 million receive Medicare benefits. Total expenditures for these two programs in 1987 were $209.1 billion and $80.2 billion, respectively (*Annual Report*, 1988b).

Social Security, Medicare, and Medicaid are, in large part, financed by current employers and employees. The ratio of retirees to active

---

[11]Calculating the costs imposed by one generation on another may be necessary when discussing current resources; however, using this approach to justify alteration of programs could be erroneous. To compare generations, it might be more appropriate to calculate lifetime present values of production and consumption for the age groups under comparison.

workers can directly affect the cost per worker or taxpayer. Employer and employee payroll taxes finance current Social Security benefits and Part A of Medicare. Federal funds finance three-quarters of Part B of Medicare and the federal portion of Medicaid expenditures. General revenues, primarily from property, sales, and income taxes, fund the state portion of Medicaid.

The decline in federal revenue associated with retirement coincides with the potential need to increase federal expenditures for public programs. As the proportion of retirees to active workers increases, the relative financial burden on active workers contributing to the financing of these programs will increase. Consequently, unless the average age of retirement increases, public programs financed by active workers on a pay-as-you-go basis will continually require either greater contributions from active employees, contributions from beneficiaries, or a combination of both. These demographic changes have already prompted a public dialogue on a variety of emerging issues.

### Social Security Solvency: The Public Policy Response

In 1975, Social Security benefit payments were greater than revenues received from payroll taxes. Reserves established by the Old-Age, Survivors, and Disability Insurance program (OASDI) for such short-run contingencies were eroding, and it appeared that the program would be bankrupt in the early 1980s. Under the Social Security Amendments of 1981, interfund borrowing from the Disability Insurance fund and the Hospital Insurance fund was authorized as an interim measure. The 1983 Social Security Amendments raised tax revenues for Social Security by forcing state and local, and then federal, employees into the program and raising the payroll tax. Concurrently, benefits were reduced in several ways. They were reduced directly for retirees receiving federal pensions and by subjecting to income tax one-half of Social Security benefits for single beneficiaries with incomes of $25,000 or more and for married couples with incomes of $32,000 or more. Benefits were also cut by altering the cost-of-living adjustment formula and by raising the age at which Social Security beneficiaries are granted full retirement benefits (normal retirement age) from age 65 to age 67 (which will be fully phased in by the year 2027) (Andrews, 1985).

The compromises that emerged staved off immediate bankruptcy and left the program financially sound until at least the year 2030.[12]

---

[12]According to Social Security Administration actuaries' intermediate assumptions, revenue for the program from payroll taxes and taxation of benefits will fail to meet

Unintentionally, these changes led to increased reserves that now exceed current benefits. This surplus of $109 billion is expected to increase to $11.8 trillion by the year 2030. Technically, Social Security financing is no longer strictly on a pay-as-you-go basis. The addition to reserves in excess of benefits paid adds a prefunding component to the financing. Since prefunding was not the intent of the framers of Social Security and the surplus reserves are held in government securities (i.e., loaned to the government) rather than loaned to private endeavors, there has been considerable discussion of this financial arrangement (Merrill Lynch & Co., Inc., 1988; Aaron, Bosworth, and Burtless, 1989).

Because this surplus is loaned to the government, federal budget deficit calculations include this surplus fund. This raises the concern that the surplus is hiding the real deficit. As this fund is spent, the deficit will loom even larger. Furthermore, with budget deficits there is always the potential for political pressure to draw upon these funds for other purposes. Social Security actuarial data suggest that the average cost per beneficiary, in real terms, will increase nearly 70 percent over the next 10 years, from $5,551 to $8,693 (in 1987 dollars; table I.2). Continued reliance on payroll taxes to keep annual revenues equal to annual expenses could necessitate an increase in the OASDI portion of the payroll tax from the current 12.1 percent (for employers and employees combined) to about 20 percent by the year 2030, using the Social Security Administration actuaries' pessimistic assumptions. Under the intermediate assumptions, the payroll tax would need to be nearly 16 percent in the year 2030.

### Meeting Medicare's Expenses: Lessons from Social Security

The financial problems the Social Security program faced in the early 1980s are expected to arise in the Medicare program within the next 10 years. With the growing number and proportion of persons aged 85 or older, Medicare program costs per beneficiary are expected to more than double by 1998 (table I.3). Reimbursements per Medicare enrollee aged 85 or over are, on average, more than twice those for persons aged 65–66 (National Center for Health Statistics, 1986). Projections of Medicare's financial status suggest that the Hospital Insurance (HI) trust fund will begin to experience a deficit under intermediate assumptions between the years 2006 and 2008, and in

costs as early as the year 2020, but the contingency fund will not be depleted until 2055. Under pessimistic assumptions, revenues will be less than costs in 2015, with the trust fund technically exhausted in the year 2030.

## TABLE I.2
## Projected Costs of the Social Security Program per Retiree

| Year | Number of Beneficiaries (in millions) | | | Disbursements (in billions of dollars)[a] | | | Cost per Beneficiary | Cost per Retiree |
|------|-------|-------|-------|-------|-------|-------|------|------|
| | OASI[b] | DI[c] | Total | OASI[b] | DI[c] | Total | | |
| *Alternative II-B* | | | | | | | | |
| 1987 | 33.9 | 4.0 | 38.0 | $188.5 | $21.1 | $209.6 | $5,514 | $5,551 |
| 1988 | 34.5 | 4.1 | 38.6 | 200.6 | 22.0 | 222.6 | 5,764 | 5,811 |
| 1989 | 35.0 | 4.1 | 39.1 | 214.9 | 23.2 | 238.1 | 6,082 | 6,137 |
| 1990 | 35.8 | 4.2 | 40.0 | 230.5 | 24.6 | 255.1 | 6,384 | 6,441 |
| 1991 | 36.3 | 4.2 | 40.5 | 247.1 | 26.1 | 273.2 | 6,741 | 6,805 |
| 1992 | 36.8 | 4.3 | 41.1 | 263.3 | 27.8 | 291.1 | 7,085 | 7,153 |
| 1993 | 37.3 | 4.3 | 41.6 | 279.9 | 29.6 | 309.5 | 7,434 | 7,507 |
| 1994 | 37.7 | 4.4 | 42.2 | 297.3 | 31.6 | 328.9 | 7,803 | 7,883 |
| 1995 | 38.2 | 4.5 | 42.7 | 315.5 | 33.9 | 349.4 | 8,191 | 8,277 |
| 1996 | 38.5 | 4.6 | 43.2 | 334.8 | 36.3 | 371.1 | 8,598 | 8,693 |
| *Alternative III* | | | | | | | | |
| 1987 | 34.0 | 4.1 | 38.0 | $188.7 | $21.6 | $210.3 | $5,528 | $5,556 |
| 1988 | 34.5 | 4.2 | 38.7 | 201.6 | 22.7 | 224.3 | 5,793 | 5,836 |
| 1989 | 35.1 | 4.3 | 39.4 | 218.3 | 24.5 | 242.8 | 6,163 | 6,215 |
| 1990 | 35.8 | 4.4 | 40.3 | 238.3 | 26.6 | 264.9 | 6,581 | 6,642 |
| 1991 | 36.5 | 4.5 | 40.9 | 258.1 | 28.9 | 287.0 | 7,010 | 7,081 |
| 1992 | 37.0 | 4.6 | 41.6 | 277.0 | 31.2 | 308.2 | 7,403 | 7,486 |

| | | | | | | | |
|---|---|---|---|---|---|---|---|
| 1993 | 37.5 | 4.8 | 42.3 | 279.1 | 33.8 | 312.9 | 7,394 | 7,435 |
| 1994 | 38.0 | 4.9 | 43.0 | 318.4 | 36.8 | 355.2 | 8,263 | 8,372 |
| 1995 | 38.5 | 5.1 | 43.6 | 340.8 | 40.2 | 381.0 | 8,729 | 8,850 |
| 1996 | 39.0 | 5.3 | 44.3 | 364.6 | 43.8 | 408.4 | 9,214 | 9,354 |

Source: Old-Age and Survivors Insurance data for all years and Disability Insurance data for 1992–1996: unpublished data from the Office of the Actuary, Social Security Administration, U.S. Department of Health and Human Services; Disability Insurance data for 1987–1991: EBRI tabulations of data from *1987 Annual Report of the Board of Trustees of the Federal Old-Age and Survivors Insurance and Disability Funds* (Baltimore, MD: Social Security Administration, 1987).

[a]Disbursements include administrative expenses and transfers to the Railroad Retirement program.
[b]Old-Age and Survivors Insurance.
[c]Disability Insurance.

**TABLE I.3**
# Projected Costs of the Medicare Program per Enrollee, 1988–2005

| Year | Number of Enrollees (in millions) | | Benefit Payments (in billions of dollars) | | Cost per Enrollee | |
|------|-------|----------|-------|----------|--------|----------|
| | Aged | Disabled | Aged | Disabled | Aged | Disabled |
| 1988 | 29.2 | 3.0 | $ 48.9 | $ 6.0 | $1,677 | $2,015 |
| 1989 | 29.7 | 3.0 | 53.9 | 6.5 | 1,814 | 2,168 |
| 1990 | 30.3 | 3.1 | 59.9 | 7.2 | 1,979 | 2,353 |
| 1991 | 30.8 | 3.1 | 66.1 | 7.9 | 2,146 | 2,541 |
| 1992 | 31.3 | 3.2 | 72.5 | 8.6 | 2,318 | 2,734 |
| 1993 | 31.7 | 3.2 | 79.1 | 9.4 | 2,494 | 2,927 |
| 1994 | 32.1 | 3.3 | 86.1 | 10.3 | 2,680 | 3,128 |
| 1995 | 32.5 | 3.3 | 93.5 | 11.2 | 2,877 | 3,347 |
| 1996 | 32.8 | 3.4 | 101.2 | 12.2 | 3,082 | 3,566 |
| 1997 | 33.1 | 3.5 | 109.1 | 13.2 | 3,301 | 3,797 |
| 1998 | 33.3 | 3.5 | 117.7 | 14.3 | 3,535 | 4,042 |
| 1999 | 33.5 | 3.6 | 126.9 | 15.6 | 3,787 | 4,306 |
| 2000 | 33.7 | 3.7 | 136.7 | 17.1 | 4,053 | 4,583 |
| 2001 | 34.0 | 3.8 | 147.1 | 18.8 | 4,327 | 4,868 |
| 2002 | 34.3 | 4.0 | 157.9 | 20.6 | 4,613 | 5,170 |
| 2003 | 34.5 | 4.1 | 169.6 | 22.6 | 4,911 | 5,489 |
| 2004 | 34.9 | 4.2 | 182.0 | 24.7 | 5,220 | 5,822 |
| 2005 | 35.2 | 4.4 | 195.2 | 27.0 | 5,539 | 6,169 |

Source: Unpublished data from the Office of the Actuary, Health Care Financing Administration, U.S. Department of Health and Human Services, October 1987.

1999 under pessimistic assumptions. Under both sets of assumptions, the trust fund will be technically bankrupt just after the turn of the century (*Annual Report, 1989*).

Even under relatively optimistic assumptions about the success of paying hospitals' prospective rates based on diagnosis, future performance of the economy, and demographic changes, the Medicare program is likely to experience an ever-widening shortfall in revenues for the foreseeable future. Assuming no changes in Medicare law, the financial shortfall in the Medicare program HI fund and Supplementary Medical Insurance (SMI) has been projected to be more than $5 billion in 1990 (Holahan and Palmer, 1987). By the year 2000, the annual revenue shortfall is expected to be nearly 0.6 percent of Gross National Product (GNP) or $34 billion (in 1990 GNP terms), and by the time the first half of the baby boom generation has become eligible for Medicare (the year 2020), the annual shortfall will be more than $90 billion (in 1990 GNP terms) (Holahan and Palmer, 1987). These projections were done prior to enactment of the Medicare Catastrophic Coverage Act of 1988. If the premiums from the catastrophic supplement as enacted are not sufficient to cover the program expansion, the shortfalls will occur even sooner.

Many factors account for the projected revenue shortfall, including health care cost inflation and advances in medical technology. But a significant factor is expected to be the growing number of Medicare beneficiaries with increased life expectancies. Increases in expenditures relative to revenues are inevitable unless per capita wages rise faster than per capita hospital costs or the payroll tax financing the HI program is increased. To avoid raising the payroll tax, labor productivity must continue to improve.

**Medicaid**

Medicaid is a welfare-based health care financing program for the poor. In 1986, more than 36 percent of the $44 billion in total Medicaid payments went to pay for nursing home care (Division of National Cost Estimates, 1987). Most of these expenditures were generated by slightly more than 6 percent of Medicaid's 21.8 million recipients. Health Care Financing Administration (HCFA) projections of Medicaid expenditures through the year 2000 indicate that Medicaid will reduce its portion of financing hospital, physician, and nursing home care but will increase its portion of financing all other care, including home care (Division of National Cost Estimates, 1987). Total Medicaid expenditures are projected to increase over the next 14 years at a slower rate than the overall increase in health care costs through the year 2000. This projection is predicated on the assumption that states will continue to contain their health care costs.

In large part, states have contained their Medicaid costs by reducing access to care. Access to care can be denied by lowering the income or asset eligibility standards necessary to receive assistance from Medicaid or by restricting the availability of services to Medicaid recipients (see chapter III). Availability of services can be restricted either directly by denying approval for the construction or license of a facility or indirectly by limiting the reimbursement rate to a level that discourages providers' participation.

Unless there are substantial improvements in the health status of the elderly, increased numbers of very old people will increase the nation's costs for long-term care services even before the baby boom generation is elderly. Increased costs for these services are likely to increase Medicaid expenditures and raise the potential for more people to become impoverished and, therefore, eligible for medical assistance through Medicaid. State legislators may find themselves in a situation in which access to long-term care requires either allocating a larger portion of the state's budget to the Medicaid program or increasing the state's budget by raising taxes.

## The Impact of Demographic Shifts on Employers

Fundamental changes have already taken place in the labor force stemming from the shifting age distribution, the changing labor force participation of women (many of whom are mothers of young children), and the propensity of workers to retire earlier. The importance of these changes is now only beginning to be realized. Declining fertility and mortality rates since the turn of the century are likely to reduce the rate of growth in labor markets. Labor market growth, which has averaged 2.2 percent per year over the last 16 years, is likely to grow at rates averaging 1.2 percent through the turn of this century (chart I.7). Consequently, there will be a dearth of entry-age workers, and for the first time the average age of the working-age population will begin to increase. The relative decline in the growth of entry-age workers is likely to increase the cost of labor.

The rapid increase in older workers will begin almost concurrently with the decline in the growth of entry-age employees. Perhaps in an attempt to maximize labor productivity with the existing work force, these two events may bring about reorganizations within firms. Employers, some of whom have offered financial incentives for older workers to retire earlier than the retirement plan's specified age, may be inclined to provide incentives to workers to retire later. The inducement may be in the form of increased pensions, retraining, and increased flexibility, such as part-time or part-year employment.

Pressure on labor costs is likely to be exacerbated by the growing number of retirees relative to active workers. Social Security benefits, Medicare, Medicaid, and most private retiree health benefits are financed by current workers. Therefore, assuming no change in either the growth in labor productivity or the benefit provisions of these programs, the larger the "dependency ratio" the larger the proportion of total output and income produced by workers that will be trans-

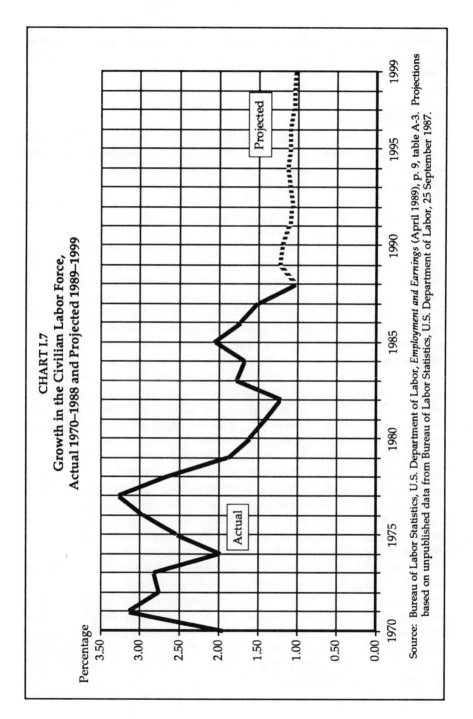

CHART I.7
Growth in the Civilian Labor Force,
Actual 1970–1988 and Projected 1989–1999

Percentage

Projected

Actual

Source: Bureau of Labor Statistics, U.S. Department of Labor, *Employment and Earnings* (April 1989), p. 9, table A-3. Projections based on unpublished data from Bureau of Labor Statistics, U.S. Department of Labor, 25 September 1987.

ferred to nonworkers. This will tend to raise the relative cost of labor directly from increases in payroll taxes and indirectly from other taxes or obligations that might be necessary to finance public programs.

## Conclusion

Long-term care encompasses the organization, delivery, and financing of care to people who are not able to function independently. The current system is fragmented and, therefore, confusing. Furthermore, efforts to contain public program expenditures have affected the availability of, and access to, long-term care. Without significant changes in morbidity (rates of disability), the growing number of elderly ensures an increasing number of people who are likely to be functionally dependent. The growing proportion of elderly to nonelderly has important implications for proposals for public financing of long-term care. As the demand for assistance increases, more and more resources will be channeled from other sectors into the long-term care market. The cost of this shift in resources will depend on the relative growth of the economy and the response of long-term care providers. Their response will depend on both the financing and reimbursement of long-term care.

Demographic shifts from a younger to an older America will affect the labor market and public programs such as Social Security, Medicare, and Medicaid. Public response to the expected financial shortfalls in the Medicare program and to the expected rise in Medicare costs will affect beneficiaries, taxpayers, and employers.

Employers and employees are an integral part of our retirement income security system. As taxpayers, they are the primary financers of the public programs that provide economic security and support to the elderly. Private pensions and postretirement medical benefits, too, are an important source of this support system. Employees and their dependents are the primary givers of long-term care as well as the potential recipients of such care.

The demographic changes upon us impose both an additional challenge and a political imperative to address issues concerning the organization, delivery, and financing of long-term care. Over the next century, the proportion of people at greatest risk of needing long-term care, relative to the proportion of people who can provide physical and financial assistance, will not be as small as it is now. The window of opportunity, in terms of public policy options, may never again be as wide open as it is today.

# II. The Risk of Needing Long-Term Care

## Introduction

Increasingly, because of improvements in medical technology, death will not be directly caused by an acute episode, such as a heart attack or stroke, or by an infection, such as pneumonia. In the early part of this century, death often occurred at a relatively young age from infectious disease. Few resources were available to interrupt the progress of infections; consequently, the need for long-term care was relatively rare (Fries, 1983). Today, medicine and technology have substantially reduced the risk of death from most acute infections, with the notable exception of acquired immunodeficiency syndrome (AIDS). Death is now more likely to occur as the result of, or in conjunction with, medical conditions that may persist for many years, such as chronic heart or respiratory conditions, arthritis, or rheumatism. These conditions may limit people's abilities to function independently. Functional limitations may also result from cognitive dysfunctions and degenerative brain diseases such as Alzheimer's disease or related dementias. While depression and other forms of mental illness are also common among the elderly, not much is known about their impact on functional limitations and death. It is known, however, that the elderly have the highest suicide rate.[1]

The causes of death in older people are often very different from the causes of death in younger ones. Heart disease, the most common cause of death among the elderly, ranks third among the population aged 25 to 44 and second among those aged 45 to 64. Accidents are the most common cause of death among the younger population, but are the seventh most common cause among the elderly. Three out of four deaths among the entire population occur from degenerative diseases, such as heart disease and cancer, primarily at advanced ages (Olshansky and Ault, 1986). While death rates from many degenerative diseases have fallen in recent years, their prevalence as chronic conditions has increased (Office of Technology Assessment, 1985; Manton, 1982).

---

[1]Experts suggest that the suicide rate among the elderly has been increasing faster than among any other age group because of the increase in the length of time older people suffer from chronic illness (Manton, Blazer, and Woodbury, 1987).

Increased life expectancy has been due primarily to a decrease in the risk of death from heart disease or stroke. Between 1968 and 1985, mortality rates from heart disease decreased 2.2 percent annually for men aged 65 to 69. Mortality rates from vascular disease declined at a 4.9 percent annual rate during the same period for the same subgroup. There were also substantial declines in mortality rates from digestive diseases and diabetes for both sexes. Only mortality rates for cancer have increased, at a 1 percent annual rate for men and a 1.4 percent annual rate for women, aged 65 to 69, between 1968 and 1980 (Poterba and Summers, 1987).

While age-specific incidence rates of heart disease and stroke have fallen, age-specific rates for cancer have not. In addition, there has been little or no decrease in age-specific prevalence rates for osteoarthritis, diabetes, physical disability, hearing impairment, vision impairment, osteoporosis-related fractures, Parkinson's disease, or other diseases commonly viewed as being closely related to aging. It is not clear, however, whether individuals are surviving heart attacks and strokes only to spend more time in poor health. Some argue that modern medicine is beginning to approach the limit of our natural life span. If this is true, gains in life expectancy in the future will become smaller while advances in medical technology will begin to reduce morbidity, causing what has been called "the compression of morbidity" (Fries, 1980, 1983). Others, however, think that there is no evidence that the natural limit of the human life span is being approached and that, therefore, life expectancy will continue to increase, with or without improvements in the quality of life (Gruenberg, 1977; Schneider and Brody, 1983; Verbrugge, 1984; Manton and Soldo, 1985; Manton, 1986b).

## Psychological Health

Loss of memory and confusion, or cognitive dysfunction, are common problems that can also lead to the need for assistance and institutionalization. Not all sources of cognitive dysfunction, however, need be permanent. There are reversible illnesses that often mimic dementia. It is estimated that of the elderly who seek medical attention because of intellectual deterioration, perhaps 10 percent to 15 percent have clinical dementia syndrome with reversible causes (Katzman, 1986). Some of the most common causes include depression, drug intoxication, hypothyroidism, anemia, alcohol abuse, metabolic disturbances, systemic illness, chronic subdural hematoma, and normal-pressure hydrocephalus.

Irreversible sources of cognitive dysfunction include vascular dementia, or multi-infarct dementia, and Alzheimer's disease. Of the people with an organic brain disease, approximately 15 percent to 30 percent have multi-infarct dementia and approximately 50 percent to 75 percent have Alzheimer's disease.[2] Nontreatable or irreversible dementia is often referred to as "senile dementia of the Alzheimer's type," or SDAT. In 1980, the number of people with Alzheimer's disease and related disorders was estimated to be 2 million (7.5 percent of the elderly). Without changes in prevention or treatment, there could be 3.8 million people with degenerative brain disease by the year 2000, and 8.5 million by the year 2050 (Brody, Brock, and Williams, 1987).

The prevalence of moderate to severe dementia increases exponentially with advancing age. Rare in people in their forties, dementia has been identified in 1 percent to 2 percent of people aged 60 to 65, 4 percent of people aged 70, 16 percent of people aged 80, and 32 percent of people aged 85. SDAT is also more common among women than men (Katzman, 1986). An estimated 2.5 million to 6.5 million people (elderly and nonelderly) suffer from moderate to severe SDAT (Office of Technology Assessment, 1987; Katzman, 1986). It is presumed that 30 percent to 50 percent of all people in nursing homes are victims of Alzheimer's disease or a related dementia (Office of Technology Assessment, 1985). The exact number of people with SDAT is unknown since certain diagnosis is impossible without a brain biopsy. Studies have found that misclassification ranges from 15 percent to 30 percent.[3]

Dementia diminishes both the quality of life and life expectancy. It gradually deprives the victims of their higher mental faculties, causing them to lose their capacity to care for themselves or to respond to their caregivers. During the course of this disease there are radical changes in personality, with the victim usually becoming irritable and unmanageable. Eventually the victim requires assistance in all bodily functions—eating, bathing, dressing—and enters into an immobile vegetative state. Death as a result of dementia is usually related to immobilization, general debilitation, and the gross personal

---

[2]The remaining cases are due to mixed Alzheimer's disease and multi-infarct dementia, or to conditions such as Pick's disease, Parkinson's disease, multiple sclerosis, chronic brain disease due to alcoholism, tumors, or Creutzfeld-Jacob's disease (Katzman, 1986).

[3]Recent advances in medical technology may make absolute diagnostic testing possible in the future (Altman, 1986; Brody, 1984).

33

incompetence that often appears late in the course of the disease. Life expectancy of victims is assumed to be one-half that of unafflicted people (White et al., 1986).

With no cure and little knowledge about the disease, it is not yet possible to distinguish the effect of the disease itself from the influence of other age-related diseases, "normal" brain aging, or social variables related to occupation, education, cultural roles, expectations, or other factors. What is known is that caring for someone with an irreversible progressive dementia is devastating. The victims will never get better; eventually, they are likely not to even recognize their caregiver. The care needed is physically demanding and emotionally exhausting. The day of a person taking care of an SDAT victim has been likened to a 36-hour day (Mace and Rabins, 1981).

Of all the illnesses commonly associated with aging, irreversible dementia creates the greatest need for long-term care. If age-specific prevalence and incidence rates remain unchanged, the number of victims can be expected to increase as more people live to advanced ages. In 1985, estimates of the full economic burden of SDAT on the U.S. economy approached $88 billion (Hu, Huang, and Cartwright, 1986; Huang, Cartwright, and Hu, 1988). Indirect economic costs accounted for nearly one-half the expenditures ($43.7 billion) and were due chiefly (99.1 percent) to the value of the life loss to society from the disease. The direct economic costs were estimated to be $44.1 billion, of which 69 percent was for community home care and 21 percent was for medical and nursing home care. The direct economic cost of SDAT alone suggests that the less than 2 percent of the population estimated to be afflicted with the disease consumed more than 10 percent of national health care expenditures in 1985. By the year 2040, as many as 7.5 million people, or 2.5 percent of the population, could be afflicted with SDAT,[4] suggesting that the share of national health care expenditures demanded by the families of SDAT victims could increase to 12.5 percent.[5] The congressional Office of Technology Assessment has estimated that in 1985, the market value of voluntarily

---

[4]Author's estimate based on the projected age distribution and current prevalence rates of SDAT. An estimate by the Office of Technology Assessment (1987) was very close (7.4 million).

[5]These estimates exclude the dementia associated with the last stages of acquired immunodeficiency syndrome (AIDS). To date, the life expectancy of patients with AIDS or even advanced AIDS-related complex (ARC) is less than two years, and the duration of dementia associated with AIDS is much less. This could change dramatically if new drug therapies prolong the lives of AIDS victims without reducing AIDS-related dementia.

provided informal care to victims of SDAT was $26.7 billion to $30.5 billion (Office of Technology Assessment, 1987).

## Health Care Utilization and Expenditures

Generally, health worsens and health care costs increase with age. Old age brings with it more aches, pains, and illness that result in physician visits, hospitalization, diagnostic tests, and medical procedures. Medications are increasingly needed, as are medical devices such as hearing aids, eyeglasses, canes, walkers, wheelchairs, and supplies such as syringes and diapers. But these expenses are relatively low compared with the expense of a hospital stay that may require the intensive use of life-sustaining technology. Not surprisingly, the elderly use a disproportionate share of health care services. In 1987, the elderly represented 12.3 percent of the population, but their medical care consumed more than 36 percent of all health care expenditures (table II.1). On a per capita basis, health expenditures in 1987 were more than four times greater for the elderly ($5,235 per person) than for the nonelderly ($1,283 per person).

A substantial proportion of health care spending, especially for the elderly, occurs in the last year or so of life. Heroic efforts to treat respiratory or heart failure, for example, are very expensive. It has been estimated that more than 1 percent of Gross National Product is consumed on health expenditures by people in their last year of life (Fuchs, 1984). In 1978, Medicare beneficiaries who died—about 5.9 percent of all beneficiaries—consumed about 28 percent of all Medicare expenditures (Lubitz and Prihoda, 1984). One study found that Medicare-covered health care expenditures for persons during their last year of life averaged more than six times the average cost among survivors (McCall, 1984). This same study also found that the cost varies tremendously by Medicare entitlement status. Those enrolled by virtue of their age consumed fewer services in their last year of life than did those enrolled in Medicare because they were disabled or because of end-stage renal disease (ESRD). In 1978, the cost of care for those in the first group averaged less than $6,000, compared with more than $7,700 for the disabled and $44,000 for those with ESRD (McCall, 1984).

Payments to hospitals constitute the largest source of health care expenditures in the United States. Of the $442.6 billion spent on personal health care in 1987, 44 percent was for hospital care and 23 percent was for physician services. Less than 10 percent of personal health care expenditures in 1987 was for nursing home care, and 2.5

## TABLE II.1
## Personal Health Care Expenditures, by Type and as a Percentage of Total Health Care Expenditures among the Nonelderly and Elderly, 1987

| Type of Care | Nonelderly | | | Elderly | | |
|---|---|---|---|---|---|---|
| | Total | Private | Public | Total | Private | Public |
| | aggregate amount (in billions) | | | | | |
| Personal Health Care | $284.3 | $213.0 | $71.3 | $158.2 | $59.9 | $98.3 |
| Hospital care | 127.0 | 84.6 | 42.4 | 65.6 | 10.2 | 55.4 |
| Physicians' services | 68.3 | 58.8 | 9.5 | 33.1 | 11.9 | 21.2 |
| Nursing home care | 8.7 | 2.7 | 6.0 | 32.9 | 19.1 | 13.8 |
| Other | 80.2 | 67.1 | 13.1 | 26.7 | 18.7 | 8.0 |
| | per capita amount | | | | | |
| Personal Health Care | $1,283 | $962 | $322 | $5,235 | $1,982 | $3,253 |
| Hospital care | 573 | 382 | 191 | 2,171 | 338 | 1,833 |
| Physicians' services | 308 | 265 | 43 | 1,095 | 394 | 702 |
| Nursing home care | 39 | 12 | 27 | 1,089 | 632 | 457 |
| Other | 362 | 303 | 59 | 884 | 619 | 265 |
| | percentage distribution by type of service | | | | | |
| Personal Health Care | 100.0% | 100.0% | 100.0% | 100.0% | 100.0% | 100.0% |
| Hospital care | 44.7 | 39.7 | 59.5 | 41.5 | 17.0 | 56.4 |
| Physicians' services | 24.0 | 27.6 | 13.3 | 20.9 | 19.9 | 21.6 |
| Nursing home care | 3.1 | 1.3 | 8.4 | 20.8 | 31.9 | 14.0 |
| Other | 28.2 | 31.5 | 18.4 | 16.9 | 31.2 | 8.1 |

Source: Unpublished data from the Office of the Actuary, Health Care Financing Administration, U.S. Department of Health and Human Services, November 1988.

percent was spent on other types of personal health care (U.S. Department of Health and Human Services, 1988). For the elderly, hospital care represented 41.5 percent of per capita health care expenditures, or $2,170 per person (table II.1). For the nonelderly, hospital care represented a slightly larger proportion, 44.7 percent, but a much smaller dollar amount ($1,283 per person), since health care expenditures for the nonelderly are, overall, so much less than those for the elderly. The rate of hospital discharges among the elderly is more than three times the rate among the nonelderly, and the average length of a hospital stay among the elderly is about 50 percent longer than that among the nonelderly.[6]

Physician services for both the elderly and the nonelderly constitute a roughly similar proportion of health care expenditures. In 1987, physician services for the elderly represented nearly 21 percent of personal health care expenditures, and 24 percent for the nonelderly. The elderly are responsible for 63 percent of physician patient revenues. In 1986, physician visits in hospitals or ambulatory settings averaged 2.5 per person for those aged 17 to 44, 3.6 for those aged 45 to 64, and 4.9 for those aged 65 or over (National Center for Health Statistics, 1987b). On a per capita basis, physician services were 3.5 times greater ($1,095 versus $308) for the elderly than for the nonelderly.

In 1987, physician services and nursing home care each consumed roughly the same proportion of the elderly's health care expenditures—around 21 percent, or $1,092 per person. But for the nonelderly, nursing home expenditures represented only 3.1 percent of personal health care and were 27 times lower per capita ($39.27) than those for the elderly. Other personal health care expenditures represented nearly 17 percent of the elderly's and 28 percent of the nonelderly's personal health care expenditures. These expenditures include measurable home- and community-based care for both post acute care recovery and long-term care and dental services, vision care, and durable and nondurable medical products and supplies. In per capita terms, the elderly spend twice as much as the nonelderly for this care ($884 versus $352, respectively).

---

[6]In 1986, the average length of stay in nonfederal short-stay hospitals was 8.5 days for all patients aged 65 and over, and 5.4 days for all patients under age 65. (Author's calculation based on data from the National Center for Health Statistics, 1987d.)

37

## Catastrophic Acute and Ambulatory Care

Out-of-pocket expenditures reflect services that are less likely to be covered by insurance. Most of the elderly (95 percent) have Medicare, and most Medicare beneficiaries (72 percent) have supplemental Medigap coverage (Bureau of Data Management and Strategy, 1989). Consequently, out-of-pocket expenditures for acute care and ambulatory care are relatively small for the elderly. In 1984, hospital care for the elderly represented 5.6 percent of total out-of-pocket spending and physician care more than 21 percent (table II.2). For the nonelderly, hospital care represented 18.4 percent of total out-of-pocket expenditures and physician care more than 23 percent.[7] These differences reflect, in part, the near-universal health insurance coverage of the elderly through Medicare and Medigap policies and the greater likelihood that this coverage is more comprehensive for acute and ambulatory care.

Depending on their source of insurance coverage, the elderly's out-of-pocket expenses differ substantially (table II.3). These differences probably reflect both the health status of the insured and the scope of coverage. In 1980, the average total charge per noninstitutionalized person was $730, of which 27 percent was paid out-of-pocket. That year total mean per capita charges of the elderly were nearly three times those of the nonelderly, but out-of-pocket expenditures as a percentage of total charges were less—19 percent as opposed to 30 percent. Although the elderly had relatively smaller responsibility for total charges, the average per capita out-of-pocket expense was greater owing to the greater amount of charges. The per capita out-of-pocket expenses of the elderly were almost twice those of the nonelderly ($327 versus $179, respectively).

Among the nonelderly, mean per capita out-of-pocket expenses were the least for those with Medicaid and the most for those with Medicare (but not also with Medicaid). This reflects the fact that the nonelderly with Medicare are likely, by virtue of their disabilities, to be heavy users of health care and because Medicaid provides relatively broad and deep coverage. Average per person out-of-pocket expenses among the nonelderly with only private insurance were less than one-half those of nonelderly persons with Medicare, but as a percentage of total charges their out-of-pocket expenses were much greater. This difference may reflect the relatively healthy nature of the privately

---

[7]Author's calculation of national health expenditure data published in Levit et al., 1985, table 2, and Waldo and Lazenby, 1984, table 11.

**TABLE II.2**

**Distribution of Out-of-Pocket Expenditures for Health Care among the Nonelderly and Elderly, 1984**

| Type of Care | Nonelderly | | | Elderly | | |
|---|---|---|---|---|---|---|
| | Total expenditures (in billions) | Distribution | Per capita expenditures | Total expenditures (in billions) | Distribution | Per capita expenditures |
| Total | $65.3 | 100.0% | $302 | $30.2 | 100.0% | $1,063 |
| Hospital Care | 12.0 | 18.4 | 56 | 1.7 | 5.6 | 60 |
| Physicians' Services | 14.5 | 22.2 | 67 | 6.5 | 21.5 | 228 |
| Nursing Home Care | 3.3 | 5.1 | 15 | 12.6 | 41.7 | 442 |
| Other | 35.5 | 54.4 | 164 | 9.5 | 31.5 | 333 |

Source: EBRI tabulations of data in Katherine R. Levit et al., "National Health Expenditures: 1984," *Health Care Financing Review* (Fall 1985), p. 9, table 2; and Daniel R. Waldo and Helen C. Lazenby, "Demographic Characteristics and Health Care Use and Expenditures by the Aged in the United States: 1977–1984," *Health Care Financing Review* (Fall 1984), p. 10, table 11.

Note: Percentages may not add to 100 because of rounding.

## TABLE II.3
## Mean per Capita Charges and Out-of-Pocket Expense, Percentage of Total Charges Paid Out of Pocket, and Coverage for Noninstitutionalized Persons, by Age and Type of Health Insurance Coverage: United States, 1980

| Age and Type of Coverage | Mean per Capita Total Charge | Mean per Capita Out-of-Pocket Expense | Percentage of Total Charges Paid Out-of-Pocket | Persons Covered Number (in millions) | Persons Covered Percentage |
|---|---|---|---|---|---|
| All Persons | $730 | $195 | 27% | 217.9 | — |
| Under Age 65 | | | | | |
| Total | 604 | 179 | 30 | 194.0 | 100.0% |
| Medicaid | 766 | 72 | 9 | 18.1 | 9.3 |
| Medicare, no Medicaid | 2,542 | 441 | 17 | 2.2 | 1.2 |
| Private, no Medicaid | | | | | |
| or Medicare | 615 | 192 | 31 | 141.8 | 73.1 |
| Other coverage | 695 | 107 | 15 | 5.9 | 3.0 |
| No coverage | 218 | 179 | 82 | 25.8 | 13.3 |
| Aged 65 or over | | | | | |
| Total | $1,760 | $327 | 19% | 23.8 | 100.0% |

| | | | | | |
|---|---|---|---|---|---|
| Medicare only | 1,104 | 319 | 29 | 4.9 | 20.5 |
| Medicare and Medicaid | 3,106 | 233 | 7 | 2.9 | 12.2 |
| Medicare and other coverage | 1,767 | 352 | 20 | 15.1 | 63.5 |
| Other coverage | 903 | 195 | 22 | 0.6 | 2.7 |
| No coverage | a | a | 67 | a | a |

Source: Embry Howell, Larry S. Corder, and Allen Dobson, "Out-of-Pocket Health Expenses for Medicaid Recipients and Other Low-Income Persons, 1980," *National Medical Care Utilization and Expenditure Survey*, Office of Research and Demonstrations, Health Care Financing Administration, U.S. Department of Health and Human Services, Series B, Descriptive Report No. 4, DHHS pub. no. 85-20204 (Washington, DC: U.S. Government Printing Office, August 1985), p. 9, table A.

aSample too small for accurate estimate.
Note: Percentages may not add to 100 because of rounding.

insured population and the greater cost sharing or relatively less complete coverage for routine ambulatory health care among the privately insured population.

Among the elderly, average out-of-pocket expenditures per person were about the same, regardless of their source of insurance coverage (table II.3). However, those with both Medicare and Medicaid (the "dually eligible") paid the smallest percentage out of pocket and those with Medicare alone paid the largest. Generally, the dually eligible are in very poor health (McMillan et al., 1983; McMillan and Gornick, 1984), but their Medicaid and Medicare coverage are substantial sources of health care financing. Those with only Medicare face the out-of-pocket expenditures often paid by Medigap policies or employer-provided retiree health benefits.

Relatively few people are intensive users of health care; therefore, differences among individuals are not fully captured in per capita averages. In 1984, only 15 percent of the population aged 45 or over was hospitalized.[8] In 1980, approximately 5 percent of all people had no out-of-pocket expenditures for health care. Nearly 83 percent of all people had out-of-pocket health expenditures of 5 percent or less of family income, 4.2 percent had 15 percent or more, and 7.2 percent had 11 percent or more. Nearly 85 percent of the nonelderly spent 5 percent or less of their family income on health care, and less than 4 percent spent more than 15 percent. More than one-third of the elderly spent 6 percent or more of their family income on health care, and 10 percent spent more than 15 percent.

In 1980, among those with only health care expenditures (excluding nursing home expenditures), out-of-pocket expenses per person averaged $229 for the nonelderly and $370 for the elderly (tables II.4 and II.5). Mean per capita expenses for hospital care were relatively similar—$669 for the nonelderly and $710 for the elderly. For the nonelderly without health insurance, however, mean per capita out-of-pocket hospital costs ($1,380) were more than twice the average of $678 (table II.4). For people with Medicaid, out-of-pocket costs for hospital care were more than one-and-one-half times the average ($1,059). Among the elderly who had been hospitalized, mean per capita out-of-pocket expenditures for the dually eligible were also more than one-and-one-half times the average ($1,204) (table II.5). For the nonelderly, the second largest source of out-of-pocket expenditures was for orthodontia care, while for the elderly it was dental care.

---

[8]EBRI tabulations of the 1984 Survey of Income and Program Participation (SIPP).

# TABLE II.4

## Mean per Capita Out-of-Pocket Expenses for Persons under Age 65 with Expenses, by Type of Health Insurance Coverage and Type of Service: United States, 1980

| Type of Service | All Persons | Persons under Age 65 | | | | | |
| --- | --- | --- | --- | --- | --- | --- | --- |
| | | Total | Private (no Medicare or Medicaid) | Medicaid | Medicare (no Medicaid) | Other coverage | No coverage |
| Total | $245.82 | $228.66 | $225.82 | $169.17 | $482.15 | $168.21 | $255.31 |
| Dental Visit | 111.25 | 107.54 | 108.05 | 92.87 | 87.22 | 119.28 | 106.49 |
| Orthodontia Visit | 462.81 | 465.22 | 468.55 | a | a | a | a |
| Doctor's Office Visit | 76.02 | 72.76 | 72.31 | 64.21 | 99.24 | 65.19 | 75.62 |
| Emergency Room Visit | 58.03 | 59.51 | 50.76 | 63.75 | a | 49.92 | 89.76 |
| Out-Patient Visit | 69.04 | 67.59 | 62.05 | 98.58 | 74.86 | 57.04 | 91.98 |
| Other Medical Provider Visit | 79.05 | 80.13 | 81.66 | 71.64 | 63.55 | 66.37 | 74.66 |
| Hospital Stay | 678.29 | 669.38 | 560.47 | 1,059.69 | 987.57 | 229.71 | 1,380.13 |
| Prescribed Medicine | 42.24 | 34.03 | 32.51 | 27.66 | 124.88 | 32.02 | 33.39 |
| Other Medical Expense | 76.06 | 72.91 | 71.72 | 66.86 | 78.77 | 80.75 | 81.76 |

Source: Embry Howell, Larry S. Corder, and Allen Dobson, "Out-of-Pocket Health Expenses for Medicaid Recipients and Other Low-Income Persons, 1980," *National Medical Care Utilization and Expenditure Survey*, Office of Research and Demonstrations, Health Care Financing Administration, U.S. Department of Health and Human Services, Series B, Descriptive Report No. 4, DHHS pub. no. 85-20204 (Washington, DC: U.S. Government Printing Office, August 1985), p. 28, table 13.

[a] Sample too small for accurate estimate.

## TABLE II.5
## Mean per Capita Out-of-Pocket Expenses for Persons Aged 65 Years or over with Expenses, by Type of Health Insurance Coverage and Type of Service: United States, 1980

| Type of Service | All Persons | Persons Aged 65 or over | | | | | |
|---|---|---|---|---|---|---|---|
| | | Total | Total Medicare | Medicare only | Medicare and Medicaid | Medicare and other coverage | Private and other insurance |
| Total | $245.82 | $369.47 | $370.23 | $380.13 | $302.21 | $378.47 | $256.63 |
| Dental Visit | 111.25 | 147.51 | 148.22 | 153.39 | 153.41 | 149.08 | 114.80 |
| Orthodontia Visit | 462.81 | a | a | a | a | a | a |
| Doctor's Office Visit | 76.02 | 97.22 | 97.57 | 97.56 | 86.95 | 98.63 | 96.29 |
| Emergency Room Visit | 58.03 | 43.84 | 44.21 | 57.90 | a | 41.44 | a |
| Out-Patient Visit | 69.04 | 77.13 | 76.57 | 53.61 | a | 85.89 | a |
| Other Medical Provider Visit | 79.05 | 72.28 | 73.19 | 96.21 | 54.10 | 69.51 | a |
| Hospital Stay | 678.29 | 710.04 | 708.94 | 769.99 | 1,204.04 | 599.64 | a |
| Prescribed Medicine | 42.24 | 89.31 | 89.75 | 98.17 | 43.22 | 94.91 | 74.18 |
| Other Medical Expense | 76.06 | 90.43 | 89.85 | 78.94 | 68.00 | 93.08 | a |

Source: Embry Howell, Larry S. Corder, and Allen Dobson, "Out-of-Pocket Health Expenses for Medicaid Recipients and Other Low-Income Persons, 1980," *National Medical Care Utilization and Expenditure Survey,* Office of Research and Demonstrations, Health Care Financing Administration, U.S. Department of Health and Human Services, Series B, Descriptive Report No. 4, DHHS pub. no. 85-20204 (Washington, DC: U.S. Government Printing Office, August 1985), p. 29, table 14.

[a]Sample too small for accurate estimate.

## Long-Term Care

Spending for nursing home care (including care provided in skilled nursing facilities, intermediate care facilities, and personal care homes that provide nursing care) represents the largest and best-measured portion of total long-term care spending in the United States. In 1985, expenditures for nursing home care were $35.2 billion. Estimates of spending on home- and community-based long-term care services for the same year were, at a minimum, $13.7 billion. Thus, long-term care expenditures for this period amounted to approximately $48.9 billion.[9] Since 1985, it has been more difficult to estimate total long-term care expenditures; however, in 1987, nursing home expenditures nationwide were $40.6 billion. If nursing home expenditures continued to represent the same proportion of total long-term care, then long-term care expenditures in 1987 may have amounted to at least $56 billion.[10]

Long-term care, in general, and nursing home care, in particular, represent the largest out-of-pocket health care expense for everyone in need of long-term care. Of the $40.6 billion spent on nursing home care in 1987, Medicare paid $600 million and private insurance paid $400 million. Most of the remainder was paid either directly by residents and their families ($20 billion) or by Medicaid ($17.8 billion). Of the $15.4 billion spent in 1987 on home- and community-based care, about 79 percent was publicly funded.[11]

Although many people enter nursing homes for a relatively short period, long-time residency can last many years. In 1985, the median

---

[9]In 1985, nursing home expenditures were $35.2 billion and public expenditures for home health care were $9 billion (Waldo, Levit, and Lazenby, 1986). In 1981, industry estimates of private insurance and out-of-pocket expenditures for home health care were $2.3 billion (Doty, Liu, and Wiener, 1985). Factoring for inflation to 1985, using the consumer price index (CPI), adds $2.7 billion to home health care costs. Medicare spending for hospice care was $15 billion in that year. Other public programs supporting community-based services spent 26 percent of $6.7 billion in 1984 (O'Shaughnessy, Price, and Griffith, 1987). Inflating this estimate to 1985 using the CPI adds $1.8 billion. Altogether, this puts the entire cost of long-term care at $49 billion in 1985.

[10]Given that community-based services have been increasing faster than the number of nursing home beds, and that nursing home residents were relatively older in 1985 than they were in 1977, it is likely that nursing home expenditures are now a smaller proportion of long-term care expenditures than they were estimated to be in 1985. This suggests that long-term care expenses are even greater. Unfortunately, data on community-based services do not exist to reestimate aggregate expenditures.

[11]Many forms of paid assistance, especially assistance not arranged through a Medicare- or Medicaid-certified home health agency, are not likely to be detected and, therefore, are less likely to be measured.

length of stay among residents was more than 20 months, for a total expense of at least $36,000 (Hing, 1987). Among all elderly with health care expenditures of $2,000 or more, more than 81 percent of the out-of-pocket expenses were estimated to be for nursing home care and 10 percent for hospital care (Rice and Gabel, 1986).

These estimates of the cost of long-term care exclude the value of care provided informally by spouses, family, and friends. It has been estimated that if informal caregiving to the population aged 18 or older were provided by paid aides, long-term care expenditures in 1978 would have been some $9.6 billion higher—two-thirds of what was spent on nursing home care that year (Paringer, 1985). Using this estimated ratio of the value of informal care to expenditures for nursing home care, the commercial value of informal long-term care in 1987 may have amounted to $27.1 billion.

## Nursing Home Residents

Most nursing home residents (86.9 percent) are elderly, but 13.1 percent are under age 65 (National Center for Health Statistics, 1989). At any point in time about 5 percent of the elderly are believed to be institutionalized (Sirrocco, 1985). This was determined in the 1972 and 1977 National Nursing Home Surveys and reconfirmed in the 1985 National Nursing Home Survey. The distribution of nursing home residents by age, however, reveals that the prevalence, or frequency, and probably the risk of admission rise dramatically with age (table II.6). In 1985, 1.2 percent of those aged 65 to 74, 5.8 percent of those aged 75 to 84, and 22 percent of those aged 85 or older were in institutions. If nursing home prevalence remains the same, by the year 2030 all the nursing home beds constructed as of 1985 could be filled with people aged 85 or older.

Nursing home residents tend to be not only very old but are more likely to be white women. In 1987, nearly two-thirds (62.8 percent) of all nursing home residents and three-quarters (74.6 percent) of all *elderly* nursing home residents were women (Hing, 1987; Sekscenski, 1987). More than 90 percent (92.8 percent of all nursing home residents and 93.1 percent of all elderly nursing home residents) were white. In 1985, 5 percent of all elderly white people were in nursing homes compared with 4 percent of all black people and 2 percent of people of all other races. These differences became more apparent the older the age group. Of the population aged 85 or older, 23 percent of the white population resided in nursing homes, compared with 14 percent of the black population (Hing, 1987). In 1985, most elderly nursing

## TABLE II.6
## Prevalence of Institutionalization among the U.S. Population, by Age, 1985

| Age | Total Population (in thousands) | Institutionalized Population (in thousands) | Percentage of Total Population Who Are Institutionalized | Distribution as a Percentage of the Institutionalized Population |
|---|---|---|---|---|
| Total | 240,228 | 1,491 | 0.6% | 100.0% |
| Under 65 | 210,372 | 173 | 0.1 | 11.6 |
| 65 or over | 29,857 | 1,318 | 4.4 | 88.4 |
| 65 to 74 years | 17,222 | 212 | 1.2 | 14.2 |
| 75 to 84 years | 9,345 | 509 | 5.4 | 34.1 |
| 85 years or over | 3,290 | 597 | 18.1 | 40.0 |

Source: Noninstitutionalized population estimates from the Bureau of the Census, U.S. Department of Commerce, "United States Population Estimates by Age, Sex, and Race: 1980 to 1987," *Current Population Reports*, Population Estimates and Projections, Series P-25, no. 1022 (Washington, DC: U.S. Government Printing Office, March 1988), pp. 24–25, table 2; institutionalized population estimates from the National Center for Health Statistics, Public Health Service, U.S. Department of Health and Human Services, "The National Nursing Home Survey: 1985 Summary for the United States," *Vital and Health Statistics*, Series 13, no. 97, DHHS pub. no. (PHS) 89-1758 (Washington, DC: U.S. Government Printing Office, January 1989), p. 25, table 18.

home residents (83.6 percent) were not married at the time of their admission. Almost two-thirds (64.2 percent) were widowed. Limitations in activities of daily living (ADLs) among nursing home residents also increased with age and tended to be greater among women (Hing, 1987).

A substantial portion of the elderly are likely to be admitted to a nursing home for a relatively short period. However, the majority of those who stay beyond three months are not likely to return home (National Center for Health Statistics, 1989). Of the estimated 1.5 million nursing home residents in 1985, 82 percent were discharged during that year (Hing, 1987; Sekscenski, 1987).[12] Nearly three-quarters (72 percent) were discharged alive. The median duration of a stay was 70 days for those discharged alive and 163 days for those who died in the nursing home that year. Among those discharged alive, almost one-third (32.3 percent) were discharged within the first month of admission, more than one-half (55.4 percent) were discharged within three months, and more than two-thirds (67.6 percent) were discharged within six months.[13] However, it is important to recognize that 77 percent of those who went home (rather than to a hospital) were discharged within three months. Nearly 90 percent of nursing home residents were discharged within six months (National Center for Health Statistics, 1989).

National data on nursing home use have some fundamental flaws. In particular, when a nursing home resident leaves, either to go to a hospital or to visit family, say over a holiday, it is counted as a discharge from the nursing home. When that resident returns, it is counted as an admission. If people essentially live in the nursing home, but do visit family or have several short trips to the hospital, then the national data would understate the long stays and overstate the short stays. Research from the 1987 National Medical Expenditures Survey indicates that 16 percent of nursing home residents as of January 1, 1987, had been discharged to a hospital and then readmitted to the nursing facility. Their findings suggest that the number of nursing home admissions was overstated by at least 25 percent (Short et al., forthcoming).

---

[12]The 1985 survey was conducted from August 1985 through January 1986 and refers to the 12 months prior to the survey date. Therefore, data actually refer to any 12-month period between August 1984 and January 1986.

[13]These data do not control for multiple admissions, so some of the admissions and discharges may be for the same individuals. Tabulations from the 1984 National Long-Term Care Survey (NLTCS) of chronically disabled elderly in the community indicate that 8.9 percent had been in a nursing home in the prior 12 months.

Between 1973 and 1985, there seems to have been a slight shift in the age distribution of nursing home residents (chart II.1). This may be due, in part, to the decline in nursing home beds relative to the growth in the elderly population, or, in part, to the increased pressure imposed on hospitals through Medicare's prospective reimbursement system to discharge Medicare patients sooner. In the 1977 National Nursing Home Survey (NNHS), about one-third of all nursing home residents were aged 85 or over (table II.7). By the time of the 1985 NNHS, 59.4 percent were aged 80 or over, and nearly 40 percent were aged 85 or over.

Due to the changing age distribution, the number of people dying in nursing homes has increased. In the 1977 NNHS, 25.9 percent of all nursing home discharges were because of death. In the 1985 NNHS, the proportion of discharges due to death had increased to 28.1 percent (Sekscenski, 1987). Between 1977 and 1985, the median stay in nursing homes increased from 597 days to 614 days. However, according to the National Center for Health Statistics, this difference was not statistically significant (Sekscenski, 1987).

The 1984 National Long-Term Care Survey (NLTCS) provides details on Medicare recipients aged 65 or older who had some impairment in either ADLs or instrumental activities of daily living (IADLs) that either lasted or were expected to last at least 90 days. The 1985 NNHS provides a good basis for the distribution of nursing home residents and nursing home discharges by age, sex, and race. But more detailed questions about limitations, how residents paid for their care, and where they were prior to their admission are found in the 1984 NLTCS.

Because of the differences in the scope and design of the two surveys, there appear to be differences in some characteristics of nursing home residents. Some of the differences could be due to the different periods covered (1984 and 1985) and because the NLTCS is based on Medicare recipiency. Most of the differences, however, are likely to be due to the survey questions, since only about 3 percent of the elderly are not eligible for Medicare. The distributions by race and age in the two surveys were similar, although the residents were slightly older in the 1985 NNHS. In the 1985 NNHS, 93.1 percent of the elderly were white; in the 1984 NLTCS, 90 percent were white. In the 1985 NNHS, 45.2 percent of the elderly were aged 85 or older; in the 1984 NLTCS, 36.5 percent were aged 85 or older. In the 1985 NNHS, 83.9 percent were aged 76 or older; in the 1984 NLTCS, 78.2 percent were aged 76 or older.

The distribution of limitations among nursing home residents, however, is quite different in the two surveys (table II.8). Measures of

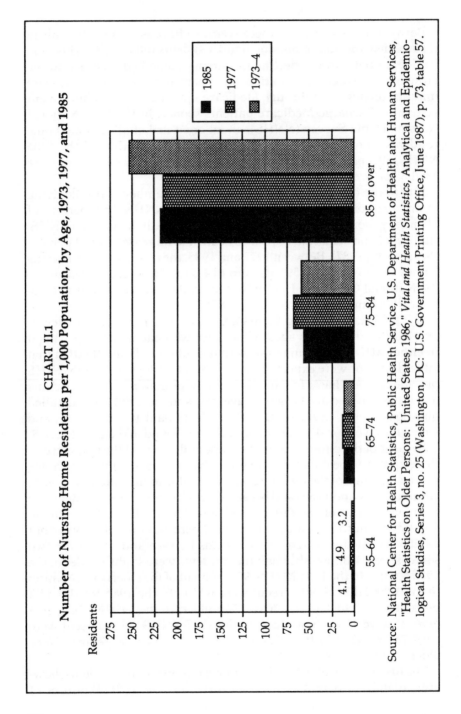

CHART II.1

Number of Nursing Home Residents per 1,000 Population, by Age, 1973, 1977, and 1985

Legend:
- 1985
- 1977
- 1973–4

55–64: 4.1, 4.9, 3.2

65–74

75–84

85 or over

Residents: 0, 25, 50, 75, 100, 125, 150, 175, 200, 225, 250, 275

Source: National Center for Health Statistics, Public Health Service, U.S. Department of Health and Human Services, "Health Statistics on Older Persons: United States, 1986," *Vital and Health Statistics*, Analytical and Epidemiological Studies, Series 3, no. 25 (Washington, DC: U.S. Government Printing Office, June 1987), p. 73, table 57.

TABLE II.7
# Median Length of Stay and Percentage Distribution of Nursing Home Residents, by Age, 1977 and 1985

| Age | 1977 | | 1985 | |
|---|---|---|---|---|
| | Percentage distribution | Median stay (in days) | Percentage distribution | Median stay (in days) |
| Total | 100.0% | 597 | 100.0% | 614 |
| Under 45 years | 2.5 | 657 | 3.0 | 551 |
| 45–54 years | 3.3 | 786 | 2.5 | 876 |
| 55–64 years | 7.7 | 632 | 6.2 | 686 |
| 65–69 years | 6.3 | 592 | 5.5 | 657 |
| 70–74 years | 10.0 | 440 | 8.7 | 510 |
| 75–79 years | 15.3 | 517 | 14.6 | 544 |
| 80–84 years | 20.4 | 513 | 19.6 | 560 |
| 85–89 years | 20.2 | 621 | 19.8 | 615 |
| 90–94 years | 10.8 | 821 | 14.2 | 684 |
| 95 years or over | 3.4 | 940 | 6.0 | 917 |

Source: National Center for Health Statistics, Public Health Service, U.S. Department of Health and Human Services, "Health Statistics on Older Persons," *Vital and Health Statistics*, Analytical and Epidemiological Studies, Series 3, no. 25 (Washington, DC: U.S. Government Printing Office, June 1987), p. 74, table 58; and National Center for Health Statistics, Public Health Service, U.S. Department of Health and Human Services, "The National Nursing Home Survey: 1985 Summary for the United States," *Vital and Health Statistics*, Series 13, no. 97, DHHS pub. no. (PHS) 89-1758 (Washington, DC: U.S. Government Printing Office, January 1989), p. 26, table 19.

Note: Percentages may not add to 100 because of rounding.

disability suggest that those in the 1985 NNHS were much more functionally dependent than those in the 1984 NLTCS. In the 1985 NNHS, 7.6 percent of the residents had no ADL limitations and 30.4 percent had six. Almost conversely, in the 1984 NLTCS, 19.3 percent had no ADL limitations and 8.5 percent had six. It is likely that these differences reflect the survey questions. In the 1985 NNHS, limitations were recorded if the resident received any assistance, while the 1984 NLTCS questions focused on the extent of an individual's dependency in terms of the number of ADLs he or she was unable to perform at all without assistance.

### TABLE II.8
## Number of Dependencies in Activities of Daily Living among the Institutionalized Population Aged 65 or over, 1984 and 1985

| Number of Dependencies in Activities of Daily Living | Institutionalized Population (1984 National Long-Term Care Survey) | Institutionalized Population (1985 National Nursing Home Survey) |
|---|---|---|
| Total | 100.0% | 100.0% |
| None | 19.3 | 7.6 |
| One | 12.7 | 11.1 |
| Two | 13.0 | 9.9 |
| Three | 13.7 | 7.8 |
| Four | 17.5 | 13.5 |
| Five | 15.4 | 19.8 |
| Six | 8.5 | 30.4 |

Source: EBRI tabulations of the 1984 National Long-Term Care Survey, Health Care Financing Administration, U.S. Department of Health and Human Services; and National Center for Health Statistics, Public Health Service, U.S. Department of Health and Human Services, "The National Nursing Home Survey: 1985 Summary for the United States," *Vital and Health Statistics*, Series 13, no. 97, DHHS pub. no. (PHS) 89-1758 (Washington, DC: U.S. Government Printing Office, January 1989), p. 38, table 28.

Note: Percentages may not add to 100 because of rounding.

Reported payment sources for nursing home care in the 1984 NLTCS included residents themselves (reported by 35.3 percent of the residents), Medicaid (31.3 percent), Medicare (12.8 percent), and a child (5.8 percent). At the time of the 1984 survey, Medicaid was indicated by 40 percent of the respondents, the nursing home resident was indicated by 36 percent, and Medicare was indicated by 8.3 percent (table II.9). When asked who was the primary payer or who paid the most at the time of entry into the nursing home, 60 percent of the residents indicated Medicaid. At the time of the interview in 1984, however, less than two-thirds (68.4 percent) of the residents indicated Medicaid paid the most. About one-half (50.7 percent) of the residents indicated that they entered without any assistance from Medicaid but were receiving assistance at the time of the interview.

For about 7.3 percent of the residents receiving assistance from Medicaid, Medicaid was not the largest source of payment upon enter-

**TABLE II.9**
# Sources of Payment for Nursing Home Residents

| All Payers | Percentage on Entering | Percentage Now |
|---|---|---|
| Self | 35.3% | 36.0% |
| Spouse | 2.8 | 2.4 |
| Child | 5.8 | 5.4 |
| Other Relative | 2.6 | 2.2 |
| Non-Relative | 0.3 | 0.4 |
| Private Insurance | 2.2 | 1.3 |
| Medicare | 12.8 | 8.3 |
| Medicaid | 31.3 | 39.9 |
| Other Payer | 1.4 | 1.7 |
| CHAMPUS[a] | 1.7 | 2.0 |
| Other | 3.8 | 0.5 |
| | | |
| Total | 100.0 | 100.0 |

| Primary Payer | Percentage on Entering | Percentage Now |
|---|---|---|
| Self | 16.8% | 16.4% |
| Spouse | 1.7 | 1.0 |
| Child | 5.0 | 3.4 |
| Other Relative | 0.5 | 0.2 |
| Non-Relative | 0.2 | 0.0 |
| Private Insurance | 0.9 | 0.6 |
| Medicare | 10.3 | 5.0 |
| Medicaid | 59.5 | 68.4 |
| Other Payer | 0.9 | 1.7 |
| CHAMPUS[a] | 1.2 | 0.8 |
| Other | 3.0 | 2.5 |
| | | |
| Total | 100.0 | 100.0 |

Source: EBRI tabulations of the 1984 National Long-Term Care Survey Institutionalized Component, Health Care Financing Administration, U.S. Department of Health and Human Services.
[a]Civilian Health and Medical Program of the Uniformed Services.
Note: Percentages may not add to 100 because of rounding.

ing the home, but was by the time of the interview. In the 1984 NLTCS about one-quarter of the elderly in nursing homes reported that prior to institutionalization they had lived at home (26.7 percent), and one-quarter (25.01 percent) reported that they had been in the hospital. But more than one-third (35.6 percent) did not know where they had been immediately prior to nursing home admission.

## Chronically Disabled Persons Living in the Community

In 1984, an estimated 15.4 million people, or 6.4 percent of the population, were living in the community and claimed to have a limitation requiring assistance from others. These limitations varied in severity from needing assistance with light housework to personal hygiene (bathing, using the toilet, etc.). Contrary to popular belief, *less than one-half* of the chronically disabled living in the community (48.8 percent) were elderly. Three-quarters (75.7 percent) were aged 45 or older, but more than 12 percent were aged 15 or younger (table II.10). Like the size of the nursing home population, the number of persons reporting limitations increased with age. Less than 3.1 percent of children under age 15 were reported to have limitations, while the prevalence rates among those aged 25 to 45 was 2.1 percent, and for those aged 45 to 65, 19.4 percent. Prevalence rates after age 65 doubled, and among those aged 75 or older, 41.2 percent reported limitations requiring the assistance of others.

Table II.11 compares the prevalence of common chronic conditions among people aged 45 to 64 with their prevalence among people aged 65 or older. Among the elderly, rates of prevalence of arthritis, hearing and visual impairments, and arteriosclerosis are twice those of people under age 65. Data from the 1977 NNHS indicated that nearly all residents of the surveyed institutions reported one or more chronic conditions. The most frequent diagnoses were arteriosclerosis (48 percent), heart trouble (34 percent), senility (32 percent), arthritis and rheumatism (25 percent), hypertension (21 percent), and diabetes (15 percent) (National Center for Health Statistics, 1981).

Table II.12 shows the distribution of people in the community aged 45 or older by marital status, age, and potential dependency. ADL limitations for this tabulation include getting into or out of bed, moving about the home inside, or looking after personal needs such as dressing, undressing, eating, or personal hygiene without assistance from others. IADL limitations include the inability to lift or carry groceries, to walk about three city blocks, or to prepare meals or do light housekeeping.

TABLE II.10
# Prevalence of Disability among the Noninstitutionalized Population, 1984

| Age Group | Total Population (in thousands) | Persons with Limitations[a] (in thousands) | Percentage among the Disabled | Percentage within Each Age Group |
|---|---|---|---|---|
| Total | 243,432 | 15,452 | 100.0% | 6.4% |
| Under 15[b] | 62,445 | 1,916 | 12.4 | 3.1 |
| 15–24 | 39,297 | 346 | 2.2 | 0.9 |
| 25–34 | 40,464 | 596 | 3.9 | 1.5 |
| 35–44 | 30,480 | 890 | 5.8 | 2.9 |
| 45–54 | 22,264 | 1,431 | 9.3 | 6.4 |
| 55–64 | 22,060 | 2,734 | 17.7 | 12.4 |
| 65–69 | 8,928 | 1,682 | 10.9 | 18.8 |
| 70–74 | 7,378 | 1,691 | 10.9 | 22.9 |
| 75 or over | 10,116 | 4,166 | 27.0 | 41.2 |

Source: EBRI tabulations of published Survey of Income and Program Participation data in Bureau of the Census, U.S. Department of Commerce, "Disability, Functional Limitation, and Health Insurance Coverage: 1984–1985," *Current Population Reports*, Household Economic Studies, Series P-70, no. 8 (Washington, DC: U.S. Government Printing Office, December 1986), pp. 4 and 9, tables C and H.

[a]Limitations for everyone aged 15 or over are based on the need for assistance from another person in doing either light housework, preparing meals, dressing, eating, personal hygiene, or getting around.

[b]Limitations for children are based on whether the child had a long-lasting physical, mental, or emotional condition that limited walking, running, playing, or learning to do regular schoolwork.

Note: Percentages may not add to 100 because of rounding.

In general, within each age group, those who were married were less likely to report ADL limitations than those who were not married. The proportion of the population both without limitations and with a spouse decreases with age. Among widowed, divorced, or separated individuals, more than 70 percent of those with ADL limitations were aged 75 or over.

In the 1984 Survey of Income and Program Participation (SIPP), more than 7.5 million elderly persons reported some level of limitation that created dependency. The 1984 NLTCS, however, found slightly fewer than 6.1 million Medicare recipients with chronic disabilities. The NLTCS used much more careful screening criteria to identify the

**TABLE II.11**

# Prevalence of Common Chronic Conditions among Persons Aged 45–64 and 65 or over, as a Percentage of Persons with the Conditions in Each Age Group

| | Age | |
|---|---|---|
| Condition | 45–64 | 65 or over |
| Arthritis | 24.7% | 46.5% |
| Hypertensive Disease | 24.4 | 37.9 |
| Hearing Impairments | 14.3 | 28.4 |
| Heart Conditions | 12.3 | 27.7 |
| Chronic Sinusitis | 17.8 | 18.4 |
| Visual Impairments[a] | 5.5 | 13.7 |
| Orthopedic Impairments (back, extremities, or other) | 11.8 | 12.8 |
| Arteriosclerosis | 2.1 | 9.7 |
| Diabetes | 5.7 | 8.3 |
| Varicose Veins | 5.0 | 8.3 |
| Hemorrhoids | 6.7 | 6.6 |
| Frequent Constipation | 2.2 | 5.9 |
| Urinary System Disease | 3.2 | 5.6 |
| Corns and Callosities | 3.6 | 5.2 |
| Hay Fever | 7.8 | 5.2 |
| Hernia of Abdominal Cavity | 2.5 | 4.9 |

Source:  Division of Health Interview Statistics, National Center for Health Statistics, as quoted in Special Committee on Aging, Senate, U.S. Congress, *Aging America: Trends and Projections* (Washington, DC: U.S. Government Printing Office, 1984), p. 59, chart 42.
[a]The category of visual impairments is a combination of blindness in one or both eyes and other vision problems.

chronically disabled, who were defined as those whose disability had lasted or was likely to last for 90 days or longer.[14]

Even among the chronically disabled elderly on Medicare who were identified in the 1984 NLTCS, only slightly more than one-quarter (28.8 percent) had ADL limitations requiring assistance from others (eating, bathing, getting into or out of bed, dressing, or getting to the bathroom or using the toilet). Nearly four-fifths (78.8 percent) of the

[14]Potential respondents to the NLTCS were screened by telephone prior to in-person interviews.

TABLE II.12
# Limitations of People in the Community, by Age and Marital Status, 1984

| Age Group | Type of Limitation by Age Group | | | |
| --- | --- | --- | --- | --- |
| | No Limitations | ADL Limitations[a] | IADL Only[b] | Total |
| Married | | | | |
| 45–54 | 93.0% | 1.4% | 5.6% | 100.0% |
| 55–64 | 87.0 | 1.9 | 11.1 | 100.0 |
| 65–74 | 80.1 | 3.6 | 16.3 | 100.0 |
| 75 or over | 64.8 | 9.6 | 25.6 | 100.0 |
| All ages | 86.0 | 2.7 | 11.4 | 100.0 |
| Widowed, Divorced, or Separated | | | | |
| 45–54 | 85.4 | 1.6 | 13.0 | 100.0 |
| 55–64 | 78.3 | 2.2 | 19.5 | 100.0 |
| 65–74 | 70.4 | 2.8 | 26.9 | 100.0 |
| 75 or over | 46.0 | 13.2 | 40.8 | 100.0 |
| All ages | 68.2 | 5.4 | 26.4 | 100.0 |
| Never Married | | | | |
| 45–54 | 86.9 | 3.7 | 9.4 | 100.0 |
| 55–64 | 82.6 | 1.9 | 15.5 | 100.0 |
| 65–74 | 74.6 | 5.1 | 20.3 | 100.0 |
| 75 or over | 62.7 | 8.5 | 28.9 | 100.0 |
| All ages | 78.0 | 4.5 | 17.5 | 100.0 |

| Age Group | Age Group by Type of Limitation | | |
| --- | --- | --- | --- |
| | No Limitations | ADL Limitations[a] | IADL Only[b] |
| Married | | | |
| 45–54 | 39.4% | 18.6% | 18.1% |
| 55–64 | 35.1 | 24.3 | 33.9 |
| 65–74 | 19.7 | 28.7 | 30.3 |
| 75 or over | 5.9 | 28.4 | 17.7 |
| All ages | 100.0 | 100.0 | 100.0 |

**(continued)**

**TABLE II.12 (continued)**

| | Type of Limitation by Age Group | | |
| Age Group | No Limitations | ADL Limitations[a] | IADL Only[b] |
|---|---|---|---|
| **Widowed, Divorced, or Separated** | | | |
| 45–54 | 24.8% | 5.9% | 9.8% |
| 55–64 | 27.8 | 10.0 | 17.9 |
| 65–74 | 27.9 | 13.7 | 27.6 |
| 75 or over | 19.5 | 70.4 | 44.8 |
| All ages | 100.0 | 100.0 | 100.0 |
| **Never Married** | | | |
| 45–54 | 31.0 | 23.2 | 15.0 |
| 55–64 | 29.8 | 12.1 | 24.9 |
| 65–74 | 24.0 | 29.0 | 29.1 |
| 75 or over | 15.1 | 35.8 | 31.0 |
| All ages | 100.0 | 100.0 | 100.0 |

Source: EBRI tabulations of the 1984 Survey of Income and Program Participation, Bureau of the Census, U.S. Department of Commerce.
[a]Activity of daily living (ADL) limitations include needing help with personal needs, such as dressing and undressing, eating, or personal hygiene, transferring into and out of bed, and moving around inside the home.
[b]Instrumental activity of daily living (IADL) limitations include having difficulty getting around the house without assistance and needing help to do light housework, prepare meals, or lift more than 10 pounds.
Note: Percentages may not add to 100 because of rounding.

chronically disabled, or 17 percent of all the elderly, had IADL limitations requiring assistance from others (including difficulties getting around outside, preparing meals, doing laundry, light housekeeping, grocery shopping, managing money, taking medication, and making telephone calls) (table II.13). Less than 8 percent of the chronically disabled had indications of dementia and less than one-quarter had indications of incontinence.[15]

While the prevalence of IADLs and ADLs increases with age, the relationship is not strong. This may indicate an increased likelihood that older people are dying or leaving the community and entering an institution. In 1984, 5 percent of all chronically disabled elderly persons had four or more ADL limitations. Only 4.1 percent of those aged 65 to 70, and 7.6 percent of those aged 85, had as many deficits.

---

[15]The question about dementia was asked only of people who answered the survey on behalf of the chronically disabled person being surveyed. Incontinence and other limitations are not mutually exclusive.

# TABLE II.13

## Distribution of IADL[a] and ADL[b] Limitations, Incontinence, and Dementia among Disabled Elderly, by Age, 1984

| Limitations | Total Population | Distribution | Distribution by Age | | | | | |
| --- | --- | --- | --- | --- | --- | --- | --- | --- |
| | | | 70 or under | 71–75 | 76–80 | 81–85 | 86 or over |
| IADLs Only | 3,253,000 | 53.8% | 54.0% | 54.3% | 55.0% | 54.4% | 50.4% |
| Number of IADLs | | | | | | | |
| 0 | 1,280,255 | 21.2 | 26.2 | 26.0 | 21.8 | 17.2 | 10.0 |
| 1 | 1,342,462 | 22.2 | 27.3 | 23.6 | 23.7 | 21.0 | 11.4 |
| 2 | 867,239 | 14.3 | 13.7 | 14.4 | 16.0 | 14.2 | 13.2 |
| 3 | 771,381 | 12.8 | 11.7 | 13.7 | 9.8 | 14.7 | 14.9 |
| 4 | 544,424 | 9.0 | 7.2 | 7.9 | 8.5 | 9.6 | 13.6 |
| 5 | 416,385 | 6.9 | 6.0 | 5.6 | 7.5 | 6.2 | 10.2 |
| 6 | 342,638 | 5.7 | 3.9 | 4.1 | 5.9 | 6.8 | 9.2 |
| 7 | 315,172 | 5.2 | 2.2 | 3.3 | 4.4 | 6.8 | 12.1 |
| 8 | 166,718 | 2.8 | 1.8 | 1.5 | 2.6 | 3.4 | 5.6 |
| Total | 6,046,674 | 100.0 | 100.0 | 100.0 | 100.0 | 100.0 | 100.0 |

(continued)

59

**TABLE II.13 (continued)**

| Limitations | Total Population | Distribution | Distribution by Age | | | | | |
| --- | --- | --- | --- | --- | --- | --- | --- | --- |
| | | | 70 or under | 71–75 | 76–80 | 81–85 | 86 or over |
| Number of ADLs | | | | | | | | |
| 0 | 4,486,326 | 74.2% | 79.5% | 79.1% | 76.2% | 70.5% | 60.1% |
| 1 | 820,689 | 13.6 | 10.1 | 10.6 | 13.4 | 15.8 | 21.0 |
| 2 | 257,664 | 4.3 | 3.8 | 3.2 | 3.0 | 5.5 | 6.9 |
| 3 | 180,260 | 3.0 | 2.4 | 2.9 | 2.9 | 2.7 | 4.4 |
| 4 | 143,336 | 2.4 | 2.0 | 2.2 | 2.2 | 2.6 | 3.2 |
| 5 | 97,134 | 1.6 | 1.4 | 1.1 | 1.8 | 1.6 | 2.3 |
| 6 | 61,269 | 1.0 | 0.7 | 0.8 | 0.5 | 1.3 | 2.1 |
| Total | 6,046,676 | 100.0 | 100.0 | 100.0 | 100.0 | 100.0 | 100.0 |
| Incontinence | 1,426,546 | 23.6 | 26.8 | 22.1 | 20.2 | 23.9 | 25.0 |
| Dementia | 464,538 | 7.7 | 3.0 | 4.6 | 7.9 | 11.1 | 15.5 |

Source: EBRI tabulations of the 1984 National Long-Term Care Survey, Health Care Financing Administration, U.S. Department of Health and Human Services.

[a]Instrumental activity of daily living (IADL) limitations include respondents who could not do household chores (moving furniture, scrubbing floors, washing windows), laundry, or grocery shopping, manage their own money, take medicine, make telephone calls, prepare meals, or get around outside.

[b]Activity of daily living (ADL) limitations include respondents who needed assistance from others with eating, transferring to or from bed or chair, moving around inside the home, dressing, bathing, getting to the bathroom, or using the toilet, or were incontinent.

Note: Percentages may not add to 100 because of rounding.

This suggests that—among the entire population—while age is an important indicator of risk of institutionalization, other factors, such as marital status, living arrangement, physical environment of the home, income, or the proximity of children, may be equally or more important than the number of IADL or ADL deficits.

Table II.14 summarizes the demographics of the chronically disabled population organized by increasing levels of dependency. The level of dependency does not increase with average age. In general, the oldest groups, "the survivors," include both the most and the least dependent. In fact, those with no ADL limitations and no problems with incontinence were on average 81.1 years old, while the average age of the chronically disabled elderly was 77. Among those missing from this chronically disabled group are those who died or entered an institution. Consequently, among the chronically disabled elderly, age per se becomes a much less significant indicator of the degree of dependency (although it is more likely that the older the person, the more functionally dependent he or she will be). Since women have a longer life expectancy, the survivor population in the community is predominantly female. The more functionally dependent the individual, the less likely he or she is to live alone. Finally, most of those living with others live with their spouses.

## Chronically Disabled Persons: Differences between Nursing Home- and Community-Based Residents

Table II.15 provides an overall comparison of elderly persons living in nursing homes with those living in the community in 1984. The elderly in nursing homes were clearly older (45 percent were aged 85 or over), as were the disabled in the community (15 percent were aged 85 or over), relative to everyone living in the community (7.6 percent). Compared with those living in the community (59 percent), those in nursing homes were most likely to be women (75 percent). The disabled in the community were more likely to be women (65 percent) as well. Disabled blacks were slightly less likely to be living in nursing homes, as were married individuals.

In the 1984 NLTCs, 1.6 million chronically disabled elderly persons on Medicare were living in nursing homes. Four times as many, or 6.1 million, lived in the community.[16] Although poor health and func-

---

[16]The 1985 NNHS estimated that there were 1.3 million elderly persons in nursing homes. This figure would place the ratio of elderly in nursing homes to chronically disabled elderly in the community closer to 5 to 1.

## TABLE II.14
## Demographic Characteristics of the Noninstitutionalized Elderly with ADL[a] Limitations, by Degree of Severity, 1984

| Limitation | Number (in thousands) | Average Age | Percentage Female | Percentage Living with Spouse | Percentage Living with Others | Percentage Living Alone |
|---|---|---|---|---|---|---|
| No ADL limitations and no incontinence | 48.1 | 81.1 | 55.8% | 51.4% | 34.3% | 13.3% |
| At least one limitation | 3,972.1 | 76.8 | 61.6 | 43.2 | 23.4 | 33.4 |
| Only one limitation | 1,453.9 | 77.0 | 73.5 | 39.5 | 24.0 | 36.4 |
| Two limitations, but not in bathing | 55.8 | 76.7 | 81.9 | 35.6 | 42.0 | 22.3 |
| Bathing and one other limitation | 345.8 | 79.1 | 69.6 | 40.4 | 35.9 | 23.7 |
| Bathing, dressing, and one other limitation | 68.5 | 78.4 | 52.1 | 51.7 | 35.8 | 12.5 |
| Bathing, dressing, and either getting to the bathroom or using the toilet and one other limitation | 67.1 | 77.1 | 58.3 | 46.1 | 39.8 | 14.0 |
| Bathing, dressing, and either getting to the bathroom or using the toilet, getting into or out of bed, and one other limitation | 33.4 | 76.0 | 65.0 | 61.5 | 31.6 | 6.9 |

| | | | | | | |
|---|---|---|---|---|---|---|
| Bathing, dressing, and either getting to the bathroom or using the toilet, getting into or out of bed, eating, and incontinence | 1.8 | 80.2 | 100.0 | 45.7 | 54.3 | [b] |
| Total | 6,046.7 | 77.0 | 64.9 | 42.4 | 24.9 | 32.7 |

Source: EBRI tabulations of the 1984 National Long Term Care Survey, Health Care Financing Administration, U.S. Department of Health and Human Services.

[a]Activity of daily living (ADL) limitations include respondents who needed assistance from others with eating, transferring to or from bed or chair, moving around inside the home, dressing, bathing, getting to the bathroom, or using the toilet, or were incontinent.
[b]Number too small to be statistically reliable.

**TABLE II.15**

# Selected Characteristics of Nursing Home and Community Residents Aged 65 or over, 1984 and 1985

| Subject | Living in Nursing Homes, 1985 | Disabled Living in Community, 1984 | Everyone Living in Community, 1984 |
|---|---|---|---|
| Total Aged 65 or over | | | |
| Number (in thousands) | 1,316 | 6,047 | 26,343 |
| Percentage | 100.0% | 100.0% | 100.0% |
| | | | |
| Age | | | |
| 65–74 | 16.1 | 46.1 | 61.7 |
| 75–84 | 38.7 | 38.9 | 30.7 |
| 85 or over | 45.2 | 15.0 | 7.6 |
| | | | |
| Gender | | | |
| Men | 25.4 | 35.1 | 40.8 |
| Women | 74.6 | 64.9 | 59.2 |
| | | | |
| Race | | | |
| White | 93.1 | 84.5 | 90.4 |
| Black | 6.2 | 11.9 | 8.3 |
| Other | 0.7 | 1.2 | 1.3 |
| Unknown | a | 2.3 | a |
| | | | |
| Marital Status | | | |
| Widowed | 64.2 | a | 34.1 |
| Married | 16.4 | 42.1 | 54.7 |
| Never married | 13.5 | a | 4.4 |
| Divorced or separated | 5.9 | a | 6.3 |
| | | | |
| With Living Children | 63.1 | 75.3 | 81.3 |

Source: Special Committee on Aging, Senate, U.S. Congress, *Aging America: Trends and Projections*, 1987–88 ed. (Washington, DC: U.S. Department of Health and Human Services, 1988), p. 119, table 4–11; and EBRI tabulations of the 1984 National Long-Term Care Survey, Health Care Financing Administration, U.S. Department of Health and Human Services.

aData not available.

Note: Percentages may not add to 100 because of rounding.

tional dependency are correlated with institutionalization (Wingard, Jones, and Kaplan, 1987), in terms of severity of dependency it is not clear that those in nursing homes are much more dependent than those in the community (table II.16). In fact, while a smaller proportion of the chronically disabled in the community were incontinent, a larger proportion in nursing homes were without any ADL deficits.

Of considerable concern is the difference between the two populations, and, more specifically, which factors explain why some chronically disabled elderly persons are in nursing homes and why the majority are in the community. It has been estimated that for every five people aged 85 or older living in an institution, there is another person still living in the community at a comparable level of disability (Soldo and Manton, 1985). While the distribution in table II.16 suggests that a larger percentage of nursing home residents had more limitations, this may be partly due to the fact that over time nursing home residents may become more dependent on others. This proportion tends to support the notion that elderly individuals living in nursing homes—especially those who have not been there for long—may not be appreciably more dependent than the chronically dependent in the community.[17]

Factors cited most often to explain nursing home residency or to predict nursing home admission include age; functional, medical, mental, and marital status; living arrangements; social supports; income; race; and sex. It is difficult to generalize the results of these studies because most of them have used different populations and different sets of risk factors (Kane and Kane, 1987). While the results tend to be consistent, the predictive power of the estimates they produce has been quite small and, therefore, limited (Kane and Kane, 1987; Wingard, Jones, and Kaplan, 1987; Cohen, Tell, and Wallack, 1986a).

Table II.16 shows the distribution of ADL limitations, which have been grouped from one or two limitations (excluding bathing) to limitations that include the inability to bathe, a factor that, along with immobility, is a very strong predictor of institutionalization (Hughes, 1986). However, less than one-quarter of the disabled elderly in nursing homes indicated that they had two or more ADL deficits, including the need for assistance in bathing.

---

[17]The findings of Soldo and Manton (1985) and this ratio are not necessarily exact correlates, since they are measuring a different, although related, phenomenon.

## TABLE II.16
# Severity of Functional Dependency among Chronically Disabled Elderly in Nursing Homes and in the Community, 1984

| Limitation | Institutionalized | | Noninstitutionalized | |
|---|---|---|---|---|
| | Number (in thousands) | Percentage | Number (in thousands) | Percentage |
| No ADL[a] limitations and no incontinence | 119.8 | 7.7% | 48.1 | 0.8% |
| At least one limitation | 834.6 | 53.8 | 3,972.1 | 65.7 |
| Only one limitation | 173.7 | 11.2 | 1,453.9 | 24.0 |
| Two limitations, but not in bathing | 66.6 | 4.3 | 55.8 | 0.9 |
| Bathing and one other limitation | 100.6 | 6.5 | 345.8 | 5.7 |
| Bathing, dressing, and one other limitation | 101.6 | 6.5 | 68.5 | 1.1 |
| Bathing, dressing, and either getting to the bathroom or using the toilet and one other limitation | 95.4 | 6.1 | 67.1 | 1.1 |
| Bathing, dressing, and either getting to the bathroom or using the toilet, getting into or out of bed, and one other limitation | 47.7 | 3.1 | 33.4 | 0.6 |
| Bathing, dressing, and either getting to the bathroom or using the toilet, getting into or out of bed, eating, and incontinence | 11.2 | 0.7 | 1.8 | [b] |
| Total | 1,551.3 | 100.0 | 6,046.7 | 100.0 |

Source:  EBRI tabulations of the 1984 National Long-Term Care Survey, Health Care Financing Administration, U.S. Department of Health and Human Services.

[a]Activity of daily living (ADL) limitations include respondents who needed assistance from others with eating, transferring to or from bed or chair, moving around inside the home, dressing, bathing, getting to the bathroom, or using the toilet, or were incontinent.

[b]Number too small to be statistically significant.

Note:  Percentages may not add to 100 because of rounding.

# The Risk of Institutionalization

Cross-sectional data suggest that about 5 percent of the elderly can be found living in nursing homes at any point in time (table II.17). These cross-sectional surveys, however, are apt to be biased because they are more likely to include long-term nursing home residents and less likely to include short-term ones. Adjusting for this bias may dramatically increase the number of elderly who are in nursing homes at some time during the year. Estimates indicate that instead of the suggested 4.7 percent of the elderly in nursing homes in 1977, a more accurate figure would have been 8.9 percent (Hughes, 1986).

The risk of institutionalization, however, is substantially higher than actual institutionalization at any point in time. Studies of obituary notices and death certificates, for example, have shown that around 20 percent of the elderly die in a nursing facility (Wingard, Jones, and Kaplan, 1987). The marked difference between the cross-sectional estimates previously mentioned and this estimate reflects the fact that many individuals die shortly after admission to a nursing home.

Cross-sectional estimates of the proportion of elderly persons residing in nursing homes are not sufficient indices of either the long-term care needs of the elderly or the risk of nursing home institutionalization faced by an individual over his or her lifetime (Liang and Tu, 1986). Implicit in these studies is the assumption that current rates of nursing home utilization are "appropriate." Distortions in the long-term care market, such as regional restrictions on the supply of nursing home beds or community-based care services, limit the ability to determine the "real" risks of institutionalization (U.S. General Accounting Office, 1983). In 1979, the U.S. General Accounting Office cited studies estimating that between 10 percent and 18 percent of all nursing home residents could live in the community, and that between 10 percent and 40 percent of residents were receiving higher levels of care than necessary (U.S. General Accounting Office, 1979).

The lifetime risk of being institutionalized is difficult to assess since it is complicated by a number of demographic, health, economic, and social factors for which data are limited. Studies of the risk of institutionalization vary with the methodology and data used. Table II.17 summarizes studies that assess the rates of institutionalization of specified populations. The studies vary widely in their methodologies, in populations surveyed, in their definitions of nursing homes, and in the periods covered. Because of these variations and limitations, no one study should be viewed as definitive.

## TABLE II.17
## Studies of Rates of Nursing Home Utilization

| Percentage Institutionalized | Type of Study | Period | Study Site | Ages | Data Source | Author (Year)[a] |
|---|---|---|---|---|---|---|
| **At Point in Time** | | | | | | |
| 4.6% | Cross-sectional | 1974 | United States | 65 or over | NCHS[b] | Ingram and Barry (1977) and others[c] |
| **At Time of Death** | | | | | | |
| 20.0% | Cross-sectional | 1971 | Detroit, MI | 65 or over | Death certificates | Kastenbaum and Candy (1973) |
| 21.0 | Cross-sectional | 1972 | United States | 55 or over | NCHS[b] | Ingram and Barry (1977) |
| 19.0 | Cross-sectional | 1975 | Springfield, IL | 65 or over | Death certificates | Lesnoff-Caravaglia (1978–1979) |
| **Prior to Death** | | | | | | |
| 26.0% | Prospective | 1955–76 | Piedmont, NC | 60 or over | Death certificates and interviews | Palmore (1976) |
| 39.0 46.0 | Prospective | 1965–75 | Alameda, CA | 55 or over, 65 or over | Death certificates and interviews | Vicente et al. (1979) |
| **Over Period** | | | | | | |
| 9.0% | Prospective | 1975–80 | Massachusetts | 65 or over | Death certificates and interviews | Branch and Jette (1982) |
| 12.0 | Prospective | 1971–77 | Manitoba, Canada | 65 or over | Nursing home records and interviews | Shapiro and Tate (1985) |
| 5.5 | Prospective | 1982–84 | United States | 65 or over | NLTSC[d] | Manton (1988) |

| Over Lifetime | | | | | | |
|---|---|---|---|---|---|---|
| 48.0% | Cross-sectional | 1976 | United States | Life span<br>65 or over | NCHS[b] | McConnel (1984) |
| 63.0 | Extrapolated | | | | | |
| 29.7 | Cross-sectional | 1976 | United States | At birth<br>65–70 | NCHS[b] | Liang and Tu (1986) |
| 35.6 | Extrapolated | | | | | |
| 43.1 | Prospective | 1977 | United States | 65 or over | Current Medicare<br>Survey | Cohen, Tell, and<br>Wallack (1986a) |
| | Extrapolated | | | | | |

Source: Adapted from Deborah L. Wingard, Denise Williams Jones, and Robert M. Kaplan, "Institutional Care Utilization by the Elderly: A Critical Review," *The Gerontologist* (April 1987). p. 158, table 3, updated by the author.

[a]See reference list for full citations.
[b]National Center for Health Statistics, Health Care Financing Administration, U.S. Department of Health and Human Services.
[c]One of many possible citations.
[d]National Long-Term Care Survey (of functionally disabled Medicare beneficiaries).

Studies that use cross-sectional data estimate the proportion of the population in long-term care facilities at a particular time. Although at any given time only about 4 percent to 5 percent of the elderly are institutionalized, studies of death certificates have found that about 20 percent of the elderly who die each year resided in nursing homes. While death certificate data suggest that risk of institutionalization increases as a person gets closer to death, death certificate data alone are inadequate for quantifying the likelihood of nursing home placement. Studies of death certificate data miss people who lived in a nursing home but died in a hospital or at home (Wingard, Jones, and Kaplan, 1987).

Prospective studies, also known as cohort or longitudinal studies, begin with noninstitutionalized people and follow them over time to determine the rate at which they are institutionalized. The prospective studies in table II.17 fall into studies that follow people until death and those that follow people for a fixed period. Both studies that prospectively measure nursing home placement over their subjects' lifetimes are geographically limited and, therefore, may not be extrapolative to the total population. In the studies estimating the lifetime risk of nursing home placement, cross-sectional data on institutionalization rates at each age were used to construct the equivalent of an actuarial life table, which was used to extrapolate lifetime risk of a typical person as he or she ages.

The estimates of lifetime risk at age 65, based on retrospective analyses of cohorts' rates of institutionalization, range from a high of 63 percent to a low of 39 percent (McConnel, 1984; Cohen, Tell, and Wallack, 1986a; Liang and Tu, 1986). Most studies assume that nursing home residents remain in the facility until they die. Since about 59 percent of nursing home residents were discharged alive in 1985, this assumption biases the estimate downward.

From these studies, it has been estimated that almost 70 percent of people aged 65 or over will die having spent less than one month in a nursing home (Scanlon, 1988). Almost 80 percent will spend less than three months in a nursing home, 13 percent will spend more than one year, and 9 percent will spend two or more years. That is, while few people will spend any time in a nursing facility, those who do are likely to spend a very long time—perhaps, in large part, due to existing financing arrangements.

## Conclusion

Chronic disabilities often accompany expanded life expectancy. Increasingly, death is likely to be associated with chronic medical conditions that may persist for many years, such as chronic heart or respiratory conditions, arthritis, or rheumatism. Three out of four deaths among the entire population now occur from degenerative diseases, primarily at advanced ages (Olshansky and Ault, 1986; Office of Technology Assessment, 1985; Manton, 1982). Many people with degenerative diseases need help that can vary from being driven to the grocery store to assistance with daily activities such as eating or using the toilet. This sort of assistance is often necessary for people with cognitive dysfunctions and degenerative brain diseases such as Alzheimer's disease or related dementias.

The increasing number of elderly persons, especially the rapid growth of those aged 85 or older, means that unless there are significant reductions in the frequency of disability, the number of elderly who will need assistance will increase. The distribution of the kinds of care sought will depend, however, on whether age-specific disability rates change. Unless future age-specific morbidity rates fall substantially below current levels, there will be tremendous increases in the number and proportion of the population afflicted with incapacitating conditions. In spite of the substantial increases in life expectancy, disability rates have not decreased. As suggested in table II.10, in 1984, one-quarter of the elderly (28.5 percent) needed some level of assistance; among people aged 75 or older, 41.2 percent needed assistance. As suggested in table II.6, among the population aged 85 or older, 18.1 percent resided in nursing homes.

If current trends of nursing home utilization continue, as indicated by chart II.1 and table II.6, all of the currently available nursing home beds could be filled with the nearly 1.2 million people aged 85 or older projected to need nursing home care in the year 2030. It has been predicted that by the year 2050 the number of people needing nursing home care will be two-and-one-half times the number of nursing home residents in 1975 (Russell, 1981). One study projected the institutionalization rates observed in the 1977 NNHS onto the projected population in the year 2000 and found a nearly 50 percent increase in the number of people in institutions over those estimated to be living there in 1985 (Weissert, 1985).

Another study estimated that in 1980 nearly 6 million episodes of long-term care service per day were given outside of institutions, and projected that the daily volume of noninstitutional services would increase to nearly 20 million by the year 2040 (Manton and Liu, 1984b). This same study estimated that the number of elderly with IADL or ADL limitations will nearly triple in 60 years, from an estimated 6.6 million in 1985 to 18.8 million in the year 2040, assuming that the prevalence of chronic conditions remains the same. The estimates suggest that by the year 2010 the demand for institutional care will increase 73 percent and the demand for noninstitutional care will increase 66 percent. Assuming that long-term care services continue to be in relatively short supply, the cost of care will increase and access to care will become even more difficult.

# III. The Organization and Delivery of Long-Term Care

## Introduction

Long-term care is provided at many different sites and consists of many different services. It is provided in hospitals, nursing homes, personal and domiciliary care homes, adult foster homes, congregate housing, adult day care centers, senior centers, and at individuals' homes by home health agencies, Visiting Nurse Associations, and many community for-profit and nonprofit firms and organizations. Community-based services or programs can include:

- Case management;
- Health assessment or screening programs that identify health problems and assist, through referral and follow-up, in obtaining necessary and appropriate care;
- Health education and wellness programs that teach patients and caregivers about maintaining health and support and programs that teach caregivers how to cope with stress;
- Hospice care, which provides specialized nursing care and counseling to terminally ill individuals and their families who no longer wish to pursue medical treatment;
- Respite care, which provides temporary care to disabled people so that caregivers can take a break;
- Congregate dining, which offers low-cost meals to older people in a group setting;
- Home-delivered meals;
- Companion services, telephone reassurance, electronic monitoring services, and transportation and escort services that can provide transportation or assist individuals in getting to their destination using public transportation; and
- Financial counseling programs, which help individuals manage their money, pay their bills, file their income and property taxes, and complete their insurance claim forms.

The scope and depth of services offered by providers may appear to be similar but may in fact be different, and providers that appear dissimilar may in fact offer similar types of care. A licensed nursing home, for example, may offer food, shelter, supervision, and personal assistance, but could also offer adult day care and home health care to clients who are not residents of the nursing home. Similarly, nursing services, supervision, congregate meals, and personal assistance, although a normal part of nursing home care, can also be obtained from a variety of sources, including adult day care centers, senior centers, or home health agencies.

Similar providers may have different goals and therefore assist different types of clients (Kane and Kane, 1987). Home health care programs, for example, may include medical diagnosis and functional assessment, health care treatments, health education, training and supervision of family caregivers, homemaking or chore services, personal care for sustained or even indefinite periods, and terminal care. These different aspects of home care require different combinations of professional and paraprofessional staff and services, including physicians; housekeepers; registered nurses (RNs); licensed practical nurses (LPNs); physical, occupational, or speech therapists; nutritionists; social workers; and other mental health professionals and aides. Nursing homes, too, may be staffed differently depending on the institution's goals and philosophy. Different goals may include prolonging life, maintaining or improving physical functioning through rehabilitation so that residents can return to the community, reducing the use of acute care facilities, improving emotional and/or social well-being, improving cognitive functions, and enhancing residents' happiness (Kane and Kane, 1987).

Long-term care is unlike most other health care services. It is difficult to discern the best alternatives, and the choice among them is not necessarily made by a physician or other health care professional. Unlike preventive, elective, or acute medical care, the decision to seek specific forms of care is not dominated by physician preferences. Because of the lack of traditional third-party financing, the demand for long-term care is sensitive to price, family preferences, and ability to pay. In contrast, the demand for most other medical services is more likely to be affected by physician preferences and the standards of medical care in the community, usually without much regard to price, ability to pay, and sometimes family preferences.

Regardless of family preferences and ability to pay for long-term care, there may be limited availability of services in a particular community. Since public programs have primarily paid for nursing home or skilled home health care, community-based services that include unskilled nursing care are less likely to be available. The breadth and depth of community-based services vary from region to region depending on the size and demographic composition of the community and on the responsiveness of state and local governments and religious, philanthropic, and other voluntary organizations. Con-

74

sequently, in some communities there may be a comprehensive menu of services, while in others there may be virtually none.

The organization and delivery of long-term care is confusing and fragmented. No single source is likely to be able to provide a comprehensive list of services or programs to which individuals are entitled in a given area or to fully assist families in choosing the best option to meet their needs. Physicians are likely to be limited by their personal and professional experience with long-term care. Professional placement services, Area Agencies on Aging, and state agencies are likely to have put together select lists of available services but may not be able to direct families to those that are most appropriate. Furthermore, these lists are likely to be randomly compiled. The list that any single individual or family puts together is likely to have been influenced by those from whom the information was obtained (both the specific agency and the individuals contacted) and will reflect the amount of time and effort undertaken in the search.

The fragmentation and dislocation that characterize the delivery of long-term care have several undesirable consequences. Programs tend to focus on what they do for the patient rather than on the patient's needs. This often leads to barriers between different sources and different sites of care that make it difficult to put together a continuum of care that meets an individual's needs in terms of specific services and their timing.

In addition to inhibiting the development of an efficient and effective care plan, the fragmentation and barriers inherent in the delivery system minimize competitive pressures of the marketplace. In most areas of health care the preponderance of third-party reimbursement disables the market, but in the market for long-term care the fragmented and confusing array of options has this effect. Long-term care providers are less likely to face competition and to feel the need to provide efficient and high-quality care to remain in business. Medicaid reimbursement policies only confound the market incentives providers face, leaving a bifurcated set of preferences that can easily lead to situations in which access to care is denied or delayed for those who are most in need of help.

## Institutionalized Care

Until 1988, federal law recognized two kinds of nursing homes, skilled nursing facilities (SNFs) and intermediate care facilities (ICFs), which were distinguished by the level of care provided. New federal laws have been enacted that will phase out the distinction between

SNFs and ICFs and make other changes. However, since data and previous law made this distinction, it is necessary to know the difference between these two types of care to understand the nursing home market. In general, SNFs were required to be staffed and equipped to provide more skilled nursing care, while ICFs were required to be staffed to provide more personal care. For example, whereas ICFs were required to have a nurse on duty only during each day shift, SNFs were required to have one on duty 24 hours a day.

In 1986, there were an estimated 17,122 nursing homes and 9,258 residential facilities providing long-term care in more than 1.7 million beds (table III.1). One-half of the nursing homes, but 66 percent of the beds, were certified as SNFs. One-third of the nursing homes were certified as ICFs only, and 18 percent were not certified as either. Skilled nursing facilities are typically larger, averaging 120 beds. ICFs average 76 beds, noncertified homes 38 beds, and residential facilities, typically the smallest, 22 beds. The 1985 National Nursing Home Survey found that 41.2 percent of SNF beds were certified for Medicare reimbursement and 72.9 percent were certified for Medicaid reimbursement that year (National Center for Health Statistics, 1989).

Most of the nursing home industry is proprietary, or for profit. Nearly three-quarters (72.1 percent) of the nursing homes were for profit, as were 85 percent of the residential facilities. About one-quarter of the nursing homes, but nearly one-third (31 percent) of the beds, were owned either by nonprofit organizations or the government. In 1985, 41 percent of the facilities and about one-half of the beds were affiliated with national nursing home chains (Strahan, 1987). The three largest—Beverly Enterprises, ARA, and Hillhaven—together accounted for 10 percent of the nursing home beds (Kane and Kane, 1987).

Although federal law distinguished SNFs and ICFs in terms of medical orientation, it has been difficult to see the difference between them in either the level of care provided or the level of care needed by the residents. In part, this is because states had a great deal of discretion in interpreting federal standards, and some states' standards were substantially more stringent. Facilities certified as SNFs in one state might have been certified as ICFs in another, and ICFs in some states could be SNFs in others. This also reflects the difficulty in evaluating and then placing individuals in the appropriate nursing facility. Determining needs that will be best served by either an SNF or an ICF is not only difficult, it has not been standardized among states or even in regions within states. Furthermore, any assessment is likely to be accurate for only a limited period.

## TABLE III.1
## Number of Hospital-Based Nursing Facilities, Nursing Homes, and Residential Care Facilities, by Type of Ownership and Certification, 1986

| Characteristic | All Facilities | | Hospital-Based | | Freestanding Nursing Homes | | Residential | |
|---|---|---|---|---|---|---|---|---|
| | Facilities | Beds | Facilities | Beds | Facilities | Beds | Facilities | Beds |
| Total | 26,380 | 1,770,206 | 734 | 60,983 | 16,388 | 1,507,392 | 9,528 | 201,831 |
| | | | | | *type of ownership* | | | |
| For-Profit | 20,286 | 1,240,213 | 63 | 4,800 | 12,336 | 1,078,952 | 7,887 | 156,461 |
| Nonprofit | 4,815 | 398,996 | 437 | 31,747 | 3,263 | 328,728 | 1,115 | 38,521 |
| Government | 1,279 | 130,997 | 234 | 24,436 | 789 | 99,712 | 256 | 6,849 |
| | | | *certification* | | | | | |
| Skilled Nursing Facility | 8,639 | 1,037,173 | 594 | 53,060 | 8,045 | 984,113 | — | — |
| Intermediate Care Facility | 5,473 | 416,703 | 98 | 5,235 | 5,375 | 411,468 | — | — |
| Uncertified Nursing Home | 3,010 | 114,499 | 42 | 2,688 | 2,968 | 111,811 | — | — |
| Residential Facility | 9,258 | 201,831 | — | — | — | — | 9,258 | 201,831 |

Source: Al Sirrocco, "Nursing and Related Care Homes as Reported from the 1986 Inventory of Long-Term Care Places," *Advancedata from Vital and Health Statistics* no. 147 (22 January 1988).

Consequently, the distribution of SNF and ICF beds among states varies widely (table III.2). These differences are less likely to reflect residents' actual needs in those states than they are to reflect the historical sources of care and Medicaid reimbursement policy. In 1986, in states such as Iowa, Oklahoma, Louisiana, and New Mexico, ICF-only facilities accounted for more than 90 percent of the nursing facilities, while in other states, such as Alabama, California, Florida, New Jersey, New York, and Pennsylvania, less than 10 percent of the facilities were ICF only.

The distribution of nursing home beds also varies with the state's share of the national elderly population. In 1986, the average number of nursing home beds per 1,000 population aged 65 or over was 57.1 nationwide, but it ranged from a high of 89.6 in Minnesota to a low of 26.7 in Florida. Among the 10 states with the largest proportions of elderly, three had lower-than-average bed rates per 1,000, and among the 10 states with the lowest proportion of elderly, four had greater-than-average bed rates.

The wide variations in staffing ratios reflect differences in state Medicaid licensing agreements (table III.3). In 1981, nursing home beds per licensed nurse ranged from a low of 4.5 in Alaska to a high of 18.8 in Oklahoma. Nineteen states had ratios of 10 or more beds per licensed nurse (either RNs or LPNs). Ratios of RNs to LPNs ranged from a high of 1.9 in New Hampshire to a low of 0.2 in Texas. Interestingly, low bed ratios, which reflect more nurses per resident, do not necessarily reflect state requirements for better-trained nurses. Two of the four best states in terms of low bed counts per licensed nurse had very low ratios of RNs to LPNs, and among states with the most beds per nurse, the ratio of RNs to LPNs varied considerably.

Nursing homes have long been an adjunct part of our welfare system. Prior to the passage of Medicare and Medicaid legislation in 1965, nursing homes received some financial support from Grants to States for Old-Age Assistance and Medical Assistance for the Aged under Title I of the Social Security Act of 1935, the Old Age Assistance program, and other cash assistance programs. Grants to aid nursing home construction were made in 1954 by amendments to the Hospital Survey and Construction Act of 1946, commonly called the Hill-Burton Act after its principal sponsors. Construction was also encouraged by public expenditure payments on behalf of residents through the Medical Assistance for the Aged program, or the Kerr-Mills Act (Vladeck, 1980).

The framers of Medicare legislation tried to avoid expanding public financing of nursing home care. However, Rep. Wilbur Mills (D-OH)

## TABLE III.2
## Nursing Home Facilities and Beds, by Type of License and Bed Rate per 1,000 Elderly in Each State

| State | Total Nursing Homes, 1986 | Percentage of Homes Certified as SNF[a] or as Both SNF and ICF,[b] 1981 | Percentage of Homes Certified as ICF Only, 1981 | Elderly as a Percentage of State Population, 1986 | Total Nursing Home Beds, 1986 | Bed Rate per 1,000 Elderly, 1986 |
|---|---|---|---|---|---|---|
| Alabama | 203 | 91% | 9% | 12.2% | 21,970 | 44.1 |
| Alaska | 10 | 77 | 23 | 3.4 | 830 | 45.7 |
| Arizona | 134 | 100 | 0 | 12.5 | 13.734 | 33.5 |
| Arkansas | 237 | 40 | 60 | 14.5 | 21,860 | 63.5 |
| California | 1,569 | 97 | 3 | 10.6 | 118,430 | 41.7 |
| Colorado | 183 | 83 | 17 | 9.0 | 18,109 | 61.9 |
| Connecticut | 256 | 89 | 11 | 13.2 | 27,198 | 64.3 |
| Delaware | 36 | 62 | 38 | 11.4 | 3,906 | 54.1 |
| District of Columbia | 19 | 50 | 50 | 12.2 | 3,760 | 49.1 |
| Florida | 649 | 98 | 2 | 17.7 | 55,225 | 26.7 |
| Georgia | 298 | 76 | 24 | 10.0 | 34,742 | 56.7 |
| Hawaii | 23 | 76 | 24 | 9.8 | 2,769 | 26.9 |
| Idaho | 60 | 90 | 10 | 11.2 | 4,910 | 43.3 |
| Illinois | 775 | 56 | 44 | 12.0 | 89,333 | 64.2 |
| Indiana | 449 | 31 | 69 | 11.9 | 48,244 | 73.5 |
| Iowa | 440 | 6 | 94 | 14.6 | 33,296 | 79.7 |
| Kansas | 342 | 15 | 85 | 13.5 | 27,024 | 81.7 |

(continued)

## TABLE III.2 (continued)

| State | Total Nursing Homes, 1986 | Percentage of Homes Certified as SNF[a] or as Both SNF and ICF,[b] 1981 | Percentage of Homes Certified as ICF Only, 1981 | Elderly as a Percentage of State Population, 1986 | Total Nursing Home Beds, 1986 | Bed Rate per 1,000 Elderly, 1986 |
|---|---|---|---|---|---|---|
| Kentucky | 277 | 47% | 53% | 12.1% | 20,424 | 45.3 |
| Louisiana | 276 | 6 | 94 | 10.3 | 33,853 | 75.1 |
| Maine | 144 | 12 | 88 | 13.3 | 9,758 | 62.2 |
| Maryland | 200 | 53 | 47 | 10.6 | 23,934 | 50.9 |
| Massachusetts | 612 | 52 | 48 | 13.6 | 47,126 | 59.4 |
| Michigan | 480 | 69 | 31 | 11.6 | 48,857 | 46.9 |
| Minnesota | 399 | 69 | 31 | 12.5 | 47,490 | 89.6 |
| Mississippi | 140 | 83 | 17 | 12.0 | 14,454 | 45.8 |
| Missouri | 552 | 37 | 63 | 13.7 | 46,892 | 67.5 |
| Montana | 57 | 88 | 12 | 12.1 | 6,531 | 65.1 |
| Nebraska | 214 | 14 | 86 | 13.6 | 16,535 | 75.5 |
| Nevada | 30 | 88 | 12 | 10.3 | 2,659 | 26.8 |
| New Hampshire | 75 | 34 | 66 | 11.6 | 6,791 | 56.6 |
| New Jersey | 356 | 91 | 9 | 12.8 | 33,214 | 34.2 |
| New Mexico | 56 | 9 | 91 | 9.8 | 5,884 | 40.8 |
| New York | 777 | 92 | 8 | 12.8 | 98,747 | 43.4 |
| North Carolina | 402 | 72 | 28 | 11.5 | 23,540 | 32.2 |
| North Dakota | 81 | 69 | 31 | 13.0 | 6,820 | 76.3 |
| Ohio | 886 | 43 | 57 | 12.3 | 83,991 | 63.7 |
| Oklahoma | 382 | 2 | 98 | 12.4 | 31,665 | 76.9 |
| Oregon | 214 | 29 | 71 | 13.4 | 15,357 | 42.2 |

| | | | | | |
|---|---|---|---|---|---|
| Pennsylvania | 788 | 94 | 6 | 14.5 | 84,338 | 48.8 |
| Rhode Island | 101 | 57 | 43 | 14.6 | 9,759 | 69.0 |
| South Carolina | 157 | 75 | 25 | 10.5 | 12,981 | 36.5 |
| South Dakota | 114 | 51 | 49 | 13.8 | 7,851 | 79.2 |
| Tennessee | 267 | 25 | 75 | 12.3 | 29,708 | 50.6 |
| Texas | 1,027 | 21 | 79 | 9.5 | 103,423 | 65.6 |
| Utah | 84 | 50 | 50 | 8.1 | 5,728 | 42.7 |
| Vermont | 47 | 52 | 48 | 11.8 | 3,367 | 51.6 |
| Virginia | 288 | 32 | 68 | 10.4 | 22,448 | 37.2 |
| Washington | 328 | 85 | 15 | 11.7 | 26,345 | 50.8 |
| West Virginia | 103 | 46 | 54 | 13.6 | 8,365 | 32.0 |
| Wisconsin | 409 | 74 | 26 | 13.1 | 53,170 | 84.8 |
| Wyoming | 27 | 65 | 35 | 8.5 | 2,081 | 48.6 |
| Total | 16,033 | 59 | 41 | 12.1 | 1,519,426 | 52.1 |

Source: Total nursing homes from National Center for Health Statistics, Public Health Service, U.S. Department of Health and Human Services, *Health United States 1987*, DHHS pub. no. (PHS) 88-1232 (Washington, DC: U.S. Government Printing Office, 1988), p. 144, table 90; percentage of SNF and ICF homes and percentage of ICF homes only from Committee on Nursing Home Regulation, Institute of Medicine, *Improving the Quality of Care in Nursing Homes* (Washington, DC: National Academy Press, 1986), appendix D, p. 357, table C; percentage of total population from Bureau of the Census, U.S. Department of Commerce, "State Population and Household Estimates with Age, Sex, and Components of Change: 1981–1987," *Current Population Reports*, Population Estimates and Projections, Series P-25, no. 1024 (Washington, DC: U.S. Government Printing Office, 1988), pp. 29–79, table 6; number of beds and bed rate from Charlene Harrington, James H. Swan, and Leslie A. Grant, "Nursing Home Bed Capacity in the States, 1978–1986," *Health Care Financing Review* (Summer 1988), pp. 87–89, tables 1 and 3.

aSkilled nursing facility.
bIntermediate care facility.

TABLE III.3
## Total Nursing Home Beds per Licensed Nurse, Total Licensed Nurses, and Ratio of Registered Nurses (RNs) to Licensed Practical Nurses (LPNs), by State, 1981

| State | SNF[a] and ICF[b] Beds per Licensed Nurse | Total Licensed Nurses | RN/LPN Ratio |
|---|---|---|---|
| Alabama | 8.4 | 2,469 | 0.3 |
| Alaska | 4.5 | 143 | 1.3 |
| Arizona | 16.2 | 199 | 1.6 |
| Arkansas | 11.0 | 1,799 | 0.3 |
| California | 9.3 | 12,308 | 0.7 |
| Colorado | 10.8 | 1,753 | 1.3 |
| Connecticut | 6.8 | 3,645 | 1.6 |
| Delaware | 7.1 | 393 | 1.5 |
| District of Columbia | 6.5 | 179 | 1.3 |
| Florida | 11.0 | 3,155 | 0.8 |
| Georgia | 9.0 | 3,405 | 0.4 |
| Hawaii | 4.8 | 524 | 1.1 |
| Idaho | 8.3 | 575 | 0.9 |
| Illinois | 12.7 | 7,095 | 1.2 |
| Indiana | 16.9 | 2,462 | 0.9 |
| Iowa | 11.8 | 2,891 | 0.8 |
| Kansas | 16.9 | 1,520 | 0.8 |
| Kentucky | 12.6 | 1,611 | 0.5 |
| Louisiana | 11.3 | 2,181 | 0.3 |
| Maine | 8.5 | 1,075 | 1.1 |
| Maryland | 9.2 | 2,273 | 1.1 |
| Massachusetts | 7.5 | 6,000 | 1.1 |
| Michigan | 10.1 | 4,582 | 0.9 |
| Minnesota | 10.1 | 4,588 | 0.9 |
| Mississippi | 5.6 | 2,195 | 0.3 |
| Missouri | 12.2 | 2,151 | 0.6 |
| Montana | 8.2 | 772 | 1.1 |
| Nebraska | 13.8 | 1,263 | 0.8 |
| Nevada | 6.6 | 344 | 1.5 |
| New Hampshire | 7.1 | 949 | 1.9 |
| New Jersey | 8.1 | 3,979 | 1.7 |
| New Mexico | 9.0 | 396 | 0.5 |
| New York | 5.8 | 16,228 | 0.9 |

**(continued)**

### TABLE III.3 (continued)

| State | SNF[a] and ICF[b] Beds per Licensed Nurse | Total Licensed Nurses | RN/LPN Ratio |
|---|---|---|---|
| North Carolina | 8.2 | 2,649 | 0.8 |
| North Dakota | 9.7 | 677 | 1.1 |
| Ohio | 9.0 | 7,867 | 0.8 |
| Oklahoma | 18.8 | 1,507 | 0.4 |
| Oregon | 11.6 | 1,282 | 1.3 |
| Pennsylvania | 7.6 | 9,075 | 1.1 |
| Rhode Island | 7.3 | 1,171 | 1.3 |
| South Carolina | 6.9 | 1,577 | 0.7 |
| South Dakota | 11.5 | 685 | 1.2 |
| Tennessee | 9.6 | 2,556 | 0.3 |
| Texas | 12.9 | 7,757 | 0.2 |
| Utah | 8.9 | 586 | 0.6 |
| Vermont | 7.0 | 426 | 1.1 |
| Virginia | 7.1 | 2,877 | 0.7 |
| Washington | 8.5 | 2,926 | 1.5 |
| West Virginia | 7.8 | 733 | 0.8 |
| Wisconsin | 10.4 | 5,155 | 1.0 |
| Wyoming | 9.7 | 196 | 1.2 |

Source: Committee on Nursing Home Regulation, Institute of Medicine, *Improving the Quality of Care in Nursing Homes* (Washington, DC: National Academy Press, 1986), appendix D, p. 362, table H.
[a]Skilled nursing facility.
[b]Intermediate care facility.

appended Medicaid to the administration's Medicare bill, thereby enabling open-ended financing of nursing homes. It has been argued that nursing home coverage was never confronted directly, and that Medicaid was hastily enacted and was a side issue in the political debate over Medicare. One review of the legislative history confirms that nursing homes have evolved without any deliberate public policy objective (Committee on Nursing Home Regulation, 1986).

When Medicare and Medicaid became law in 1965, federal and state authorities had to certify health care providers quickly. Only 740 of 6,000 nursing home operator applicants could meet federal standards for Medicare participation in the first year (Committee on Nursing Home Regulation, 1986). Existing state standards were temporarily adopted for Medicaid nursing homes. But concern about the quality of nursing home care resulting from the temporary standards led to federal standards, known as the Moss amendments. Under these amendments, Medicaid was to impose standards by January 1, 1969, that required nursing homes to disclose ownership and maintain standards for recordkeeping, dietary services, drug dispensing, medical services, and environment and sanitation. In addition, the amendments required transfer agreements with hospitals, created a program of medical review, and established requirements for nursing services. The regulations promulgated by the U.S. Department of Health, Education, and Welfare (HEW) to meet these standards, however, turned out to be weaker than many consumer advocates would have liked. One troubling issue—the level of staffing—allowed LPNs to be in charge of the afternoon and night shifts. LPN certificates are granted to high school graduates with 12 to 18 months of training.

Regardless of the arguments over the strength of the new HEW standards, many nursing homes had trouble meeting them. Nursing home interests responded by developing the concept of a lower-level nursing facility, the ICF. They proceeded to sell the ICF concept to legislators by arguing that many residents did not need the level of nursing provided by SNFs and that these less-expensive facilities could save money. The so-called Miller amendment proposed paying for ICFs, but did not include any standards other than the life safety and sanitation standards required of SNFs. Some states felt that even these few standards were only meant to be advisory. Almost overnight, states simply reclassified patients and facilities from SNFs to ICFs to save money, an action that established the legitimacy of ICFs (Vladeck, 1980).

**How Medicaid Affects Access to Nursing Homes**

Medicaid is the largest payer of long-term care. Consequently, state Medicaid eligibility and reimbursement policies have had a considerable impact on nursing homes, affecting the availability of nursing home beds for Medicaid recipients, ownership of the homes, and the quality of care provided. Initially, states based Medicaid reimbursement on facilities' costs. Finding that they were unable to control these costs, many states moved toward prospective reimbursement methods. Prospective pricing is usually based on the previous year's costs, inflated to a specified ceiling. Rates may vary depending on a wide range of factors including number of beds, type of ownership, and geographical area or by the level of each Medicaid recipient's impairment. The underlying principle, however, is that a nursing home is paid a set amount regardless of its actual costs. The closer this payment is to actual costs, the greater the incentive for nursing homes either to cut their costs or to avoid accepting Medicaid recipients.

For the most part, reimbursement policies have been effective in controlling investment in nursing facilities. The expansion of nursing homes in the 1960s and early 1970s was in large part due to excessive rates of return to investors (Baldwin and Bishop, 1984). When reimbursement policies were changed to control nursing home expenditures, and in response to "scandals" concerning excess profits and underhanded schemes developed to maximize profits, the rate of return on nursing home investments declined and so did the growth of nursing home beds available to Medicaid patients (Baldwin and Bishop, 1984). Between 1981 and 1986, Medicaid nursing home expenditures increased 5.7 percent per year and the number of beds increased 1.3 percent per year. In sharp contrast, from 1967 to 1981, Medicaid nursing home expenditures increased at an annual rate of 18 percent and the number of beds increased at the annual rate of 3.7 percent.

Nursing homes prefer private paying patients, especially if they are relatively easy to manage (Special Committee on Aging, 1986). Medicaid and Medicare reimbursement tends to run 18 percent less than charges (Harrington and Swan, 1984). This discourages nursing homes from admitting patients who exhibit a "behavior problem," have bed sores, or in other ways suggest that they will require extraordinary or "heavy" care. To help overcome this bias, at least 10 state Medicaid programs are experimenting with reimbursement policies that pay nursing homes more for "heavy care" patients. Minnesota has attempted to thwart this disincentive by requiring nursing homes that accept Medicaid patients to charge private paying residents at the same rates.[1]

In addition to reimbursement policies, states have used regulations to limit the growth of nursing home beds to control Medicaid nursing home expenditures. In 1980, all except three states had laws requiring that to build or expand a nursing home a proprietor had to prove the need for it and receive a "certificate of need" (CON) from the state (Harrington, Swan, and Grant, 1988). A 1984 survey of 32 states found that nine had some form of moratorium on the construction of new nursing home beds and five required consideration of how the beds would be paid for before issuing a CON. The CON process explicitly favored issuing certificates for beds that were less likely to be occupied by Medicaid patients rather than issuing them on the basis of need (Isaacs and Goldman, 1984). Since 1981, the number of Medicaid

---

[1]Medicaid rates were relatively high in Minnesota; therefore, to date only six nursing homes have dropped their participation in the Medicaid program since the law went into effect in 1983.

recipients in nursing homes, and Medicaid spending as a proportion of all nursing home expenditures, has declined.[2]

While the supply of nursing home beds per person varies widely from state to state, occupancy rates do not. Occupancy rates range from 80 percent to 100 percent (Neuschler, 1987). Many nursing homes regularly maintain waiting lists for admission. With the population growing faster than the number of nursing home beds, most observers have concluded that there is an excess demand for nursing home services (Scanlon, 1980; Swan and Harrington, 1985; Committee on Nursing Home Regulation, 1986).

The question of whether states have an under- or oversupply of nursing home beds is controversial. A few studies have suggested that some states may have an oversupply. Looking at factors showing how difficult it was to transfer Medicare hospital patients to nursing homes, one study found five states with above-average hospital-to-nursing-home transfers. Interviews with state Medicaid officials in these five states indicated that two of the states (Colorado and Nebraska) had a surplus of nursing home beds (ICF Incorporated, 1982). A similar study found that in 1982, only 20 states had an undersupply of nursing home beds (Swan and Harrington, 1986). In another study, based on interviews of state health planning and development agencies in 45 states, officials in 18 states reported that they had an oversupply of beds while 9 states reported an undersupply (Swan and Harrington, 1986). A survey of state Medicaid program managers showed that only 28 had difficulties placing Medicaid patients (Neuschler, 1987).

Two studies, in 1986 and 1987, that compared an estimate of the state population requiring personal care in relation to the number of nursing home beds in 49 states yielded similar results for 36 states but not for 13 others. The 1987 study suggested that access to nursing homes was above average in three states that the 1986 study had identified as having an undersupply of nursing home beds, and that access was below average in 10 states for which the 1986 study had indicated no undersupply of beds (Swan and Harrington, 1986; Rohrer, 1987).

The 1987 study found the number of beds *per expected* proportion of disabled elderly to be relatively similar in each state. This suggests that access to nursing homes, whether difficult or simple, is also similar in each state, and that if there is a shortage of nursing homes

---

[2]For more information on the relative impact of various efforts to reduce Medicaid nursing home expenditures, see Holahan and Cohen, 1987; Cohen and Holahan, 1986; Kolb and Krueger, 1984; and Lave, 1985.

it is not as much state-specific as it is nationwide—an interpretation that contradicts the conclusions of the 1986 study. On the other hand, the high occupancy rates, waiting lists, and documented evidence of limited access for publicly financed patients and patients in need of a great deal of nursing care suggest discrimination in nursing home access. This would reconcile some of the seemingly contradictory results of the 1986 and 1987 studies and those of ICF Incorporated and others.

The general preference of nursing homes to admit private paying clients over Medicare or Medicaid clients as a way to maximize revenues suggests a dual consideration in deciding whom to accept as residents (Scanlon, 1980). In most states, private paying patients who do not need extensive care may be more likely to obtain care that they are willing and able to pay for, while those with severe disabilities have more difficulty obtaining care. Medicaid and Medicare patients, too, are likely to have difficulty gaining admission, and the more disabled the patient, the more difficult it may be to find placement.

The exception may be in those 10 states in which Medicaid programs provide additional payments for patients who have relatively greater needs.[3] In those states, if the reimbursement has been sufficient, nursing homes have established the capacity to provide needed care to heavier-care Medicaid patients and, therefore, heavier-care private and Medicare patients. But even in those 10 states there is limited evidence that the case-mix adjustment has more than a modest effect on increasing access to care (Kane and Kane, 1987).

**Responding to Concerns about Quality**

The quality of a nursing home resident's life is usually a reflection of the quality of care he or she receives. Inadequate care, neglect, and abuse can lead to premature death, permanent injury, increased disability, and unnecessary fear and suffering. But quality of life also includes less-measurable factors such as a sense of well-being and feelings of self-worth and self-esteem. For nursing home residents this is directly related to their satisfaction with the care received, personal

---

[3]Holahan and Dubay (1987) indirectly provide additional evidence for this thesis in a study examining the effects of bed supply on hospital discharge delays for Medicare patients awaiting placement in a Medicare-approved SNF. Because Medicare is such a small component of the nursing home market, Medicaid reimbursement policies were found to be much more important in explaining delays in different states. In the states in which Medicaid adjusts reimbursement for heavier-care patients, Medicare had fewer patients in hospitals awaiting nursing home placement (8.6 percentage points fewer, holding other factors constant).

achievement or purpose, and dignity. Much of this is related to their sense of control over their lives.

For most nursing home residents, however, personal autonomy has been the exception, not the rule (Vladeck, 1980; Committee on Nursing Home Regulation, 1986).[4] Many nursing homes do not provide residents any opportunity to participate in fundamentally important— much less even relatively unimportant—decisions. Residents are not likely to be included in the planning of their own care or to have any say in their roommates or the placement of furniture or personal belongings. They are not likely to have much choice in what or when they eat, what activities they participate in, what they wear, or even when they get up or retire. Furthermore, residents are not likely to have any privacy. Basic choices that we not only take for granted but that define us as individuals are usually taken away from nursing home residents.

Studies have shown that the quality of a nursing home's food and the quality of the interaction between the staff and the resident significantly affect a resident's perception of quality of life and his or her sense of well-being (Committee on Nursing Home Regulation, 1986). However, when nursing home reimbursement does not increase with costs, the first thing nursing homes tend to cut is the quality of the food (Vladeck, 1980), followed by patient-care-related expenses such as nurses and professional staff (Holahan and Cohen, 1987). Nursing homes seem more reluctant to cut administration, laundry, housekeeping, operations, and maintenance (Holahan and Cohen, 1987). In general, the larger the percentage of private paying patients in a nursing home, the stronger the incentives to improve or maintain the quality of care. Conversely, the greater the percentage of revenues a nursing home derives from Medicaid, the more Medicaid reimbursement policies will affect its quality. The stronger the cost containment strategy inherent in the Medicaid reimbursement program, the more likely nursing homes are to cut patient care and services to contain their expenses.

Concern over the quality of care in nursing homes has led to many official inquiries. For example, in May 1986, the staff of the U.S. Senate Special Committee on Aging completed a two-year investigation of nursing homes. In summarizing their findings they identified five problems: (1) that "tens of thousands of patients in nursing homes suffer from poor nutrition, inadequate nursing care, and squalid living

---

[4]However, this could change if the new laws governing conditions of participation in Medicare and Medicaid are effectively enforced.

conditions"; (2) that federal inspection reports show that between 600 and 800 SNFs fail to meet minimum quality standards year after year; (3) that finding a nursing home at all, let alone one that offers quality care, is extremely difficult and is a process over which the consumer has little or no control; (4) that the U.S. Department of Health and Human Services has failed to ensure that nursing homes receiving public funds provide high-quality medical and rehabilitative care; and (5) that existing federal penalties for use against substandard nursing homes are ineffective because of the limits on the number of enforcement actions that can be taken against substandard nursing homes (Special Committee on Aging, 1986). The staff recommended new federal legislation and additional regulations to address these problems. In particular, they called for a report by the Secretary of Health and Human Services on requiring state Medicaid programs to pay nursing homes more for heavy-care patients, to authorize more immediate sanctions and even public receivership when homes are found to be substandard, to define nursing home residents' rights, and to provide a mechanism to strengthen those rights.

An Institute of Medicine report issued in 1986 dealt with quality of care. It noted the difficulty in quantifying grossly inadequate care and indicated that although conditions have probably improved substantially since the 1970s, the quality of care and the quality of life in many nursing homes were not satisfactory (Committee on Nursing Home Regulation, 1986). The study also concluded that encouraging nursing homes to provide quality care would require a more significant federal role in their regulation. Among the study's 41 recommendations, 9 were aimed at changing the criteria used to license nursing homes and 21 were aimed at monitoring their performance. Many of these recommendations, as well as others, were incorporated in the Omnibus Budget Reconciliation Act of 1987 (OBRA '87).

OBRA '87 made substantial changes in the laws regulating nursing homes. As of October 1, 1990, there will no longer be any regulatory distinction between SNFs and ICFs. The new law establishes minimum standards for nurse aides and stricter standards for nursing and staffing, elevates the rights of residents, requires patient assessment and proactive planning for their welfare, and stipulates a larger federal regulatory role. OBRA '87 amends section 1819 of the Social Security Act to define a Medicare SNF as an institution that is primarily engaged in providing skilled nursing care and related services for residents who require medical or nursing care or rehabilitation services. The law also amends section 1919 of the Social Security Act to eliminate any distinction between Medicaid SNFs and Medicaid

ICFs by establishing identical criteria for all nursing facilities. Under this section all Medicaid-approved nursing facilities perform the same functions as Medicare SNFs (although the institution need not be certified to accept Medicare payments).

Although there are some specific differences owing to the dissimilarities between the Medicare and Medicaid programs, the basic requirements for participation are the same. In general, a facility must maintain a quality assessment and assurance committee; have a transfer agreement with at least one hospital; provide a written plan of care for each patient; and reassess each patient's functional capacity every 12 months, or with any significant change in his or her condition. The facility must provide a wide range of professional services, including that of a licensed RN for at least eight consecutive hours a day, seven days a week. In addition, nurse aides must hold state certificates of approved training. Among other requirements, facilities with more than 120 beds must have at least one full-time social worker on their staffs.

The new law, which will be fully effective in September 1990, dramatically strengthens the rights of nursing home residents by establishing a bill of rights and giving patients redress, with civil penalties of up to $10,000. Patients will be free to choose their own attending physician, participate in the planning of their care and treatment, and be fully informed of any changes. The law requires that patients be free of physical restraints unless their physician certifies that they are necessary for the patient's safety. Residents will have a right to privacy in their own rooms; a right to confidentiality in treatment, test results, and medical records; and a right to be granted their personal preferences in living arrangements and roommates. Finally, the law guarantees residents rights to submit grievances without fear of reprisal; form and participate in family and/or resident groups; participate in social, religious, or community activities that do not interfere with the rights of others; and examine the results of state surveys on the quality of care provided by the facility in which they reside.

These provisions in OBRA '87 are likely to raise the cost of nursing home care at least 2 percent, in large part due to increased staffing requirements for professional and paraprofessional staff and new minimum standards for certifying nurse aides. Many facilities licensed for intermediate care will require increased staffing of RNs, LPNs, and dietitians as well as staff to provide rehabilitation and pharmaceutical services and routine and emergency dental services. In the short run, states will have to reorganize their licensing and evaluation procedures, and nursing homes will have to provide the necessary training to get their nurse aides certified. The Congressional Budget Office estimated that recertification and compliance will cost the federal government $447 million and state governments $345 million during the phasing-in period between federal fiscal years 1988 and 1990.[5]

## Other Facilities

Other facilities in addition to nursing homes provide long-term care. These include personal care and domiciliary care facilities, foster homes, congregate housing, and retirement communities. Since there are no federal guidelines for state licensing of these types of facilities, defining them is even more difficult than distinguishing between skilled and intermediate care nursing facilities (Scanlon, Difederico, and Stassen, 1979).

There is a wide array of housing programs, ranging from assisting individuals in maintaining their independent residences to shared living arrangements in which individuals receive some assistance. Many of these programs offer financial assistance with rent (low-rent public housing, section 8 of the 1974 Housing and Community Development Act, and section 202 of the Housing Act of 1959). In 1985, there were approximately 1.6 million housing units occupied by the elderly under these three programs (Kane and Kane, 1987).

Boarding houses, retirement homes, domiciliary care homes, adult foster care homes, sheltered care facilities, and halfway houses generally provide food, shelter, oversight, and personal care. It is virtually impossible to determine the number and types of facilities or the characteristics of residents. A 1982 survey of regulatory authorities found 142 distinct programs administered by 92 state government agencies nationwide (Kane and Kane, 1987). A 1983 study identified 30,000 such homes (5,000 of which were unlicensed) housing 370,000 elderly, and a 1985 survey found 382,207 residential care beds, 28,638 foster care beds, 6,396 free-standing beds that provide board plus care, and 41,272 unclassified beds.

These facilities focus on providing personal care and assistance, including supervision and housekeeping services. They are similar to nonmedical nursing homes that could meet neither the staffing nor

---

[5]Congressional Budget Office (1987) estimates of H.R. 3188, the Omnibus Budget Reconciliation Act of 1987. The state portion was estimated by applying the proportion of estimated federal expenditures related to this section of the bill to the total increase in state and local outlays.

the physical plant standards of ICFs. Personal care homes are likely to provide assistance with bathing, using the toilet, eating, transferring from bed to chair, and moving about. Medications and treatments may also be administered in accordance with physician orders. Domiciliary care facilities are likely to provide less personal care, focusing instead on providing room, board, housekeeping, and supervision to those who are not able to live by themselves and maintain a home but are able to eat, move about, and tend to their personal hygiene. Estimates made in 1973 indicate that there were fewer than 10,000 residents in fewer than 500 personal care or domiciliary care facilities (11,107 beds). Most (three-quarters) of the homes had fewer than 25 beds and were for-profit institutions (73.4 percent). Less than one-quarter (22.3 percent) were nonprofit, and 4.3 percent were government facilities (Scanlon, Difrederico, and Stassen, 1979).

**Life Care Communities**

Life care communities, or continuing care retirement communities, merge the financing and delivery of housing and long-term care. They can provide long-term care insurance, or long-term care itself, as well as a residence. The community is typically located in a campus-like setting that includes apartments or townhouses, a central eating and recreation facility, and a nursing facility. The arrangement enables individuals to remain independent in their own apartments. If cooking becomes too difficult, meals can be taken in the central facility. Home health aides can deliver meals, and full-time nursing care can be obtained in the nursing home. Social activities are included, and the centers are often governed by the residents. People are attracted to life care communities because the integrated delivery and financing of long-term care within the community *guarantees* access to long-term care services. In addition, residents feel their spouses are protected from impoverishment (Cohen et al., 1988).

Estimates of the current number of life care communities vary due to inconsistent definitions. The American Association of Homes for the Aging estimates that there are 700 communities. Nearly all are operated by nonprofit organizations (97 percent), and most are affiliated with a religious organization (87 percent) (Tell, Wallack, and Cohen, 1987). Generally, life care communities are financed by a substantial entrance fee (which may be refundable at death) and a monthly fee that together guarantee housing, nursing, and social services. In approximately one-third of the communities the contract is "all inclusive," meaning that monthly fees do not increase if the resident moves into the nursing facility. In another one-third of the communities this basic agreement is modified by charging for stays in the nursing facility, typically 80 percent or more of the per diem nursing home cost, after a stay of specified length. In these modified contracts, the amount of financial risk residents face varies inversely to the number of nursing home days covered under the contract. The number of days covered can range from as few as 5 to more than 180, depending on the facility (Raper and Kalicki, 1988).

The remaining one-third of the communities, called fee-for-service communities, have available all of the services found in the all-inclusive plans but include only a fraction of them in the monthly fee. The services not included can be purchased as needed or preferred. In particular, although nursing home care is available, it must be paid for as used. While these communities guarantee access to a nursing home bed, the individual is at financial risk for the cost of using that bed; the fee-for-service life care community is not at risk for the costs of long-term care and therefore is not an insurance plan. In the modified plan the costs are shared, in part, by nursing home residents, while in the all-inclusive plan they are shared by the entire community. This latter type of community gave rise to the concept of life care communities in the early decades of the 20th century. Modified and fee-for-service plans are more recent developments, starting in the mid to late 1970s.

Among 365 life care communities listed in the National Continuing Care Directory, 37.8 percent, or 33,765 dwelling units, were all-inclusive. The average entrance fee for a single person was $60,811, and ranged from a low of $35,000 in Indiana to a high of $128,000 in Massachusetts. Monthly fees in the two states were $1,205 and $653, respectively, and averaged $892 for all the communities (table III.4). For a couple, the average entrance fee was $65,648 (ranging from a low of $35,000 in Indiana to a high of $128,000 in Massachusetts). Monthly fees for two persons averaged $1,327 among all states ($1,205 and $1,117 in Indiana and Massachusetts, respectively). The average size of single units was 659 square feet. Not all states had communities, but among the 31 that did the average number of units available per 1,000 elderly varied from a high of 8.4 in Delaware to a low of 0.38 in Washington, with an average of 1.16 nationwide.

Life care communities may tend to use nursing homes less than the general community.[6] One study found evidence that suggests that the use of nursing homes is systematically different in life care commu-

---

[6]People who join life care communities may be at a different risk of institutionalization prior to joining the community than the general population.

# TABLE III.4
## Averages of All-Inclusive Continuing Care Retirement Communities for States with Facilities, 1988

| State | Entrance Fee for One Person[a] | Entrance Fee for Two Persons[a] | Monthly Fee for One Person[a] | Monthly Fee for Two Persons[a] | Average Square Feet per One-Bedroom Unit | Total Number of Units[b] | Number of Rooms per 1,000 Elderly |
|---|---|---|---|---|---|---|---|
| Alabama[c] | | | | | | | |
| Alaska[c] | | | | | | | |
| Arizona | $57,125 | d | $938 | d | 800 | 250 | 0.61 |
| Arkansas | 48,000 | 51,000 | 750 | 1,150 | 600 | 248 | 0.72 |
| California | 80,808 | 89,508 | 1,051 | 1,618 | 708 | 2,781 | 0.97 |
| Colorado | 53,494 | 64,193 | 559 | 779 | 658 | 743 | 2.52 |
| Connecticut | 81,663 | 85,700 | 1,236 | 1,766 | 693 | 420 | 1.00 |
| Delaware | 50,000 | 50,000 | 1,491 | 1,855 | 689 | 606 | 8.42 |
| District of Columbia[c] | | | | | | | |
| Florida | 59,681 | 61,405 | 695 | 1,000 | 709 | 6,040 | 2.92 |
| Georgia | 90,063 | 94,690 | 1,070 | 1,422 | 720 | 270 | 0.44 |
| Hawaii[c] | | | | | | | |
| Idaho | 45,000 | d | 539 | d | 600 | 157 | 1.40 |
| Illinois | 59,291 | 63,228 | 962 | 1,513 | 601 | 1,986 | 1.43 |
| Indiana | 35,000 | 35,000 | 1,205 | 1,205 | d | 283 | 0.43 |
| Iowa | 45,865 | 46,647 | 676 | 898 | 649 | 732 | 1.76 |
| Kansas | 52,000 | 52,000 | 1,098 | 1,468 | 613 | 179 | 0.54 |
| Kentucky[c] | | | | | | | |
| Louisiana | 55,400 | 58,900 | 702 | 1,041 | 711 | 190 | 0.41 |

| State | | | | | | |
|---|---|---|---|---|---|---|
| Maine[c] | | | | | | |
| Maryland | 71,674 | 80,849 | 1,205 | 1,821 | 678 | 1,236 | 2.62 |
| Massachusetts | 128,000 | 128,000 | 653 | 1,117 | 688 | 341 | 0.43 |
| Michigan | 51,000 | 58,500 | 694 | 813 | 518 | 477 | 0.46 |
| Minnesota[c] | | | | | | | |
| Mississippi[c] | | | | | | | |
| Missouri | 45,824 | 50,911 | 835 | 1,185 | 553 | 1,028 | 1.48 |
| Montana[c] | | | | | | | |
| Nebraska | 43,648 | 43,648 | 529 | 662 | 583 | 437 | 2.00 |
| Nevada[c] | | | | | | | |
| New Hampshire[c] | | | | | | | |
| New Jersey | 65,300 | 74,244 | 1,207 | 1,850 | 617 | 1,100 | 1.13 |
| New Mexico | 45,500 | 48,500 | 704 | 1,094 | 576 | 256 | 1.77 |
| New York[c] | | | | | | | |
| North Carolina | 40,438 | 41,688 | 820 | 1,472 | 628 | 674 | 0.92 |
| North Dakota[c] | | | | | | | |
| Ohio | 50,950 | 52,950 | 669 | 990 | 602 | 469 | 0.36 |
| Oklahoma | 60,000 | 60,000 | 616 | 950 | 610 | 192 | 0.47 |
| Oregon | 38,167 | 38,167 | 740 | 859 | 711 | 470 | 1.30 |
| Pennsylvania | 63,349 | 67,176 | 952 | 1,480 | 673 | 7,140 | 4.12 |
| Rhode Island[c] | | | | | | | |
| South Carolina[c] | | | | | | | |
| South Dakota[c] | | | | | | | |
| Tennessee | 63,150 | 65,150 | 597 | 904 | 576 | 375 | 0.64 |
| Texas | 45,406 | 47,031 | 638 | 959 | 632 | 959 | 0.61 |
| Utah[c] | | | | | | | |

(continued)

**TABLE III.4 (continued)**

| State | Entrance Fee for One Person[a] | Entrance Fee for Two Persons[a] | Monthly Fee for One Person[a] | Monthly Fee for Two Persons[a] | Average Square Feet per One-Bedroom Unit | Total Number of Units[b] | Number of Rooms per 1,000 Elderly |
|---|---|---|---|---|---|---|---|
| Vermont[c] | | | | | | | |
| Virginia | 76,906 | 88,389 | 1,131 | 1,669 | 657 | 2,267 | 3.75 |
| Washington | 37,000 | 37,000 | 883 | 1,178 | 600 | 200 | 0.38 |
| West Virginia[c] | | | | | | | |
| Wisconsin | 46,981 | 56,069 | 592 | 824 | 628 | 1,259 | 2.02 |
| Wyoming[c] | | | | | | | |
| All States | $60,811 | $65,648 | $892 | $1,327 | 659 | 33,765 | 1.16 |

Source: Ann Trueblood Raper and Anne C. Kalicki, eds., *National Continuing Care Directory: Retirement Communities with Nursing Care*, 2nd ed. (Washington, DC: American Association of Homes for the Aging, 1988).
[a]Prices are based on the average cost of a one-bedroom unit.
[b]Total units include units of all sizes in all-inclusive continuing care complexes, not just one-bedroom units.
[c]No facilities reported for these states.
[d]Not reported.

nities and that this process seems to change as the community matures. This study attempts to determine whether the delivery of long-term care in life care communities is different from that of the general community (Bishop, 1988). The study found, for example, that when nursing care in the nursing facility was covered in full, nursing home use was less than when it was not covered in full. In addition, communities with personal care services were also found to have substantially lower nursing home use. This would corroborate the work of another study that found that the risk of institutionalization was less among life care community residents than among others (Cohen, Tell, and Wallack, 1988).

## Community-Based Care

Community-based care encompasses a long list of services and providers, including home health agencies, adult day care centers, and senior centers. Together, these services represent the options available in the community to ensure that functionally dependent people are able to remain at home rather than be institutionalized. Home health care provided by a service was established as early as 1796 in Boston to help provide care to the indigent. The growth of home health care services was slow, largely because they relied on private funds. Insurance, introduced in the early 1930s, may have discouraged their expansion because benefits were limited to inpatient hospital care (Ginzberg, Balinsky, and Ostow, 1984). Substantial growth, however, was encouraged by the enactment of Medicare in 1965, which not only increased the number of programs but changed their focus and scope of services. When Medicare was enacted, there were an estimated 1,275 home health agencies (HHAs) in the United States (Foundation for Hospice and Homecare, 1988). Most of them offered nursing services only, but Medicare required physical, occupational, and speech therapy; medical and social services; and homemaker home health aide services as well. If agencies wanted to participate in Medicare, they had to expand their services.

It has been estimated that in 1987 there were 10,848 HHAs in the United States, more than one-half of which (53.5 percent) were certified by Medicare. Total payments to HHAs in 1985 were estimated at between $4.2 billion and $6 billion. It has been estimated that total expenditures in 1986 were $5 billion, of which 44 percent was financed by Medicare and 28 percent by Medicaid (Foundation for Hospice and Homecare, 1988). About 80 percent of the costs of running an HHA are for staff compensation. Among the 5,800 Medicare-certified HHAs, there were an estimated 130,628 full-time equivalent employees, more than one-half of whom were RNs or nurse aides (Foundation for Hospice and Homecare, 1988).

As indicated in table III.5, the number of HHAs relative to each state's population varies widely. Unfortunately, without better data we cannot make any generalizations about differences in access among states. The capital required to expand home health services is relatively small. It is more than likely the unavailability of appropriate professionals and paraprofessionals and the lack of third-party reimbursement that constrain the growth of HHAs, rather than the required licenses or certificates of need.

Quality of care includes whether the services are appropriate to the needs and preferences of the person receiving assistance as well as whether the service meets acceptable standards. While acceptable standards for nursing home care have received a great deal of attention, the issue of acceptable standards for care at home has barely been addressed. Given the difficulties with assuring standards in the already highly regulated nursing home industry, the prospects for assuring quality of care in the home are poor. The integrity of the caregivers will be of utmost importance. Quality care may depend on the adequacy of the compensation paid to caregivers and on the value we place on their services.

### Adult Day Care

Adult day care includes many long-term care services that are usually provided in a central location but for less than 24 hours a day. Services may include physical therapy and other forms of rehabilitation, assistance with ADL supervision, and social and recreational activities (Kane and Kane, 1987). Adult day care centers differ from senior centers in that activities are prescribed on the basis of an initial assessment of each individual. Centers can be found in hospitals, nursing homes, and social service agencies, or they may be freestanding. A few centers were started initially to provide day care for children but have expanded to include care for adults. Although most of these centers have found it necessary to keep the two populations separate and to hire different staffs for each, there may be savings associated with the sharing of the administration and overall maintenance of the two programs.

Data on adult day care are limited. It seems that as of 1983 there were 980 centers (Kane and Kane, 1987), most of which were sponsored by nonprofit human services organizations. Among 353 centers surveyed in detail, the average center served 21.7 clients a day, was

TABLE III.5
# Number of Home Health Agencies and Ratio of Agencies to Elderly Population, by State, 1987

| State | NAHC-Identified Agencies[a] | Medicare-Certified Agencies[b] | Elderly Population (in thousands) |
|---|---|---|---|
| Alabama | 217 | 118 | 505 |
| Alaska | 27 | 8 | 19 |
| Arizona | 129 | 59 | 430 |
| Arkansas | 194 | 164 | 348 |
| California | 730 | 356 | 2,944 |
| Colorado | 222 | 109 | 305 |
| Connecticut | 183 | 106 | 429 |
| Delaware | 33 | 20 | 75 |
| District of Columbia | 33 | 10 | 77 |
| Florida | 487 | 191 | 2,140 |
| Georgia | 150 | 71 | 623 |
| Guam | 1 | 1 | c |
| Hawaii | 43 | 17 | 109 |
| Idaho | 41 | 30 | 115 |
| Illinois | 478 | 259 | 1,405 |
| Indiana | 250 | 134 | 670 |
| Iowa | 240 | 157 | 421 |
| Kansas | 185 | 132 | 336 |
| Kentucky | 138 | 101 | 457 |
| Louisiana | 232 | 163 | 481 |
| Maine | 27 | 19 | 159 |
| Maryland | 188 | 88 | 486 |
| Massachusetts | 295 | 144 | 800 |
| Michigan | 373 | 174 | 1,058 |
| Minnesota | 289 | 200 | 534 |
| Mississippi | 179 | 113 | 318 |
| Missouri | 254 | 188 | 703 |
| Montana | 68 | 42 | 101 |
| Nebraska | 77 | 41 | 220 |
| Nevada | 37 | 18 | 106 |
| New Hampshire | 79 | 38 | 121 |
| New Jersey | 238 | 61 | 994 |
| New Mexico | 90 | 50 | 150 |
| New York | 821 | 169 | 2,309 |

(continued)

TABLE III.5 (continued)

| State | NAHC-Identified Agencies[a] | Medicare-Certified Agencies[b] | Elderly Population (in thousands) |
|---|---|---|---|
| North Carolina | 235 | 121 | 754 |
| North Dakota | 87 | 34 | 90 |
| Ohio | 451 | 245 | 1,346 |
| Oklahoma | 188 | 86 | 418 |
| Oregon | 109 | 61 | 373 |
| Pennsylvania | 379 | 273 | 1,764 |
| Puerto Rico | 63 | 42 | c |
| Rhode Island | 56 | 13 | 145 |
| South Carolina | 153 | 45 | 367 |
| South Dakota | 57 | 23 | 100 |
| Tennessee | 342 | 327 | 602 |
| Texas | 806 | 454 | 1,627 |
| Utah | 41 | 34 | 138 |
| Vermont | 27 | 17 | 65 |
| Virgin Islands | 5 | 1 | c |
| Virginia | 234 | 158 | 623 |
| Washington | 156 | 60 | 536 |
| West Virginia | 85 | 53 | 264 |
| Wisconsin | 287 | 160 | 633 |
| Wyoming | 59 | 27 | 44 |
| Total | 10,848 | 5,785 | 29,837 |

Source: EBRI tabulations of data in Foundation for Hospice and Homecare, *Basic Home Care Statistics: The Industry, 1988* (Washington, DC: National Association for Home Care, 1988); and Bureau of the Census, U.S. Department of Commerce, "State Population and Household Estimates with Age, Sex, and Components of Change: 1981–1987," *Current Population Reports*, Population Estimates and Projections, Series P-25, no. 1024 (Washington, DC: U.S. Government Printing Office, 1988), pp. 29–79, table 6.

[a]Certified and noncertified agencies identified by the National Association for Home Care (NAHC).
[b]Agencies that are certified to participate in Medicare.
[c]Unknown.

not full, and had five participants for every staff person; the staff usually included both nurses and social workers. In 1983, the average daily fee was just over $20 (Kane and Kane, 1987). The typical participant was 75.5 years old and attended 3 to 3.2 times a week. The participants usually had, among other health problems, heart disease, diabetes, and Alzheimer's disease and suffered from depression, loneliness, or isolation (Kane and Kane, 1987).

Studies of the effectiveness of adult day care have many of the same limitations as studies of home health care. The programs vary in terms of intervention, services, goals, and populations served. In a highly visible study, adult day care participants were found to use fewer inpatient hospital services and to have fewer nursing home days than similar people not receiving adult day care, but the results were not statistically significant. Despite the savings in hospital and nursing home costs, the cost of adult day care meant that the care of program participants was nearly $2,700 more expensive per year than care for similar individuals not in the program. These findings suggest that adult day care in the program under study was not a cost-effective substitute for nursing home care (Kane and Kane, 1987).

Another study suggests that people with irreversible dementia seem to enjoy life more, sleep better, and to be more manageable once they are established in an adult day care program (Mace and Rabins, 1981). Empirical studies, however, have not fully supported this contention. Some studies have found that most clients were initially wary and reluctant. Other studies have indicated that transportation is an integral and necessary part of the program. Adult day care centers have been criticized because clients often spend an inordinate proportion of the day getting ready and being transported to and from the center. People living alone, who might benefit most from adult day care, are unlikely to attend even when transportation is provided, unless there is someone who can help them prepare to leave home.

## Substituting Home Health Care for Nursing Home Care

Home health care allows recipients to receive care without leaving the security of their home and neighborhood. Advocates argue that home health care may save dollars that otherwise would go to pay for nursing home care. It seems implausible, however, that the type of 24-hour care provided in a single facility could be replicated as efficiently in individuals' homes. The more dispersed the geographic setting, the more implausible it seems. Intermediate care nursing homes are able to provide food, shelter, supervision, aides, nursing, and a variety of other services and organized activities for about $48 a day, or $2 an hour. In a survey returned by 673 Medicare-certified HHAs, the House Select Committee on Aging found that the median cost per hour to the HHA was $31 to $35 for an RN and $21 to $25 for a home health aide (Select Committee on Aging, 1985b).

101

Unlike nursing home care, home care can be tailored to the needs of the patient, in terms of both services rendered and the patterns of his or her daily life, both complementing and substituting for the care provided by family or friends. This type of care may keep some individuals who might otherwise have entered a nursing home from doing so, but more likely it will simply enhance the long-term care of the chronically disabled and assist the primary caregiver. Nearly all studies of the costs and effects of home and community care have found that home care is not a cost-saving substitute for nursing home care (Kane and Kane, 1987; Weissert, 1988).

To save money, in relation to what would be spent without home health care, the care must be targeted to specific situations and denied to many who need it. In particular, when targeted to individuals with a relatively time-limited or episodic condition, such as a broken bone or terminal cancer, home health care is probably a cost-effective substitute for some hospital and some skilled short-term nursing home care (Hughes, 1985; Nocks et al., 1986; Kane and Kane, 1987). Thus far, demonstration projects have been unsuccessful in making the necessary distinctions among the chronically ill, those for whom community care would be a bargain relative to nursing home care, and those for whom nursing home care would be less expensive.

Relatively few people who need long-term care actually enter a nursing home. Consequently, the stronger a patient's desire to avoid institutionalization and the family's willingness and ability to assist, the more likely home care will supplement rather than substitute for nursing home care. Among people receiving home health care services who eventually enter a nursing home, the services received at home have generally not reduced nursing home stays. On the contrary, for some people home health care may merely delay entry, but the extra cost associated with keeping someone out of a nursing home is likely to be greater than the cost of a nursing home stay (Weissert, 1988; U.S. General Accounting Office, 1982 and 1987b; Kane and Kane, 1987; Kemper et al., 1986).

There are many difficulties in measuring the effects of home health care, not the least of which is the fact that there are likely to be many people in the community with unmet health and social needs. Any experimental program is likely to serve as a safety valve for either an insufficient supply of, or difficulty in obtaining access to, nursing home beds. A review of 13 studies of the effects of home health care found that home care tended to provide assistance to those with severe functional limitations, including people who were more disabled than some nursing home residents; that a small percentage of home health care clients tended to consume a disproportionate amount of care; that those receiving home health care also received informal care; and that homemaking chores were not only valued by clients but were truly needed (Kane and Kane, 1987).

The measurable value of home health care in terms of improving the quality of beneficiaries' lives is also relatively modest to negligible. The National Long-Term Care Channeling Demonstration, or "channeling," was a large project funded to evaluate, among other things, home health care. The channeling demonstration found that the home health care services provided did not increase life expectancy or reduce recipients' ability to function, relative to similar people in the community who did not benefit from the program.[7] The channeling demonstration did suggest that those receiving care were more likely to be satisfied with their lives while enrolled in the program, especially during the first six months. Under one of the two case management strategies employed, the measurement of social and psychological well-being was no longer statistically significant after 6 months, and under the second approach, after 12 months. Informal caregivers were generally happy with the channeling program, although in only one of the two case management models tested were these indications statistically significant. Perhaps the most significant result from the channeling demonstration was that under both case management approaches the primary informal caregivers were more satisfied with their lives during the first six months than those not in the program (Applebaum et al., 1988).

Further research may eventually lead to the establishment of protocols for specific situations that will enable home health care to substitute for acute or nursing home care. On the other hand, policymakers may decide that effective long-term care should include home health care as part of a continuum of care that for many does not substitute for nursing home care. What is clear is that many people—in particular, caregivers—are aided by home health care and that many are willing to pay the premium necessary to maintain

---

[7]There was one notable exception. Some of the ADL limitations were found to increase relative to the untreated or control group, and were statistically significant in more than one type of limitation under one of the two case management approaches tested. This result, however, may have come from the wording of the questionnaire which asked whether someone helped, rather than whether the respondent had the capacity to do the task. On the other hand, the home health care provided may have led to situations in which, because individuals were doing less for themselves, psychological dependence developed or skills were lost, actually leaving the individuals less capable of caring for themselves (Applebaum et al., 1988).

control over both their lives and their dignity by staying in their own homes or in the homes of their children (Branch, 1985; Kane, 1988).

## Family Support

Long-term care is very much a family affair and is therefore complicated by the fragmented and complex process of family decision-making. This process is even further complicated by the confusion over the choice of services and available sources of financing. Once options have been identified, choices must be made. This is likely to involve a difficult process of conflict, negotiation, and consensus among the family members. The process is usually enmeshed with feelings of guilt and ambivalence (Moody, 1987).

Sometimes, however, there is no time to conduct a search. If the patient is in the hospital, the decision must often be made in a matter of days or even hours. In these circumstances, there is often little choice among facilities since typically only a few beds are available. The more "desirable" nursing homes usually have waiting lists. In general, nursing homes tend to prefer not to accept a patient who might require a great deal of care or whose stay is likely to be financed by Medicaid.

Most people who need long-term care live in the community. In 1984, there were an estimated 17.5 million disabled people of all ages needing assistance to perform activities considered essential to daily living. About 9 percent of this population resided in nursing homes and another 3 percent to 4 percent resided in other institutions. The remaining 89 percent of the functionally disabled lived in the community and relied on formal community-based services and the informal services of family and friends for assistance. In the same year, approximately 27 percent of the elderly population aged 65 or over had chronic disabilities that required assistance. While almost 12 percent of the approximately 7.1 million disabled elderly lived in nursing homes and other institutions, more than 6 million disabled elderly Medicare beneficiaries lived in the community. Nearly all of these individuals received assistance from their family, friends, and available community services. Less than 10 percent received any assistance from paid helpers; only 0.62 percent received all their care from paid providers.[8]

The amount and scope of help varies tremendously, but without the assistance of family and friends many in the community would not

---

[8]Author's calculations from the 1984 National Long-Term Care Survey.

be able to remain independent. Help may come from family members living in the same household but is equally likely to come from outside. In 1984, more than two-thirds (67.5 percent) of the chronically disabled elderly in the community lived with others, 42 percent lived with a spouse, and 13 percent lived with their children (table III.6). Most of the chronically ill elderly (87.8 percent), regardless of living arrangement, identified a helper either in or outside of the household who regularly provided assistance.

Slightly more than one-half of the chronically disabled elderly (54 percent) needed assistance from others with one or more IADLs, one-quarter (25.8 percent) needed human assistance with ADLs, and 97 percent also needed help with IADLs. The remaining 20.1 percent had

**TABLE III.6**
# Distribution of IADL[a] and ADL[b] Limitations among Chronically Disabled Elderly, by Living Arrangement, 1984

| Living Arrangement | Distribution of Population | Limitations | | | Total |
| --- | --- | --- | --- | --- | --- |
| | | IADL Only[c] | ADL[c] | Other[c,d] | |
| Alone | 32.5% | 58.5% | 18.8% | 22.7% | 100.0% |
| Spouse | 42.1 | 51.3 | 25.3 | 23.4 | 100.0 |
| Children | 13.0 | 53.2 | 37.0 | 9.9 | 100.0 |
| Parent | 0.3 | 48.9 | 24.0 | 27.1 | 100.0 |
| Other Relative | 7.1 | 55.8 | 32.0 | 12.2 | 100.0 |
| Others | 4.1 | 49.9 | 39.0 | 11.1 | 100.0 |
| Unknown | 0.6 | 40.2 | 28.4 | 31.5 | 100.0 |
| Total[e] | 100.0 | 54.1 | 25.8 | 20.1 | 100.0 |

Source: EBRI tabulations of the 1984 National Long Term Care Survey, Health Care Financing Administration, U.S. Department of Health and Human Services.
[a]Instrumental activity of daily living (IADL) limitations include respondents who could not do household chores (moving furniture, scrubbing floors, washing windows), laundry, or grocery shopping, manage their own money, take medicine, make telephone calls, prepare meals, or get around outside without assistance from others.
[b]Activity of daily living (ADL) limitations include respondents who needed assistance from others in eating, transferring to or from bed or chair, moving around inside the home, dressing, bathing, getting to the bathroom, or using the toilet, or were incontinent.
[c]Mutually exclusive.
[d]Other limitations may include IADL or ADL limitations defined in alternative ways.
[e]Percentage of the chronically disabled elderly population.
Note: Percentages may not add to 100 because of rounding.

105

other limitations not defined using our criteria of IADLs or ADLs, but still needed assistance for some difficulty. About one-quarter (23.6 percent) of the chronically disabled elderly were incontinent and less than 8 percent (7.68 percent) had indications of dementia (table III.7).[9]

Chronically disabled elderly Medicare recipients living alone were less likely to have either IADL or ADL limitations. Nearly 59 percent had only IADL limitations and less than 19 percent had ADL limitations. Analysis reveals that chronically disabled elderly persons living alone were more likely than other disabled persons living in the community to be poorer, older women, and were less likely to have living children. Nearly one-third of those indicating incontinence lived alone.

TABLE III.7

**Distribution of Chronically Disabled Elderly with Dementia or Incontinence, by Living Arrangement, 1984**

| Living Arrangement | Distribution of Elderly with Dementia[a, c] | Distribution of Elderly with Incontinence[b, c] |
|---|---|---|
| All Elderly[d] | 7.7% | 23.6% |
| Alone | 17.3 | 32.0 |
| Spouse | 32.8 | 40.5 |
| Children | 28.9 | 14.5 |
| Parent | 0.1 | 0.2 |
| Other Relative | 12.6 | 8.4 |
| Others | 6.7 | 3.4 |
| Unknown | 1.5 | 0.8 |
| Total | 100.0 | 100.0 |

Source: EBRI tabulations of the 1984 National Long-Term Care Survey, Health Care Financing Administration, U.S. Department of Health and Human Services.
[a]Diagnosis of dementia was ascertained from the primary caregiver.
[b]The respondents indicated that bladder or bowel problems had caused them to wet or soil themselves.
[c]Not mutually exclusive.
[d]Percentage of the chronically disabled elderly population.
Note: Percentages may not add to 100 because of rounding.

---

[9]The result with respect to dementia may be specious due to the subjective nature of assessing the problem. Helpers may be more inclined to attribute dementia-like behavior to their elderly dependents, while spouses and chronically disabled individuals are much more likely to deny the possibility.

Seventeen percent of those who may have a form of dementia were living alone.

The chronically disabled elderly in the community who lived with their spouses were more likely to have ADL limitations and less likely to have IADL limitations than other disabled elderly in the community. They also tended to be relatively younger. Missing from this analysis is the ability to distinguish whether the relatively younger age is attributable to the increased likelihood of death of the spouse or to a greater propensity for the caregiving spouse to admit the dependent spouse to a nursing home. More than one-half (51.3 percent) had IADL deficits only, and one-quarter (25.3 percent) had ADL limitations. Those living with their spouses were more likely to have children and tended to be financially better off than the rest of the chronically disabled elderly Medicare population. Nearly one-third (32.8 percent) of those identified with some form of dementia, and more than 40 percent of those with incontinence, were living with their spouses.

Children are a very important source of care. More than 13 percent of the chronically disabled elderly live with their children. More than one-third (37 percent) of this number had ADL limitations. Analysis does not support the notion that the elderly who live with their children are necessarily more disabled, but they are more likely to have IADLs. More than one-half (53.2 percent) had IADL limitations only. More than one-quarter (28.9 percent) had indications of dementia, but only 14.5 percent who were incontinent lived with children. Those living with children were less likely to have other living children.

Assistance is not likely to be shared among more than two principal caregivers. Most (87.8 percent) of the chronically disabled in the community, regardless of living arrangement, identified at least one regular helper, but relatively few identified more than three helpers. Slightly more than one-half (51.6 percent) had two helpers. Nearly 90 percent of the helpers identified accounted for the first three helpers listed by each of the disabled in the community. Most of the helpers (80.5 percent) had been providing assistance for more than one year, and 33.8 percent had been providing assistance for more than five years. The amount of help provided during the week varied, with 43 percent providing one day or less and 34.4 percent providing seven days of care each week. However, less than one-third of the helpers assisted with ADLs. Among the eight IADLs asked about, 61 percent of the caregivers assisted with two or more deficits.

More than one-half (57 percent) of those identified as providing regular care to chronically disabled elderly were immediate family members (spouse, parents, siblings, children, and children by marriage). Other relatives provided 12.4 percent of the care, friends provided 8.6 percent, and volunteers provided 7.8 percent. The largest single source of care was provided by children, who make up 35.3 percent of all helpers. Daughters and daughters-in-law were more likely to help (22.8 percent) than sons and sons-in-law (12.5 percent). Eleven percent of all the helpers identified, however, were hired assistants (chart III.1).

Spouses are an important source of assistance, but from all measures children and other relatives are equally important and may be critical to keeping functionally dependent parents living in the community. In a study focusing on the decision to admit a dependent adult to a nursing home, caregivers, in general, and children, in particular, had provided an exhaustive amount of care but had reached a point where "there was nothing else to do." Children, siblings, and other relatives were more likely to have delayed a nursing home admission than spouses and friends (Smallegan, 1985).

The same study found that caregivers had devoted a tremendous amount of care to the recipient and that the decision to place the individual in a nursing home was difficult to make. In nearly two-thirds (66 percent) of the new admissions, the patient needed either 24-hour care or 24-hour supervision. The most frequently reported reason for the institutionalization was the dependent's worsening health, and the most common medical conditions precipitating admission were frequent falls, general debility, confusion, fractures, stroke, incontinence, and difficult behavior. Among those needing care prior to admission to the nursing home, 65 percent had received care from their children. Of the group with children, only 12 percent did not receive care from them. Forty-six percent received assistance from a spouse, and 15 percent received care from other relatives. Other studies of nursing home admissions suggest that incontinence and difficult behavior, which are usually related to dementia, are often the two factors that break the stamina and spirit of the caregiver.

Hired assistance is a relatively more important source of care in terms of the percentage of helpers for chronically disabled elderly who live with their parents (28 percent), for those living with nonrelatives (21.7 percent), and for those living alone (14.8 percent) (charts III.2 through III.7). Except for those living with parents, hired help never fully dominates the source of caregiving. Among those living with parents, 22.3 percent of the helpers identified are female friends, and 14.5 percent are the elderly person's mother. Children account for 11.1 percent, and siblings and volunteers each account for 8.2

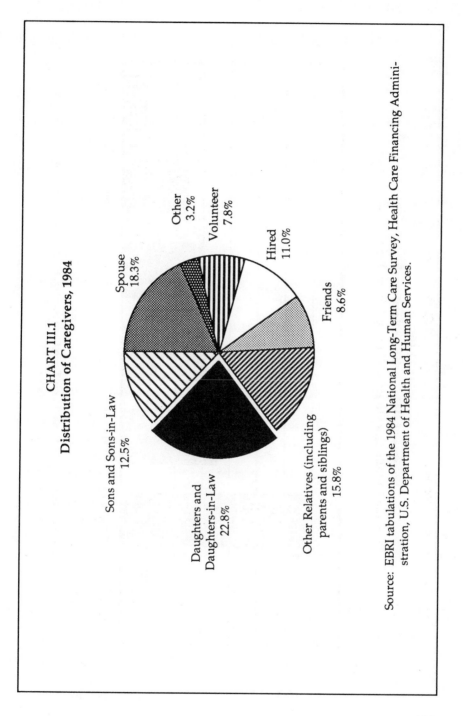

CHART III.1
Distribution of Caregivers, 1984

Other
3.2%

Volunteer
7.8%

Spouse
18.3%

Hired
11.0%

Sons and Sons-in-Law
12.5%

Friends
8.6%

Daughters and
Daughters-in-Law
22.8%

Other Relatives (including
parents and siblings)
15.8%

Source:  EBRI tabulations of the 1984 National Long-Term Care Survey, Health Care Financing Administration, U.S. Department of Health and Human Services.

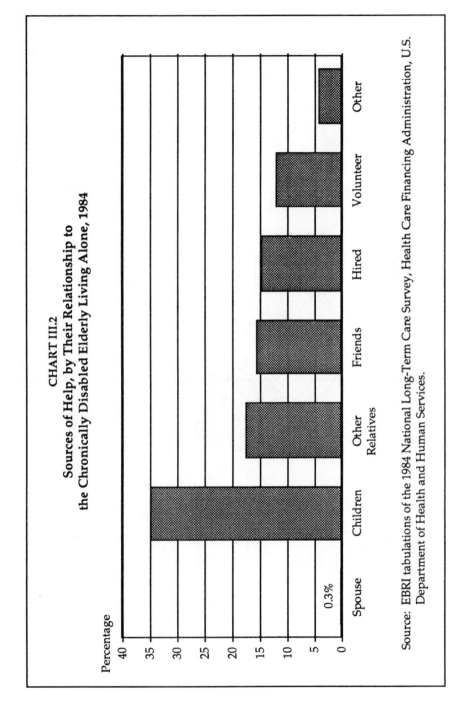

CHART III.2
Sources of Help, by Their Relationship to
the Chronically Disabled Elderly Living Alone, 1984

Percentage

40
35
30
25
20
15
10
5
0

0.3%

Spouse    Children    Other      Friends    Hired    Volunteer    Other
                      Relatives

Source:  EBRI tabulations of the 1984 National Long-Term Care Survey, Health Care Financing Administration, U.S.
         Department of Health and Human Services.

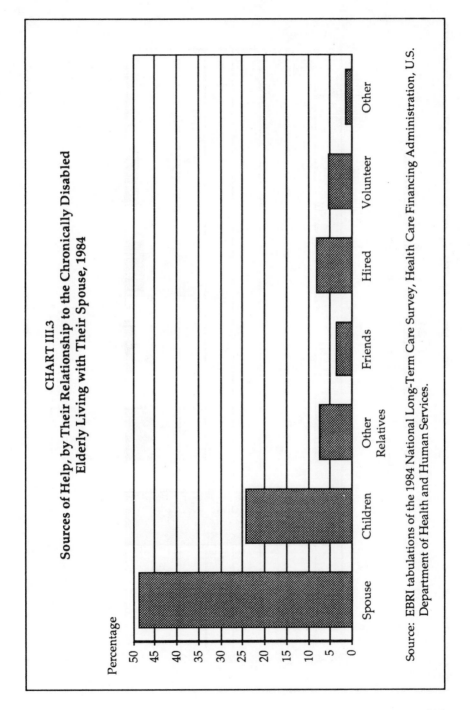

**CHART III.3**

**Sources of Help, by Their Relationship to the Chronically Disabled Elderly Living with Their Spouse, 1984**

Percentage

Spouse | Children | Other Relatives | Friends | Hired | Volunteer | Other

Source: EBRI tabulations of the 1984 National Long-Term Care Survey, Health Care Financing Administration, U.S. Department of Health and Human Services.

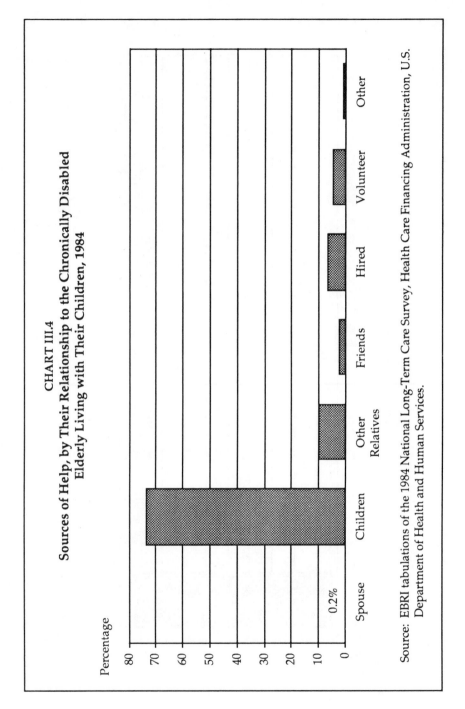

**CHART III.4**

**Sources of Help, by Their Relationship to the Chronically Disabled Elderly Living with Their Children, 1984**

Percentage

80
70
60
50
40
30
20
10
0

Spouse    Children    Other Relatives    Friends    Hired    Volunteer    Other

0.2%

Source: EBRI tabulations of the 1984 National Long-Term Care Survey, Health Care Financing Administration, U.S. Department of Health and Human Services.

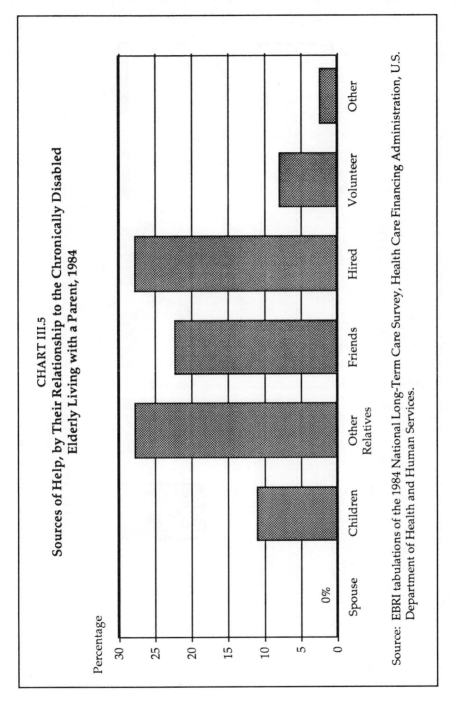

**CHART III.5**

**Sources of Help, by Their Relationship to the Chronically Disabled Elderly Living with a Parent, 1984**

Percentage

Spouse   Children   Other Relatives   Friends   Hired   Volunteer   Other

Source: EBRI tabulations of the 1984 National Long-Term Care Survey, Health Care Financing Administration, U.S. Department of Health and Human Services.

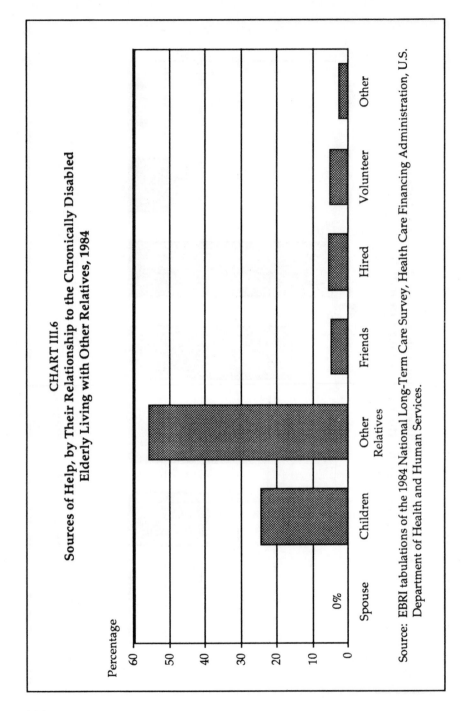

**CHART III.6**

**Sources of Help, by Their Relationship to the Chronically Disabled Elderly Living with Other Relatives, 1984**

Percentage

Spouse  Children  Other Relatives  Friends  Hired  Volunteer  Other

Source: EBRI tabulations of the 1984 National Long-Term Care Survey, Health Care Financing Administration, U.S. Department of Health and Human Services.

114

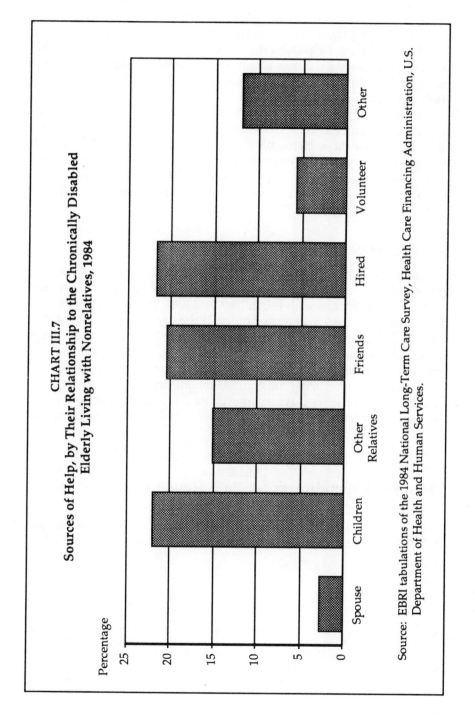

**CHART III.7**

**Sources of Help, by Their Relationship to the Chronically Disabled Elderly Living with Nonrelatives, 1984**

Percentage

Source: EBRI tabulations of the 1984 National Long-Term Care Survey, Health Care Financing Administration, U.S. Department of Health and Human Services.

percent. Among those receiving paid assistance, less than 27 percent receive all of their help from the hired helpers. The average monthly cost of paid assistance was about $146, ranging from $85 for those with no ADL limitations to $763 for those with five to six ADL limitations (table III.8).

Children are the most frequently identified sources of care for the chronically disabled elderly living alone (35.1 percent of their caregivers), and for those living with their children (73.9 percent of their caregivers). They are also important for the chronically disabled elderly living with other relatives (24.8 percent of their caregivers), living with others who are not relatives (22.1 percent of their caregivers), or living with their spouses (24.3 percent).

## Consequences of Caregiving

Caregiving carries with it social and psychological stress and requires physical and emotional endurance on the part of caregivers and their families. Care brings with it conflicts and compromises since there is less time for oneself and one's family. If the dependent adult is taken into the home, everyone in the family will have to adjust to new living arrangements and perhaps to less space. Physical and emotional endurance are especially likely to be tested if the dependent has paralysis, requires care during the night, is incontinent, becomes confused, and behaves in a disruptive manner. Caregivers often express feelings of worry, burden, frustration, and being "tied down," and complain

### TABLE III.8
# Mean of Expenditures for Paid Help, by ADL Category

| Number of ADL Limitations[a] | Mean Monthly Expenditure |
|---|---|
| None | $ 85.07 |
| 1 or 2 | 195.46 |
| 3 or 4 | 337.66 |
| 5 or 6 | 762.59 |

Source: EBRI tabulations of the 1984 National Long-Term Care Survey, Health Care Financing Administration, U.S. Department of Health and Human Services.
[a]Activity of daily living (ADL) limitations include respondents who needed assistance from others in eating, transferring to or from bed or chair, moving around inside the home, dressing, bathing, getting to the bathroom, or using the toilet, or were incontinent.

116

about social isolation (Verbrugge and Madans, 1985; Mace and Rabins, 1981; Doty, 1986a; Select Committee on Aging, 1987b).

The frustration engendered by caregiving can create the potential for abuse. There is evidence of elder abuse, neglect, and overmedication throughout the literature on the quality of nursing home care. Understanding of elder abuse in the home is much murkier. A widely cited statistic, that 4 percent of the elderly are abused, was derived from a biased sample of 73 people and was based on questions about knowledge of abuse rather than experienced abuse. A study based on interviews with 2,020 elderly people living in the Boston metropolitan area indicated that approximately 32 out of every 1,000 elderly people had experienced maltreatment in the form of either physical violence, verbal aggression, or neglect. Underreporting is quite likely and, therefore, the researchers speculate that for every incidence of abuse known, 14 incidences are likely to go unreported (Pillemer and Finkelhor, 1988).

In addition, the researchers found that 58 percent of the abusers were spouses, compared with 24 percent who were children. They point out, however, that the underlying dynamics of abuse have more to do with whom the elderly person is living and not necessarily with the relationship of the caregiver. More elderly persons in the community live with a spouse than with a child. Maltreatment was more likely to be in the form of physical violence. Age, race, religion, economic status, or educational background were not good predictors of abuse; however, health status, sex, and living arrangement were. In general, the abused were more likely to be in poor health, to be men, and to be living with others.

Despite the focus on the burden of caregiving, there may be many benefits. It can substitute for a failed marriage or an unfulfilled career, or can fill the loneliness of widowhood (Doty, 1986a; Select Committee on Aging, 1987b). In 1982, almost three-quarters (72 percent) of responding caregivers reported that caregiving made them feel useful. Nearly two-thirds (62 percent) said that caregiving was beneficial because the recipient provided company. Only 12 percent of responding caregivers indicated that the dependent did not in any way contribute to the caregiver. Dependents were reported to help with household chores (27 percent), to contribute gifts or money (25 percent), and to help care for the caregivers' children (5 percent) (Select Committee on Aging, 1987b).

In reviewing the research on caregiving, one study found that, "in the main, having an elderly parent is gratifying and helpful" (Brody, 1985). Older people are a resource to their children, providing many forms of assistance. Most people help their parents willingly when needed and derive satisfaction from doing so. Some adult children negotiate this stage of life without undue strain and experience personal growth during the process. That is not to say that caregiving is not stressful and that some people do not experience real hardship, but rather that care of a dependent parent has become a normal part of life. What makes caregiving problematic, however, is that although it is a normal part of life, it is not as well-defined by age as other life stages. It cannot be fit into a neat, orderly, sequential stage of life such as getting an education, marrying, having children, facing the "empty nest," or retiring from employment.

Individuals will vary in the extent to which they are capable of responding to the dependency of their parents. The dynamics are not well understood but are known to be more complicated than merely those of an adult child becoming the parent to an elderly dependent. One anticipates that children will reduce their dependence, but the dependency of an adult is likely to continue or increase. How the child reacts will depend in large part on the past relationship between parent and child, including unresolved childhood conflicts. These conflicts can sometimes lead to excessive caregiving, where the caregiving itself becomes an illness that can affect the well-being of the entire family.

Despite much evidence to the contrary, the myth persists that adult children today do not take care of their elderly parents as they did years ago. Many reasons have been suggested that would lead reasonable people to believe the myth. One paper summarizes these reasons as increased mobility and distance between parents and children, the proliferation of living facilities specifically for the elderly, the concentration of elderly in favorable climates, fear of escalating costs of publicly financed formal care programs, the tendency of professionals to see only problem situations, and the tendency to romanticize and idealize about a vague time in the past. The paper, however, hypothesizes that while all these factors play a role, the persistence of the myth probably lies at a deeper, subconscious level (Brody, 1985).

The paper argues that the myth does not die because it is fundamentally true. At some level all generations may expect that the devotion and care given by the young parent will need to be, and should be, reciprocated, and the indebtedness repaid in kind when the parent grows old and becomes dependent. The "truth" is that ". . . adult children cannot and do not provide the same total care to their elderly parents that those parents gave to them in the good old days of their infancy and childhood" (Brody, 1985). That is, the myth exists because of the disparity between expectation and reality. The disparity leads to guilt, and the guilt persists but is exacerbated by the persistence of the myth.

## Substituting Formal Care for Informal Care

The high price of formal care, the limited number of services available, and the dislike of nursing homes may explain why so much long-term care is provided by family and friends. Critical to insurers and to public policy decisions is the question of how much care already provided by the family would be replaced by formal or paid services if these services were affordable or subsidized and available. This important question is difficult to answer. At best there may be a few select examples of what happens to informal care when services become available. In the United States, the experience with the National Long-Term Care Channeling Demonstration and, in Canada, the addition of long-term care to the national health plan offer some indication of what may happen.

The channeling demonstration was implemented by the federal government over a five-year period commencing in 1980 to evaluate the use of comprehensive case-managed, community-based care to contain long-term care costs. Two fundamentally different case management approaches were used in ten sites (five sites for each model) throughout the country. Frail elderly at risk of needing nursing home care were either assigned to one of the two case management programs or became a part of the control group. The control group did not receive the services provided in the demonstration project but continued to use those available in the community.

Compared with those in the channeling program, the control group received substantially fewer in-home services. The increase in services in the channeling program resulted in a small amount of substitution for informal care in one of the two case management approaches used in the study. However, the substitution of formal for informal care occurred due to the withdrawal of friends and neighbors, not of spouses, children, siblings, or other relatives, who continued to provide the same amount of care regardless of whether or not their dependent was in the program (Kemper et al., 1986).

After six months in the program, one of the two case management approaches did lead to some minor substitutions among services. Meal preparation, housework, laundry, and/or shopping, other in-home care, delivered meals, and transportation were found more

119

likely to be replaced with formal care. However, therapy, help with taking medicine, personal care, general supervision, chores, and other medical treatments were not decreased and, therefore, recipients received more care. Altogether, the total amount of community care from formal and informal caregivers combined increased as a result of the channeling program (Kemper et al., 1986).

A similar result was observed in Minnesota, where applicants to Medicaid-certified nursing homes and related facilities must undergo a health and psychosocial needs assessment prior to admission. The recommendation based on the assessment is not binding, but if the individual chooses to remain in the community, the assessment team will develop a care plan and assess financial eligibility for services within their community-based program. This program includes adult day care, respite care, homemaker services, home health aide services, foster care, personal care, and case management.

One study attempted to evaluate the extent to which the availability of informal caregivers influenced the care plan provided and the extent to which the services provided affected the amount of care given. The simultaneity of these two decisions, however, created some measurement problems, which may have affected their findings. Overall, the study found that the availability of informal caregivers did not alter the allocation of formal services and that the amount of informal caregiving was not affected by the amount of formal services provided in a manner that was statistically significant. This suggests that formal services tended to supplement, rather than substitute for, informal services (Moscovice, Davidson, and McCaffrey, 1988).

The experience of Canada, which has, under the direction of each province, universal health insurance that includes federal funding for long-term care, has led to a similar conclusion (Fletcher, Stone, and Tholl, 1987). Examining the implementation of publicly financed long-term care in three Canadian provinces (Ontario, Manitoba, and British Columbia), one study found that from 1977 to 1980, health care expenditures as a percentage of Gross National Product declined, as did the percentage of public expenditures (except for 1980). In general, the changes in health care use through 1982 have led researchers to conclude that there was a stronger case for the substitution of long-term care beds for hospital beds than for the substitution of community-based care for nursing home beds. The growth in community-based services that did emerge enabled communities to restrain the growth in nursing home beds that might otherwise have occurred based on the growth of the elderly population (Kane and Kane, 1985a).

120

More notably, providing community-based homemaker and nursing services did not lead to runaway utilization.[10] There was no evidence of overinstitutionalization; in fact, the elderly in Canada may be less likely than those in the United States to use long-term care facilities (5.5 percent compared with 5.6 percent in 1985) (Doty, 1986b). Families in Canada are just as dedicated as those in the United States to maintaining the independence of the elderly, who are just as desirous of remaining independent as are elderly Americans (Doty, 1986b).[11]

## Conclusion

The organization and delivery of long-term care is not systematic. Sources of care and the services provided vary considerably. The best-organized delivery system, however, is the nursing home. But even nursing homes vary tremendously, as evidenced by the wide range of types of facilities and of bed and staffing ratios that exist among states. Furthermore, despite the fact that nursing homes are relatively well-financed and are the most regulated and best understood source of long-term care, there is widespread concern about the quality of life they offer to residents.

Formal in-home care services have not been found to be a cost-effective substitute for nursing home care. Furthermore, *additional* services have not demonstrated substantial improvements in the recipient's quality of life. Nevertheless, home health services are highly desirable. The absence of any informal services makes formal in-home services imperative, and these services do improve the quality of life of the primary caregiver. This suggests that private or public coverage of in-home care should be flexible enough to assist primary caregivers in providing long-term care. The evidence is limited, but it suggests that children and spouses will not substitute formal services for their

---

[10]It should be noted that the use of these services in two of the three provinces (at the time of the study) was controlled by a case management approach. Case management is discussed in detail in chapter VII.

[11]It is quite conceivable that the moral hazard arising from a publicly financed program is different from that arising within an environment of private insurance. (See chapter VI for a discussion of moral hazard.) If individuals feel compelled to "get their premiums' worth of services," then it might not be relevant that within public programs individuals show little, if any, tendency to substitute formal services for informal services. However, there is no evidence that the attitude concerning publicly financed services would be considerably different, since, after all, beneficiaries did pay their taxes.

care but more than likely will use formal services to complement and supplement their own assistance. More importantly, enhanced financing should improve access to such assistance.

The organization and delivery of formal long-term care services has developed by historical accident and is largely influenced by the financing of public welfare programs. Medicaid, in particular, and Medicare currently dominate both the supply and structure of the system. Virtually nothing in the current delivery system is regulated by the market forces of supply and demand. Control of public expenditures is primarily based on limiting construction and eligibility for Medicaid, or redirecting incentives in reimbursement programs.

The long-term care market fails to efficiently and effectively distribute the best services to those who need this care. Gaps in information, barriers between providers, and Medicaid and Medicare reimbursement policies can all be blamed for the market failure. Enhanced public or private financing will not by themselves ensure that long-term care will be effectively and efficiently provided. Addressing the structure and organization of the delivery system is necessary as well.

Much more research is needed on the organization and delivery of long-term care to determine what is effective. Once that determination is made, the delivery and financing of long-term care can be organized so that care is efficiently delivered. But public policy decisions about the financing of long-term care are not likely to wait until we understand how best to deliver care. Failure to recognize the need to develop an infrastructure that can assist families in sorting options and choosing appropriate care will result in either a waste of public dollars or serious inefficiencies in the private financing of long-term care. This infrastructure must be flexible enough to permit experimentation with the organization and delivery of care and to incorporate the lessons learned from the successes and failures of this effort.

# PART TWO
# FINANCING LONG-TERM CARE

PART TWO

# IV. Current Long-Term Care Financing

## Catastrophic Health Care and Health Insurance Coverage

Public attention to long-term care financing increased significantly during the 100th Congress (1987–1988). Perhaps not since the period just prior to the passage of Medicare and Medicaid in 1965 has the issue been the subject of so much official scrutiny. Public commissions were established to study the issue. Heightened press coverage was created by the 1988 presidential campaign as candidates vied for votes. The 100th Congress passed legislation to extensively expand Medicare coverage. The Medicare Catastrophic Coverage Act of 1988 (MCCA), signed into law on July 1, 1988, provided Medicare recipients with comprehensive inpatient care, limited their out-of-pocket expenses for Medicare-covered services, and, among other new benefits, provided coverage for prescription drugs. Despite the title of law, the single most likely event faced by the elderly that would lead to a financial catastrophe—the need for long-term care—was not included. Furthermore, despite the recommendations of various commissions and the attention of Congress, the press, and the public, no other legislation directed at either private or public financing of long-term care has become law.

Within a year of enacting the Medicare Catastrophic Coverage Act, and before most of the expanded benefits were scheduled to go into effect, Congress received a very clear message from the elderly that they did not want to pay for the additional benefits. Whether the elderly were misinformed about the benefits or the surtax or whether they were unhappy with the exclusion of long-term care and/or the financing mechanism is not clear. What is clear is that Congress was overwhelmed by the opposition, primarily by Medicare beneficiaries.

### Defining Catastrophic Health Care Expenses

The term "catastrophe" refers to an event or episode that is financially ruinous, suggesting that personal resources are reduced and that the individual and his or her family must significantly alter their standard of living. If the goal of public policy is to provide financial

---

Editor's note: On November 22, 1989—days before this book went to press—Congress voted to repeal the Medicare catastrophic coverage provisions of MCCA. As noted in the foreword, the author's discussion of the law has been retained in the belief that examination of MCCA's scope with regard to long-term care is valuable and relevant to policy debates during the 1990s.

protection for families with a member who is in need of medical attention, then catastrophic health care expenditures must be defined in terms of the ability of families to pay for needed health care. The ability to pay for care has to do with the absolute cost of the care as well as the patient's economic situation.

It has been convenient to define catastrophic health care expenditures simply as all out-of-pocket expenditures above some fixed threshold. Catastrophic expenses defined in this way change the relative number and distribution of people who, based on income and age, would be considered to have had these expenditures relative to the number and distribution of people who, based on ability to pay, would be considered to have them. Changing the size and distribution of the population likely to have catastrophic out-of-pocket expenditures could lead to different public policy decisions (Wyszewianski, 1986; Berki, 1986; Chollet and Betley, 1987). Defining catastrophic expenditures in terms of a fixed absolute out-of-pocket expenditure suggests that in 1980 more than one-third of families with health care expenditures in excess of $2,000 had family income of at least four times the poverty level (table IV.1).[1] If, instead, catastrophic expenditures are defined as out-of-pocket health care expenditures in excess of 10 percent of family income (as a measure of ability to pay), only 4.1 percent of families with income of at least four times the poverty level would be considered to have had catastrophic health care expenditures.[2]

Regardless of the definition used, people with catastrophic health care expenditures for acute and ambulatory care are more likely to be under age 65 (table IV.1). In 1980, more than 71 percent of all people with out-of-pocket expenditures in excess of 10 percent of family income had incomes within 200 percent of poverty. Most of these people (75 percent) were under age 65. Almost 89 percent of all people with out-of-pocket expenditures in excess of 10 percent of family income had income within 300 percent of poverty. By comparison, using an absolute dollar threshold of $2,000, 49 percent of people with out-of-pocket expenses in excess of that threshold had family income within 300 percent of poverty.

In 1980, three-quarters or more of people with out-of-pocket expenditures of $2,000 or more were under age 65, but when ability to pay

---

[1] These data exclude spending for nursing home care.
[2] Using out-of-pocket health care expenditures as a percentage of income as the measure of ability to pay can also be misleading. Assessing a family's ability to pay may necessitate evaluating income during and after the episode of care as well as assets and family size.

## TABLE IV.1
## Distribution of People with Catastrophic Out-of-Pocket Expenditures for Acute Care Services, under Different Definitions, by Age and Family Income, 1980[a]

| Age | Number of People (in millions) | Family Income as a Percentage of Poverty | | | | | Total |
| --- | --- | --- | --- | --- | --- | --- | --- |
| | | Below poverty[b] | 100% to 200% | 200% to 300% | 300% to 400% | 400% or more | |
| out-of-pocket expenditures over $2,000[c] | | | | | | | |
| Under 65 | 22.3 | 6.2% | 16.5% | 18.0% | 15.8% | 30.8% | 87.2% |
| 65 or over | 3.3 | 3.4 | 3.7 | 2.2 | 2.8 | 12.8 | |
| Total | 25.6 | 7.0 | 19.9 | 21.7 | 18.0 | 33.5 | 100.0 |
| out-of-pocket expenditures over 5 percent of family income | | | | | | | |
| Under 65 | 27.9 | 18.5 | 25.4 | 17.9 | 8.0 | 6.7 | 76.5 |
| 65 or over | 8.6 | 4.8 | 10.0 | 5.3 | 2.1 | 1.2 | 23.5 |
| Total | 36.5 | 23.4 | 35.4 | 23.2 | 10.1 | 7.9 | 100.0 |
| out-of-pocket expenditures over 10 percent of family income | | | | | | | |
| Under 65 | 10.9 | 27.7 | 25.6 | 11.7 | 5.2 | 3.2 | 73.5 |
| 65 or over | 3.9 | 6.9 | 11.2 | 5.5 | 2.2 | 0.9 | 26.5 |
| Total | 14.8 | 34.6 | 36.8 | 17.2 | 7.4 | 4.1 | 100.0 |

(continued)

**TABLE IV.1 (continued)**

| Age | Number of People (in millions) | Family Income as a Percentage of Poverty | | | | | |
| | | Below poverty[b] | 100% to 200% | 200% to 300% | 300% to 400% | 400% or more | Total |
|---|---|---|---|---|---|---|---|
| | | out-of-pocket expenditures over 20 percent of family income | | | | | |
| Under 65 | 4.4 | 43.4 | 25.4 | 3.8 | 1.6 | 0.7 | 75.0 |
| 65 or over | 1.5 | 10.3 | 10.9 | 2.1 | 1.7 | 0.0 | 25.0 |
| Total | 5.9 | 53.7 | 36.4 | 5.9 | 3.3 | 0.7 | 100.0 |

Source: EBRI tabulations of the 1980 National Medical Care Utilization and Expenditure Survey, Health Care Financing Administration, U.S. Department of Health and Human Services.

[a]Excludes institutional nursing home and community-based long-term care.
[b]Poverty income is adjusted for age and family size. For example, in 1980, poverty income was $8,414 for a family of four, $4,290 for a nonelderly single individual, and $3,949 for an elderly individual.
[c]The $2,000 threshold is in 1986 dollars.
Note: Percentages may not add to 100 because of rounding.

is used to define catastrophic health care expenditures, the prevalence of catastrophic expenditures is substantially greater among the elderly. In 1980, more than 15 percent of people aged 65 or over had out-of-pocket expenditures for health care in excess of 10 percent of family income. Fewer than 5.4 percent of people under age 65 were in similar circumstances. Using $2,000 in annual out-of-pocket expenditures as a threshold of catastrophic health care expenditures, the prevalence was 13 percent among the elderly and 11 percent among those under age 65.

In the United States in 1986, 84.4 percent of all people had some source of private or public health insurance, but 15.6 percent did not (table IV.2). For the 37.4 million people without any health insurance, what is catastrophic is determined by their ability to pay for health care. For the 201.4 million people with health insurance, the breadth and depth of their insurance coverage reduces the financial consequences of health care, and their ability to pay becomes a secondary issue.

### TABLE IV.2
## Health Insurance Coverage among the U.S. Population, by Source of Coverage, 1986

| Source of Coverage | Number (in thousands) | Percentage |
|---|---|---|
| Total Population | 238,789 | 100.0% |
| Employer-Provided Insurance | 138,510 | 58.0 |
| Individually Purchased Insurance | 8,335 | 3.5 |
| Medicare | 25,141 | 10.5 |
| Medicaid | 16,124 | 6.8 |
| CHAMPUS[a] | 8,610 | 3.6 |
| Medicare and Medicaid | 3,379 | 1.4 |
| Medicare and CHAMPUS[a] | 1,105 | 0.5 |
| Medicaid and CHAMPUS[a] | 228 | 0.1 |
| No Coverage | 37,357 | 15.6 |

Source: EBRI tabulations of the March 1987 Current Population Survey, Bureau of the Census, U.S. Department of Commerce.
[a]Civilian Health and Medical Program of the Uniformed Services.
Note: Percentages may not add to 100 because of rounding.

**Catastrophic Coverage Provided by Employer Plans**

Employer-provided health plans are the primary source of health insurance coverage in the United States. More than one-half (58 percent) of the U.S. population had an employer-sponsored health insurance plan in 1986 (table IV.2). Among the nonelderly, the percentage of people with employer-provided insurance was 65 percent.[3] Among families with at least one worker, the percentage of people with employer-provided health insurance was 80 percent, and if the largest wage earner in the family was not unemployed during the year, the proportion increases to 85 percent.

The scope of coverage provided by employer-provided health insurance varies. Sources of out-of-pocket costs for employer plan participants include uncovered services, copayments, deductibles, and all health care expenses beyond plan maximums. While many plans cover nursing home care (79 percent of health plan participants in medium-sized and large establishments in 1988) and home health care (76 percent of participants), this is usually for recuperative care, not long-term care for a chronic disability. Virtually no participants have coverage for long-term care. All participants in employer-provided health plans from medium-sized and large establishments have coverage for hospital care, intensive care, outpatient care, and diagnostic x-ray and laboratory services. Some participants (2 percent) have no coverage for physician office visits or for prescription drugs (6 percent), but some have these services covered in full (Bureau of Labor Statistics, 1989a).

Depending on the extent of health care use and family income, copayments and deductibles can become financially burdensome. Most plans, however, limit annual out-of-pocket payments for the copayments and deductibles of covered services (table IV.3). In 1988, more than one-half of health plan participants in medium-sized and large establishments were in plans with copayments limited to $1,200 or less, and three-quarters participated in plans that limited out-of-pocket expenses for covered services to $2,000 or less.

Generally, plans of smaller firms had higher out-of-pocket limits than plans of larger firms. Of firms with more than 500 employees, 88 percent limited liability to less than $2,000, and 68 percent of firms with fewer than 25 employees limited liability to under $2,000 (ICF Incorporated, 1987a). In 1988, 61 percent of the workers in medium-

[3]Unless otherwise noted, all 1986 health insurance coverage figures are from EBRI tabulations of the March 1987 Current Population Survey, Bureau of the Census, U.S. Department of Commerce.

130

TABLE IV.3

# Percentage of Full-Time Workers in Medium-Sized and Large Establishments in Employer-Sponsored Major Medical Plans with Various Plan Provisions Related to Participant Cost, 1988

| Plan Provision | Percentage of Participants |
|---|---|
| **Plan Deductible** | |
| $50 or less | 10% |
| $51–$100 | 41 |
| $101–$150 | 13 |
| $151–$200 | 18 |
| More than $200 | 9 |
| No deductible | 5 |
| Based on earnings | 3 |
| Summary: $200 or less | 82 |
| **Plan Coinsurance[a]** | |
| Health plan pays all expenses when covered expenses reach: | Maximum participant coinsurance[b] |
| $2,000 | $400 | 10% |
| $4,000 | $800 | 22 |
| $6,000 | $1,200 | 30 |
| $8,000 | $1,600 | 6 |
| $10,000 | $2,000 | 9 |
| more than $10,000 | more than $2,000 | 4 |
| coinsurance reduced or unchanged | unlimited | 19 |

(continued)

**TABLE IV.3 (continued)**

| Plan Provision | Percentage of Participants |
|---|---|
| **Plan Maximum** | |
| Lifetime maximum | |
| $100,000 or less | 4% |
| $100,001–$250,000 | 11 |
| $250,001–$500,000 | 17 |
| $500,001–$1,000,000 | 40 |
| greater than $1,000,000 | 1 |
| Lifetime and annual or disability maximum | 2 |
| Annual or disability maximum | 4 |
| No maximum | 23 |
| Summary: | |
| maximum greater than $100,000 | 92 |
| maximum greater than $250,000 | 81 |

Source: Bureau of Labor Statistics, U.S. Department of Labor, *Employee Benefits in Medium and Large Firms, 1986* (Washington, DC: U.S. Government Printing Office, 1987), p. 41, table 35; and Bureau of Labor Statistics, U.S. Department of Labor, *Employee Benefits in Medium and Large Firms, 1988* (Washington, DC: U.S. Government Printing Office, 1989), pp. 47 and 49, tables 37 and 40.

[a]Plan coinsurance numbers are from 1986 because the survey did not update these numbers for 1988. In 1986, 86 percent of participants in employer-sponsored major medical plans at medium-sized and large establishments were in plans that paid 80 percent of the cost of covered services after the deductible was met.

[b]Assumes 80 percent copayment.

sized and large establishments participating in a health plan had a deductible for covered services that was less than $100, 31 percent had a deductible of between $100 and $200, and 9 percent had a deductible of more than $200.

While most employer-sponsored health insurance plans limit employees' out-of-pocket expenses for covered services in any given year, there may be limits on the amount covered over the life of the plan. The lifetime maximum benefit varies considerably, from $50,000 or less to none. In 1986, 23 percent of the participants in health insurance plans of medium-sized and large establishments had no lifetime maximum, 4 percent had lifetime maximums of less than $100,000, and 28 percent had lifetime maximums of between $100,000 and $500,000.

### Catastrophic Coverage Provided by Public Insurance Programs

Medicare, Medicaid, and veterans health programs are the most important sources of publicly financed health care services. Eligibility for these programs and the scope and depth of coverage vary. Service veterans with service-related disabilities are entitled to care in the Department of Veterans Affairs system (which includes hospitals, nursing homes, and outpatient clinics). Veterans in need of medical assistance who were not disabled during their service but are of limited financial means may also obtain access to the system.

Medicare is an entitlement program for people aged 65 or over, the long-term disabled, and for those with end-stage renal disease. MCCA significantly limited most Medicare recipients' out-of-pocket costs for hospital care, Medicare-approved skilled nursing care, and a large portion of physical services outside of the hospital. However, beneficiaries remain exposed to risks of out-of-pocket expenditures for services that are not covered, such as long-term nursing home stays, physician charges beyond the amount Medicare determines to be reasonable, deductibles for a hospital admission and Part B services, copayments for Part B services, and premiums.

Medicaid provides health care for very low-income people in specific categories. Eligibility rules are established by each state within broad federal guidelines and are, therefore, not uniform among states. In 1986, 8.3 percent of the U.S. population was covered by Medicaid at some time during the year. Although most recipients are under age 65, Medicaid is an important source of insurance for the elderly. About 10 percent of the elderly and 3.5 percent of the nonelderly were covered in 1986. Medicaid covered about 40 percent of the poor (13.8

133

million people) and about 14 percent of the near poor[4] (1.6 million people).

In general, low-income families qualify for Medicaid either as "categorically needy" or "medically needy." The categorically needy are people who qualify for cash assistance under the Aid to Families with Dependent Children (AFDC) program or the Supplemental Security Income (SSI) program for the aged, blind, and disabled, and states must provide coverage for them.[5] At their option, states may also cover the medically needy, who are people who would qualify for either AFDC or SSI except that (1) their income levels are slightly above the categorically needy program standard but below the medically needy standard,[6] or (2) their income is higher than the medically needy standard but falls below it after subtracting medical expenses (over a specific period).[7] Thirty-eight states cover the medically needy. In addition, states have the option of including specific "state-only" eligibility groups of low-income people—those who receive cash assistance from the state but are not categorically eligible for AFDC or SSI.

By federal law, Medicaid must provide hospital care, physician services, and skilled nursing care, but states may include coverage for drugs, intermediate nursing home care, and dental services. States can impose a nominal copayment for benefits (26 did so in 1986). Except for hospital care, copayments did not exceed $3 per service in 1986 (Health Care Financing Administration, 1987). In 1985, there were 21.8 million Medicaid recipients and total state and federal expenditures for services were $39 billion. Hospital and nursing home care account for the two largest Medicaid expenditures, together totaling three-quarters of program costs. More than 37 percent of expenditures were for hospital care, and 37 percent were for nursing home care.

---

[4]The "near poor" are defined as those with family income between the federal poverty income standard and 125 percent of that standard.

[5]Technically, receipt of SSI payments is a necessary requirement, but not a sufficient criterion, for Medicaid eligibility. Fourteen states use more restrictive rules than the federal SSI standard (so-called 209(b) states). In 1989 the federal SSI income standard was $368 a month for single people and $553 for a couple; countable assets could not exceed $2,000 for individuals and $3,000 for couples.

[6]A monthly income amount between the AFDC standard and 133 1/3 percent of this standard. The actual standard among states varies from $108 to $475 a month for single people (Tilly and Brunner, 1987).

[7]This is the "spend-down" test. To become eligible, income, medical expenses, and assets are examined over a period that varies by state from one to six months. If during that time an individual qualifies, he or she is determined eligible for Medicaid (until the test is repeated). After becoming eligible, a separate calculation is made to determine how much the individual will have to contribute toward his or her care.

The Medicare Catastrophic Coverage Act of 1988 required that Medicaid pay the Part B premium and cost sharing for Medicare-covered services for elderly people with incomes below the poverty level and with assets that are no more than twice the limit for SSI eligibility. This, however, does not make elderly people below the poverty level eligible for Medicaid.

## People without Health Insurance

In 1986, more than 15 percent of the U.S. population reported that they had no health insurance. Although some of the 37.4 million people without insurance are uninsured only part of the time, 20 million to 25 million people seem to be permanently without coverage (Reinhardt, 1987).

In 1986, more than three-quarters (77.5 percent) of the uninsured were employed or were dependents of workers. About one-half were members of families headed by someone who worked full time and was *not* unemployed at any time during the year. Most uninsured workers had relatively low earnings. More than 73 percent earned less than $10,000, and nearly 93 percent earned less than $20,000 (Chollet, 1987a). Uninsured workers tend to work in smaller firms, primarily in the trade and service sectors. In 1983, 38.2 percent worked in firms of less than 25 employees, and 27.3 percent were self-employed. More than 50 percent were in retail trade or other services (Chollet, 1987a).

When tabulated by family income relative to the poverty level, in 1986 almost two-thirds of the uninsured (61 percent) were members of families with income less than twice the federal poverty income level. About one-third of the uninsured were members of families with income below poverty. Nearly 35 percent of all people with family income below poverty (14.4 percent of the population) had no health insurance in 1986; 65.3 percent, however, had either public or private health insurance (table IV.4). Medicaid, the single largest source of health care coverage, covered 40 percent of the very poor. Employer plans covered 11 percent of the very poor and Medicare covered less than 8 percent.

The near poor, people with family income between the poverty standard and twice the poverty standard (19 percent of the population), were more likely to have private insurance coverage and less likely to have public health insurance coverage in 1986. Medicaid accounted for about 30 percent, Medicare for 10 percent, and employers for nearly 41 percent of health insurance coverage. By comparison, among the one-third of the U.S. population with family income four

## TABLE IV.4
## Health Insurance Coverage, by Source and Distribution by Family Income as a Percentage of Poverty, 1986

| | Percentage of Poverty Level | | | | | | | |
|---|---|---|---|---|---|---|---|---|
| | Less than 100% | | 100%–199% | | 200%–399% | | 400% or greater | |
| Source of Coverage | number (in thousands) | percentage | number (in thousands) | percentage | number (in thousands) | percentage | number (in thousands) | percentage |
| Private Only | 5,439 | 15.8% | 20,863 | 46.3% | 59,162 | 71.5% | 61,343 | 80.2% |
| Public Only | 15,008 | 43.5 | 7,754 | 17.2 | 5,603 | 6.8 | 2,630 | 3.4 |
| Public and Private | 2,046 | 5.9 | 5,605 | 12.4 | 8,777 | 10.6 | 7,202 | 9.4 |
| Total People with Coverage | 22,492 | 65.3 | 34,221 | 75.0 | 73,542 | 88.8 | 71,175 | 93.1 |
| Total People without Coverage | 11,974 | 34.7 | 10,832 | 24.0 | 9,254 | 11.2 | 5,297 | 6.9 |

Source: EBRI tabulations of the March 1987 Current Population Survey, Bureau of the Census, U.S. Department of Commerce.
Note: Poverty income is adjusted for family size and age. For example, in 1986 poverty income was $11,203 for a family of four, $5,701 for a single nonelderly person, and $5,225 for a single elderly person.

times the poverty standard or greater, health insurance coverage was 93 percent, 80 percent of which was from private sources.

## How Long-Term Care Is Currently Financed

Medicare and private insurance are not the primary sources of financing for long-term care. Most long-term care is paid for directly by people who need assistance, their families, and public programs, particularly the Medicaid program. Medicare's fundamental purpose is to cover acute and ambulatory care and, for the most part, recuperative care following an acute episode. Except for hospice care, both the nursing home care and the home health care covered require that the care needed be at the skilled level. Medicaid does not require that the care be skilled or that it be for recuperative acute care and, therefore, covers most of the nursing home care that is publicly financed and a large share of the community-based programs. However, Medicare and Medicaid, and probably to a lesser extent private insurers, pay for long-term care provided in hospitals while people are waiting for a nursing home bed to become available. There is no estimate of the size of this hidden cost.

Nursing home care is the elderly's second largest source of formal health care (chart IV.1) and their largest out-of-pocket expense (chart IV.2). The average costs of nursing home care can range from $1,500 to $2,000 a month. Total long-term care expenses for the elderly are not readily available, but the author estimates that in 1985, 72 percent of the elderly's health care expenditures were for nursing home care (Chollet and Friedland, 1988a). In 1984, nursing home expenditures on behalf of the elderly were $25.1 billion, of which 50.1 percent was paid directly by nursing home residents and their families, 41.5 percent was paid by Medicaid, and 4.4 percent was paid by federal, state, and local programs (other than Medicaid or Medicare). Medicare financed 2.1 percent, private insurance financed 1.1 percent, and philanthropic sources financed 0.7 percent (chart IV.3).

More than 70 percent of the long-term care population live in the community, and the largest portion of their care is provided by family and friends. An estimated 60 percent to 85 percent of disabled elderly receive significant support from family and friends, and perhaps 80 percent to 90 percent of the health care provided in their homes is provided by family members (Callahan et al., 1980; Doty, Liu, and Wiener, 1985). Most of the care and services purchased to supplement informal care are not covered by either private insurance or public programs. In 1982, out-of-pocket expenditures for the most frail elderly

137

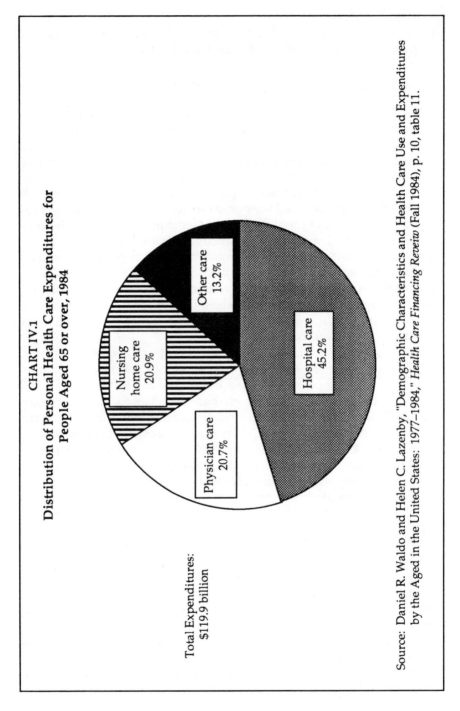

CHART IV.1

**Distribution of Personal Health Care Expenditures for People Aged 65 or over, 1984**

Other care
13.2%

Nursing home care
20.9%

Physician care
20.7%

Hospital care
45.2%

Total Expenditures:
$119.9 billion

Source: Daniel R. Waldo and Helen C. Lazenby, "Demographic Characteristics and Health Care Use and Expenditures by the Aged in the United States: 1977–1984," *Health Care Financing Review* (Fall 1984), p. 10, table 11.

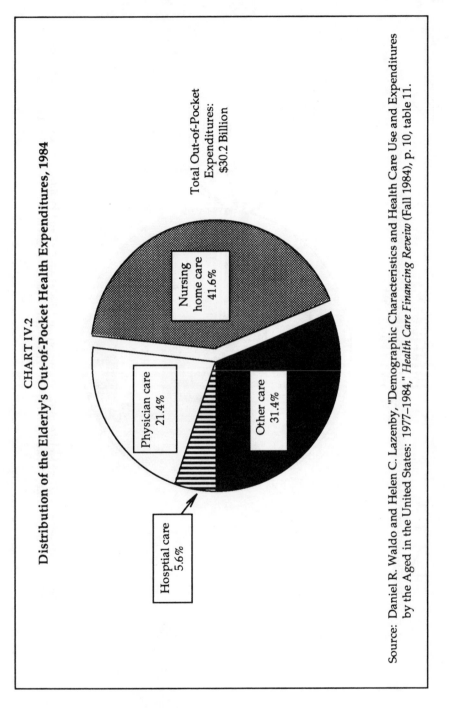

CHART IV.2

Distribution of the Elderly's Out-of-Pocket Health Expenditures, 1984

Nursing home care 41.6%

Physician care 21.4%

Other care 31.4%

Hosptial care 5.6%

Total Out-of-Pocket Expenditures: $30.2 Billion

Source: Daniel R. Waldo and Helen C. Lazenby, "Demographic Characteristics and Health Care Use and Expenditures by the Aged in the United States: 1977–1984," *Health Care Financing Review* (Fall 1984), p. 10, table 11.

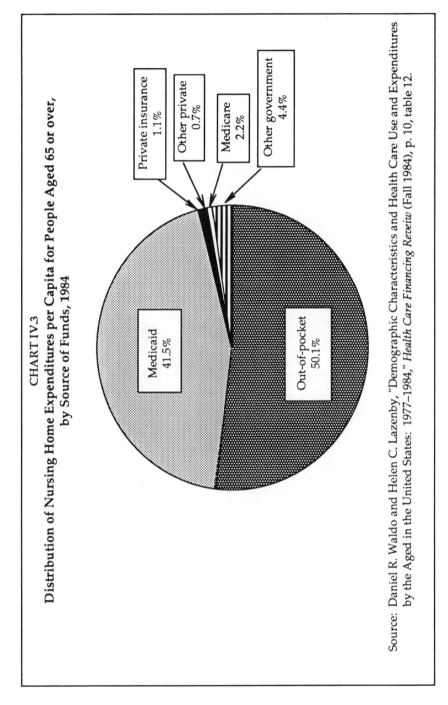

CHART IV.3

**Distribution of Nursing Home Expenditures per Capita for People Aged 65 or over, by Source of Funds, 1984**

Private insurance
1.1%

Other private
0.7%

Medicare
2.2%

Other government
4.4%

Medicaid
41.5%

Out-of-pocket
50.1%

Source:  Daniel R. Waldo and Helen C. Lazenby, "Demographic Characteristics and Health Care Use and Expenditures by the Aged in the United States: 1977–1984," *Health Care Financing Review* (Fall 1984), p. 10, table 12.

in the community averaged $164 per month, ranging from $88 per month for those with instrumental activity of daily living (IADL) limitations only to $439 a month for the most severely disabled (five or more activity of daily living (ADL) limitations) (Liu, Manton, and Liu, 1985).[8] EBRI tabulations of the 1984 National Long-Term Care Survey suggest that the average monthly cost of paid assistance was slightly less ($146), however; it ranged from $85 for those with no ADL limitations to $763 for those with five or more limitations (see table II. 8).

### Public Financing of Long-Term Care

As suggested in chapter III, the organization, delivery, and availability of long-term care services has been directly influenced by the major public programs financing long-term care. Medicaid, not Medicare, is the primary source of public financing of long-term care. Consumer ignorance of the acute-care emphasis of Medicare, and that of the many private insurance policies sold to supplement Medicare coverage ("Medigap" insurance, including employer-provided postretirement medical benefits), as well as Medicaid income and asset limitations, may be an important barrier to the development of private long-term care insurance. When American Association for Retired Persons (AARP) members were asked how they would pay for an expected nursing home stay, 79 percent of those who felt they might need more than one month of such care mistakenly believed the cost would be covered by Medicare (Abramowitz, 1987).[9] Recent surveys suggest that while more people are now aware that Medicare does not pay for long-term care, a large number of Medicare beneficiaries still do not clearly understand their coverage (Rice et al., n.d.).

*Medicare*—Medicare was created in 1965 under Title XVIII of the Social Security Act to finance acute care for the elderly entitled to Social Security benefits. In 1973, it was extended to people under age 65 who were entitled to federal disability benefits for at least two years and to individuals with end-stage renal disease (ESRD). Eligibility and scope of benefits are not subject to any income test and are uniform throughout the country.

---

[8]Individuals with IADL limitations include those who are not able to do household chores (move furniture, scrub floors, wash windows), do laundry or go grocery shopping, manage their own money, take medicine, make telephone calls, prepare meals, or get around outside. Persons with ADL limitations include those who need assistance eating, transferring from bed or chair, moving about inside, dressing, bathing, or using the toilet.

[9]This issue is discussed in detail in chapter VI.

Medicare consists of two separate programs, Hospital Insurance (HI), also known as Part A, and Supplementary Medical Insurance (SMI), known as Part B. Most Medicare beneficiaries are covered by both HI and SMI, but because eligibility is obtained in different ways a few are covered by only Part A or only Part B. In 1988, more than 31 million people, or nearly 13 percent of the U.S. population, were covered by Part A, Part B, or both; total Medicare expenditures were $85.5 billion (Bureau of Data Management and Strategy, 1989). Medicare coverage among the noninstitutionalized elderly was more than 96 percent, and among the nonelderly about 1 percent.

Part A covers unlimited stays in acute care hospitals, extended care to recuperate from an acute illness for up to 150 days in certified skilled nursing facilities (SNFs), home health care, psychiatric hospital stays of up to 190 days in the beneficiary's lifetime, and hospice benefits. People over age 65 receiving Social Security benefits, the disabled who have received Social Security payments for 24 months, and federal, state, and local government retirees who were not otherwise eligible for Social Security but who paid the Medicare payroll tax during their working years are automatically enrolled. People over age 65 or the disabled who are not entitled to Medicare coverage under one of these provisions may purchase coverage upon payment of a premium equal to the actuarial value of the Part A benefit. To finance the extended coverage limiting out-of-pocket costs for acute catastrophic illness that was enacted by MCCA, people who are entitled to Part A coverage and who also pay income tax in excess of $150 are subject to a premium based on their income tax liability ($22.50 per $150 of 1989 federal income taxes).[10]

Part B is an optional insurance program available to anyone aged 65 or over, regardless of their Social Security eligibility, or to the disabled receiving Social Security disability payments, upon payment of a monthly premium ($31.90 in 1989). Part B covers physicians' services, hospital outpatient care, home health services for beneficiaries who are not covered under Part A, durable medical equipment, laboratory services, and various other medical services.

MCCA limited Medicare beneficiaries' out-of-pocket liability and expanded the scope of coverage. It did not change the program into a long-term care insurance plan. Medicare still covers acute and recuperative care, not care specifically for chronic disabilities that limit people's capacity to function without the assistance of others. Impor-

---

[10]For 1989 it is estimated that nearly 59 percent of the elderly would not pay any of the surtax and only 5.6 percent would pay the maximum surtax.

tantly, however, the law changed the philosophical foundation of financing entitlements by requiring beneficiaries to finance the expanded benefits and by basing the additional premium on income.

Nursing home coverage under Medicare is still limited to stays in a Medicare-certified SNF for post-acute care recuperation. Prior to the MCCA, coverage of nursing home stays was restricted to beneficiaries who had been in a hospital 3 or more consecutive days within the previous 30 days. Coverage was limited to 100 days per benefit period (or spell of illness). Copayments were not required until the 21st day, when a daily copayment of $65 was applied through the 100th day. In 1980, Medicare covered an average of 30 days of skilled nursing care, much less than the average 456-day stay for nursing home care (Doty, Liu, and Wiener, 1985).

Effective January 1, 1989, Medicare coverage of nursing home care no longer required a prior hospitalization. Nursing home coverage, however, is still limited to Medicare-certified SNFs for recuperative care. A physician must certify, by providing a care plan, that there is potential for the patient's improvement. While the concept of a "spell of illness" is no longer used, coverage is still limited to 150 days per calendar year (as opposed to 100 days per spell of illness). Copayments are only required for the first eight days and are limited to 20 percent of the national average per diem hospital charge ($25.50 in 1989).[11]

Medicare also pays for recuperative home health care provided by a Medicare-certified home health agency. Prior to the MCCA of 1988, coverage was provided to the homebound who needed part-time, intermittent skilled nursing care or physical, speech, or occupational therapy as prescribed by a physician. Individuals who needed more care and purchased home health care visits with their own funds were often denied any Medicare coverage of home health care, since their purchase in effect proved that long-term care, not intermittent care, was needed.

---

[11]In April 1988, the Health Care Financing Administration (HCFA) issued a new instruction manual to the insurance carriers that administer Medicare. Designed to clarify the SNF eligibility requirements, the manual contained detailed specifications and a number of examples of cases of persons who would be eligible for the Medicare SNF benefit. HCFA data indicate that monthly SNF spending rose nearly 60 percent between January 1988 and December 1988. For the first six months of 1989, when MCCA SNF benefits changed, monthly SNF spending more than doubled. SNF benefit payments were $12 million for the month of January 1988; one year later, in January 1989, they were $97 million; and for May 1989, they were $283 million (Muse and Seagrave, 1989).

Under MCCA, effective January 1, 1990, Medicare will pay for more recuperative home health care. Medicare currently covers recuperative home health care for only up to five days a week. When the new law goes into effect, coverage can be provided for up to seven days a week for 38 days in any qualifying period, but the care needed must still be "intermittent." The care must still be provided by a Medicare-certified home health agency, and the beneficiary must still be homebound and need part-time, skilled nursing care or physical, speech, or occupational therapy as prescribed by a physician.

Although they are a relatively small portion of the Medicare budget (3.3 percent), expenditures for home health care have been growing rapidly. From 1974 to 1980 the annual growth rate was 30 percent. One study estimated that almost one-half of this increase was due to an increase in the proportion of beneficiaries utilizing home health care services, one-third was due to inflation, 8 percent was due to an increase in the number of visits per person, and 10 percent was attributable to the growth in the number of Medicare beneficiaries. Expenditures have doubled from $648 million in 1980 to $1.9 billion in 1988, an annual compound growth rate of 16.6 percent (Doty, Liu, and Wiener, 1985).

Medicare also covers hospice care. To obtain coverage for services provided by a Medicare-certified hospice program, the patient must be diagnosed as terminally ill with less than seven months to live, and the patient must choose hospice care instead of standard Medicare benefits for treatment of the illness. Care includes up to five consecutive days of inpatient respite care for caregivers (paid assistance to allow caregivers time off from their responsibilities), for which a 5 percent copayment is charged up to $520. Drugs are covered, although for outpatient care the lesser of a 5 percent copayment or $5 per prescription is charged. From the beginning of hospice coverage in November 1983 through October 1987, Medicare spent about $278 million on behalf of 91,000 hospice recipients (Committee on Ways and Means, 1988).

MCCA provides respite care of up to 80 hours in any 12-month period after a beneficiary has met the limit on out-of-pocket costs for Part B coverage ($1,370) or the prescription deductible ($600). Reimbursement under the respite care benefit would be allowed for certified homemaker or home health services, personal care services, and nursing care to Medicare recipients who are dependent on a primary caregiver who is living with them and performing, without monetary compensation, assistance with at least two ADLs on a daily basis.

*Medicaid*—Medicaid was established in 1965 under Title XIX of the Social Security Act to provide medical assistance for certain low-income people. Programs are initiated and administered by each state, and services that meet federal guidelines are partially financed by the federal government. The federal share is determined by a formula based on state per capita income, but is, at a minimum, 50 percent of state program costs. The federal government pays up to 78 percent of the costs in states with the lowest per capita income. Eligibility and covered services vary from state to state, and in some cases from area to area within each state. Each state also determines provider reimbursement rates.

To receive federal funds, a state's Medicaid program must cover the "categorically needy," which includes all people receiving assistance under the AFDC program and most people receiving cash assistance under the SSI program. States have the option to include as categorically needy people who would be eligible for cash assistance except that they are residents of medical institutions such as SNFs or intermediate care facilities (ICFs).

States can also cover the "medically needy" whose incomes and resources are large enough to cover daily living expenses, according to income levels set by the state, but are not large enough to pay for Medicaid-covered medical care. If the income and resources of a medically needy person are above a state-prescribed level, the individual must "spend down;" that is, he or she must incur medical expenses until the remaining income and assets have been reduced to specified levels.

State variations and complexities in welfare eligibility rules lead to situations where people with identical circumstances may be eligible to receive Medicaid benefits in one state but not in another. This is because each state has flexibility in defining income and assets in choosing the provisions of the guidelines they opt to use, and because there may be specific amendments or waivers to Medicaid laws specific to the state. Furthermore, individuals with similar income in the same state might not be equally eligible for Medicaid because of slightly different circumstances (O'Shaughnessy, Price, and Griffith, 1987).

Federal law requires states to cover services provided in SNFs for Medicaid recipients over age 21. In addition, states can cover SNF care for recipients under age 21, the service of ICFs and ICFs for the mentally retarded (ICFMRs), and institutional care for mental disease for people under age 21 and for those aged 65 or over. Eligibility is complicated and depends on income, assets, and categorical eligibility.[12]

Section 2176 of the Omnibus Budget Reconciliation Act of 1981 (OBRA '81) authorizes states to apply for a waiver that enables Medicaid programs to provide a variety of home- and community-based programs for individuals who, without such services, would require the level of care provided in an SNF or ICF. Out of concern about the cost, however, Congress required that states demonstrate that the costs of services to individuals receiving home- and community-based care do not exceed the cost to Medicaid of care in institutions. This provision enables the Secretary of Health and Human Services to waive state requirements that Medicaid services be available throughout the state and that covered services be equal in amount, duration, and scope for certain Medicaid recipients. It gives states the flexibility to offer selected home- and community-based services in specific geographic jurisdictions to certain individuals who meet state-defined eligibility requirements for Medicaid assistance, including the aged, blind, disabled, mentally retarded, and mentally ill, rather than to offer such services to all people in particular groups. States have been able to extend to people participating in the waiver program the more liberal Medicaid income eligibility rules that may be applied to people in institutions (O'Shaughnessy, Price, and Griffith, 1987).

Prior to the section 2176 waiver program, Medicaid services to the chronically ill or disabled living in the community were generally restricted to medical and medically related services. Through the waiver, states may expand services to include social services, including case management, homemaker and chore services, personal care, the services of home health aides, rehabilitation, adult day care, and respite care. As of February 1988, the Health Care Financing Administration (HCFA) had approved 86 waivers in 42 states (Committee on Energy and Commerce, 1988). However, those services are not widely available—50 percent of the expenditures for these programs were concentrated in five states.

Although more than 70 percent of Medicaid recipients are children and their parents, one-half (49.7 percent) of Medicaid expenditures in fiscal year 1985 were for long-term care services for the elderly (Neuschler, 1987). Medicaid has been the fastest growing component of many state budgets, and long-term care has been the fastest growing portion of Medicaid spending. Between 1975 and 1980, Medicaid

---

[12]That is, belonging to a group identified by statute as eligible. People aged 65 or over are categorically eligible.

spending for long-term care rose at an annual rate of 17 percent, compared with 15 percent for all Medicaid spending. By 1983, Medicaid spending for long-term care was $15.4 billion, or 48 percent of total Medicaid spending. Nursing home spending was the largest component of long-term care aggregate spending, accounting for more than 36 percent of Medicaid expenditures (Letsch, Levit, and Waldo, 1988).

In 30 states, eligibility for assistance with nursing home expenses is reached once Medicaid-defined assets decline to around $2,000 for single elderly and $3,000 for married couples and income is less than the cost of the nursing home. The remaining 20 states have income limits that deny medical assistance to nursing home residents regardless of the cost of the nursing home care relative to their income. For 13 of these 20 states this limit is set at three times the basic SSI payment. In the remaining 7 states the limit is less. In 1988, the basic SSI payment was $354 a month. This places the income limit at $1,062 per month.[13] That is, in 20 states, when a nursing home resident has spent all of his or her assets and income is in excess of $12,744 a year (or less in 7 states), Medicaid will not assist in the nursing home bills despite the fact that they exceed the resident's income.[14]

One study showed that one-half (50.7 percent) of nursing home residents entered without any assistance from Medicaid but were receiving assistance at the time they were interviewed in 1984. Recent data suggest that the number of people who deplete their assets while in a nursing home is not as large as was once thought. Using the 1985 National Nursing Home Survey, one study reported that while 40 percent of all nursing home discharges were receiving Medicaid assistance, only 10 percent of those who entered the nursing home as private paying residents left receiving Medicaid (Spence and Wiener, 1989). Data from the Michigan Medicaid program suggest that one-quarter of the 1984 nursing home residents on Medicaid had become eligible for Medicaid assistance after entering the nursing home (Burwell, Adams, and Meiners, 1989). Finally, using data from the 1982-1984 National Long-Term Care Survey, another study found that 31 percent of elderly people who had been in a nursing home sometime between 1982 and 1984 (but were back in the community) were receiving Medicaid assistance, while less than 7 percent of chronically dis-

[13]In 1987, the two lowest were Delaware, for which the monthly income limit was $632, and Texas, for which monthly income had to be $658.65 or less (Neuschler, 1987, table 3).

[14]Arizona does not cover nursing home care under its Medicaid program because of federal waiver.

abled elderly in the community who had no nursing home stays between 1982 and 1984 also went on Medicaid (Liu, Doty, and Manton, 1989). These three studies raise additional questions about the dynamics of the asset depletion process. It seems that movement in and out of nursing homes, the cost of prescription drugs, and low income all contribute to asset depletion *before* people become permanent nursing home residents.

The promise of Medicaid eligibility after depletion of one's assets may provide incentives for transferring personal assets to others before long-term care is needed. The frequency of asset transfer is unknown, but anecdotal evidence suggests it is not rare.[15] Attorneys advertise expertise in transferring or sheltering resources to assist families in qualifying for Medicaid. But state laws governing asset transfers have grown increasingly strict, regulating asset valuation and lengthening the required waiting period between asset transfer and application for Medicaid benefits. States must include among the Medicaid applicant's assets all assets sold or transferred at less than their fair market value during the previous 30 months. State and federal inheritance and gift taxes may also encourage people to transfer assets prior to needing long-term care. The effect of Medicaid program incentives and state and federal gift and inheritance taxes is probably complementary, but the relative impact of each is not fully understood.

The absence of private insurance that most elderly can afford may encourage them to seek ways to become eligible for Medicaid. Paradoxically, the Medicaid program may make it more difficult for private insurers to market coverage for catastrophic chronic care costs. Misconceptions about the coverage now provided by private health insurance plans, Medicare, and Medicaid and failure to recognize the risk of high health care costs associated with aging may foster an illusion that the probability of needing long-term care is unlikely, and that if it is needed, the financing will come "from somewhere." On the other hand, some contend that because surveys have found that few elderly are aware of Medicaid coverage, it is not likely to be a deterrent to private insurance (Rivlin and Wiener, 1988).

Medicaid's preeminence in long-term care financing has influenced the long-term care services that are available and how they are delivered. Medicaid programs are less likely to cover home- or community-based services and therefore encourage the provision of care in nursing

[15]The U.S. Inspector General reported that in the state of Washington, 58 percent of Medicaid nursing home residents who were initially denied assistance because their assets were too high became eligible within a few months by transferring or sheltering their assets (Kusserow, 1989).

homes. Furthermore, because an individual must expend his or her assets before becoming eligible for Medicaid, individuals in institutions may lose their financial independence and be more likely to remain institutionalized for the rest of their lives.

Medicaid reimbursement, which prohibits states from paying more than nursing homes charge private residents, encourages a two-class system of care. Not all facilities accept Medicaid recipients, and those that do tend to prefer private paying patients. Facilities that accept Medicaid patients often have long waiting lists, while nursing homes that accept only private paying patients are more likely to have beds readily available. Moreover, traditional methods of reimbursing nursing homes (flat-rate or cost-based reimbursement) have encouraged nursing homes that accept Medicaid payment to prefer patients who are the least ill and to provide excessive billable services and supplies. These incentives have resulted in instances where too many services were provided to those in lesser need of institutional care, while not enough services were provided to those in greater need (Knickman et al., 1986).

Because of Medicaid's procedures for using assets and income to determine eligibility, the financial consequences of nursing home admission depend in part on the legal arrangement of assets, sources of income, and which spouse is admitted. Jointly held income and assets are deemed to belong to the spouse in the nursing home. This means that if the spouse who enters a nursing home has direct access to family assets and income, the spouse remaining in the community may be left impoverished. Moreover, if the spouse who enters the nursing home does not have direct access to the assets and income, he or she will be able to obtain assistance from Medicaid without imposing any financial cost on the spouse remaining in the community. In a simulation based on the elderly population in Massachusetts in which one of the spouses was assumed to enter a nursing home, 57 percent were estimated to have expended their assets sufficiently to become eligible for Medicaid in 1 year (Branch et al., 1988a). Among single individuals, 74 percent were estimated to be sufficiently impoverished to become eligible for Medicaid in 6.5 months, and 83 percent were estimated to be sufficiently impoverished in 1 year.[16]

---

[16]Branch et al. assumed that for couples, Medicaid eligibility would occur once jointly held *liquid* assets were below $5,000 and income was less than $3,000. For individuals, Medicaid eligibility was assumed once liquid assets were below $4,000 and income was less than $1,000. This calculation was done using annual income rather than on a monthly basis.

MCCA revised these provisions to allow the spouse remaining in community to keep more of their combined assets and thus to decrease the time the spouse in the nursing home must wait for state assistance. Effective September 30, 1989, states are required to divide all nonexempt assets (the most important exempt asset being the home) held by either spouse equally. The spouse remaining in the community may keep a minimum of $12,000 in nonexempt assets, and the states have the discretion to allow a maximum of $60,000 if total nonexempt family assets exceed $120,000. Employee Benefit Research Institute (EBRI) simulations using 1984 income and assets data suggest that if a spouse were to enter a nursing home leaving only his or her home to the spouse remaining in the community, nursing home costs would exceed all of the remaining income and assets for 16 percent of elderly couples in one year.[17] Under the new law more than 30 percent of elderly couples could be receiving state assistance.[18] EBRI simulations for single individuals indicate that nearly 13 percent of single men and 23 percent of single women aged 65 or over could be receiving Medicaid assistance 6 months after entering a nursing home; 53 percent of the men could be on Medicaid in 2 years, and 50 percent of the women could be on Medicaid within 1.5 years.[19]

*Other Federal Programs*—In 1984, more than 80 smaller federal programs together financed 5.6 percent ($6.7 billion) of the elderly's total health care expenditures. These programs included nursing home and personal care for elderly veterans provided by the Veterans Administration (VA); home-delivered meals, congregate meals, and some in-home support services financed under Title III of the Older Americans Act; social services financed under Title XX of the Social Security Act; a variety of programs financed through the alcohol, drug abuse, and mental health block grant; and programs funded through the Developmental Disabilities Assistance and Bill of Rights Act. Of this $6.7 billion, nearly three-fourths, or 73.2 percent, went for purchasing hospital services, 16.5 percent for nursing home care, 7.9 percent for other types of care, and 2.4 percent for physician services (Doty, Liu, and Wiener, 1985). Many of these programs are small, but in some communities they are vital sources of service to frail elderly.

---

[17]This simulation assumes that the house is excluded but that all other assets and income are compared to the cost of nursing home care (at $480 per week).

[18]This simulation compares the cost of nursing home care to remaining assets and income after removing home equity and the community spouse allowance (deflated to 1984 levels).

[19]For single individuals, home equity is assumed to be liquidated and all assets spent.

OBRA '81 amended Title XX of the Social Security Act to establish the Social Services Block Grant (SSBG) program. This program enables states to provide a number of home- and community-based long-term care services for diverse groups including children, the disabled, and the elderly. The purpose of the program is to achieve or maintain economic self-support and self-sufficiency; to prevent or remedy neglect, abuse, or exploitation; to prevent or reduce inappropriate institutional care by providing for community-based care; to secure referral or admission for institutional care when other forms of care are not appropriate; and to provide certain services to individuals in institutions (excluding room and board). The SSBG program is primarily for social services, but medical care is covered when such care is "integral but subordinate" to the provision of a social service.

States have nearly complete discretion over which social services to provide; however, homemaker services, particularly for the elderly, have represented the second or third largest services expenditure category under the program, increasing nearly 5 percent between fiscal years 1979 and 1980 from $391.6 to $410.9 million. For fiscal year 1980, the average number of people receiving this service was more than 275,000 per quarter (Committee on Energy and Commerce, 1986). Fiscal year 1985 pre-expenditure reports suggest that SSBG funds were expected to be used for home care services in virtually all states, for adult day care in 26 states, and for adult foster care in 16 states. The American Public Welfare Association compiled data for a limited number of states and found that in 1983 home-based services were provided to 11 percent of Title XX recipients, or about 307,000 people of all ages. Home-based services accounted for about 14 percent of total expenditures, or $555 million (out of a total estimated $4 billion of federal and state funds) (O'Shaughnessy, Price, and Griffith, 1987).

The Older Americans Act (OAA) carries a broad mandate to improve the lives of the elderly in the areas of income; emotional and physical well-being; housing; employment; social services; and civic, cultural, and recreational opportunities. Home care, including homemaker, chore, and personal care services, is one of the major service categories under Title III of the act. For fiscal year 1984 it was estimated that the program would support more than two million home care visits to the elderly. OAA also authorizes a home-delivered meals program, with $62 million appropriated for fiscal year 1984. An estimated 67 million home-delivered meals were served under the auspices of the program during that year (O'Shaughnessy, Price, and Griffith, 1987).

Title III of the OAA authorizes formula grants to states for services to foster the development of a comprehensive and coordinated service system for older people. The purpose of such a system is to secure and maintain maximum independence and dignity in a home environment for older people capable of self-care, to remove individual and social barriers to economic and personal independence, and to provide a continuum of care for the vulnerable elderly. Grants are made to state agencies on aging which in turn award funds to 664 Area Agencies on Aging nationwide to plan, coordinate, and advocate a comprehensive service system for older people. Each Area Agency on Aging is required to spend a portion of its supportive services allotment on in-home services, such as homemaker and home-health aide, visiting and tele-phone reassurance, and chore assistance. Other community-based services may also be provided, including case management, assess-ment, adult day care, and respite care. Services are to be provided without regard to income, although special efforts are to be made to assist those in greatest social or economic need. Older people may contribute to the cost, but cannot be denied services for failure to do so. Total fiscal year 1985 appropriations for Title III were $669 million, with 50 percent of this amount ($336 million) designated for congre-gate nutrition services, and 40 percent ($265 million) for supportive services. Only about 10 percent of the federal appropriation ($68 million) was devoted to home-delivered nutrition services (Committee on Energy and Commerce, 1986).

In 1972, Title XVI of the Social Security Act established the federally administered income assistance program, Supplemental Security Income. SSI replaced previous programs of state income assistance for the aged, blind, and disabled and provides a minimum income level for aged, blind, and disabled whose countable income does not exceed the federal maximum monthly SSI benefit. In 1989, this benefit was $368 for an individual and $553 for a couple with no other income. In October 1988, an estimated 4.4 million people received federal SSI payments (1.4 million aged and 3 million blind or disabled) (Social Security Administration, 1989).

States are allowed to supplement federal SSI payments with optional supplemental payments. All but eight states and jurisdictions provide some form of optional payments (Arkansas, Georgia, Kansas, Missis-sippi, the Northern Mariana Islands, Tennessee, Texas, and West Vir-ginia do not). Furthermore, as of January 1985, 35 states supported a diverse range of community-based long-term care services through their optional state supplement programs (Social Security Adminis-tration, 1985; Committee on Energy and Commerce, 1986). Payments are made to people to support their residence in a variety of housing arrangements such as adult foster care homes, domiciliary care homes, and shared homes for adults. Some states also covered personal care and home health and other home care services.

The VA also offers nursing home care, domiciliary care, outpatient clinic services, and adult day health services, as well as cash payments for aid and attendants for certain severely disabled veterans. Services are offered directly by the VA and also on a contract basis in non-VA hospitals and community nursing homes, and on a grant basis in state veterans home facilities. By the year 2000, approximately two out of every three males aged 65 or older will be veterans, and the VA is predicting dramatic increases in the need for, and utilization of, various long-term care services by the veteran population (Committee on Energy and Commerce, 1986).

### Private Financing Options

Private options for financing long-term care prior to needing assistance currently include long-term care insurance, life care or continuing care retirement communities, and a few social health maintenance organizations.[20] In addition, there are a variety of programs that enable individuals to obtain their home equity without actually having to leave their home. Not all of these options are available in all areas. More importantly, while their availability has increased substantially since the mid-1980s, not many people know about or can afford them.

*Long-Term Care Insurance*—Most major health insurers are now either marketing or testing a long-term care product. In 1986, there were an estimated 13 to 15 large insurers selling long-term care policies of some type; by 1989, there were over 100 companies marketing policies (Van Gelder and Johnson, 1989). An estimated 423,000 people held long-term care insurance policies in 1987 (Task Force on Long-Term Health Care Policies, 1987). By 1989, there were more than 1.3 million policyholders (Van Gelder and Johnson, 1989).

The market is currently dominated by individual products that provide a fixed daily benefit amount, depending on whether care is obtained in a nursing home or at home from a home health agency. These types of insurance products reflect insurers' considerable concern about moral hazard.[21] Although newer products are less likely to

---

[20]Life care communities are described in chapter III.

[21]The term "moral hazard" refers to the increased tendency by caregivers to opt for paid help because of the very existence of coverage; it does not imply a moral judgment. A fuller discussion of moral hazard and private long-term care insurance is found in chapter VI.

require a prior hospitalization or prior skilled level of care and are likely to have inflation-adjusting features and lifetime benefits, the vast majority of policies currently outstanding have so many limiting features that many who need long-term care are unable to collect on their policies (Firman, Weissert, and Wilson, 1988; Consumers Union, 1988).

The pricing of these first generation insurance products also reflects the fact that they are marketed primarily to retirees or people who are close to retirement age, and marketed as individual (rather than group) products. Annual premiums are relatively high, reflecting the greater imminent risk of long-term care needs among the older population. Coverage sold to younger people would average individual risk over a longer period and reduce the present value of expected long-term care costs, thus reducing the annual cost of insurance premiums. This is the premise of whole or universal life insurance, compared with term insurance, for that risk.

Employment-based group products would have several advantages over those marketed for individuals. For example, the same amount of coverage could be 20 percent to 30 percent less expensive, in large part due to lower marketing costs, efficiencies in administration, and less adverse selection (i.e., individuals purchasing insurance who know in advance that they will be filing a claim). Employees would also save by having the employer conduct the search for the "best" policy. Individuals afforded this opportunity are likely to become aware of the value of long-term care insurance protection once it is explicitly recognized as important by the employer.

*Social HMOs*—Social health maintenance organizations (S/HMOs) extend the HMO model of acute care case management and prepaid financing to long-term care (Leutz et al., 1985). The S/HMO is at financial risk for both acute and long-term care services and, therefore, has every incentive to encourage the most appropriate utilization of services. Four S/HMOs are currently in their fifth year of operation. These S/HMOs are part of a HFCA-supported demonstration project.

The financial success of S/HMOs relies on enrolling members who are similar to the population average in terms of their chronic care needs. However, since membership is voluntary, adverse selection is likely to be a problem (i.e., those in immediate need of care are most likely to enroll). Therefore, S/HMOs screen individual applicants for enrollment. Current experiments, however, should provide enrollment information that could be used in the development of private commercial S/HMOs.

*Access to Home Equity*—For most elderly, the single most important asset is their home. More than 60 percent of the elderly own their homes.[22] However, the illiquidity of home equity and the importance of a home as shelter create problems in converting home equity to finance large health care expenditures. A forced sale can produce a low return. In addition, people who sell their homes to finance health care may face major changes at a time when they are physically or emotionally incapable of coping with them. Converting home equity into income without requiring the family to leave their home offers one option for overcoming these problems. Two basic types of home equity conversion are reverse mortgages and sale lease-backs (Peckman, 1982).

Reverse mortgages provide monthly loan advances to the homeowner. Repayment of these advances is deferred until the homeowner moves or dies. In the meantime, the elderly homeowner retains the title. Appreciation in the home's value during the loan period typically belongs to the homeowner or family estate. Some reverse mortgages, however, allow the loan grantor to share in the appreciation.

In a sale lease-back plan the home is sold to an investor and the former homeowner retains the right to rent the home for life. Each month the investor pays the former owner and in exchange receives a rent payment. Upon the former homeowner's death or change of residence, all rights associated with the house belong to the investor. Appreciation during this rental period also belongs to the investor, as does the responsibility of maintenance and taxes.

Only a few private- and public-sector programs facilitate home equity conversions, and participation in these programs has been negligible (Jacobs and Weissert, 1984). Poor response to them may be due to the attitudes many older people have toward selling their homes or because of regulatory uncertainty. A major difficulty in home equity conversion availability is finding lenders for whom the repayment pattern matches the lender's liabilities. Lenders are also concerned that they will be blamed if there is any misunderstanding when they finally take possession of the home. Lenders may also be reluctant to enter reverse mortgage contracts without assurance that they will not be put in the position of requiring the elderly to sell their homes when the loan term has expired. Mortgage guarantee insurance structured for this type of reverse mortgage is not widely available.

In addition, uncertainty about federal taxation may engender reluctance to enter a sale lease-back arrangement. Home equity conver-

---

[22]EBRI tabulations of the 1984 Survey of Income and Program Participation (SIPP).

sions are relatively new and extremely complicated, and homeowners may be unwilling to relinquish their homes under unfamiliar contracts. Even without these uncertainties, home equity conversion may have little potential for helping people purchase long-term care services. A $50,000 home, for example, may produce an annuity value of between $195 and $475 per month, depending on the conversion plan and the homeowner's age (ICF Incorporated, 1985b). For a 75-year-old, a $100,000 home may produce a lifetime annuity of $450 per month (Harney, 1988). Nationwide, among those with no outstanding mortgage, 56 percent of the homeowners, or 28 percent of the elderly, have between $30,000 and $75,000 in home equity. Another 10 percent of the elderly have more than $75,000 in home equity.

To assist in the development of these programs, however, the U.S. Department of Housing and Urban Development (HUD) initiated a demonstration project in 1989 to insure up to 2,500 home equity conversions. HUD plans to insure both fixed-term and lifetime home equity conversions and home equity lines of credit to individuals aged 62 or older who have little or no mortgage debt on their homes.

Programs for state-subsidized and insured lines of credit to low-income elderly homeowners have been developed in Virginia and Maryland. Under its Senior Home Equity Account, Virginia will lend between 20 percent and 65 percent of the home's equity, depending on the individual's age. The minimum age is 62 and the maximum income for borrowers is 80 percent of the area median (Virginia Housing Development Authority and Virginia Department for the Aging, 1988). Because of the income limits and below-market interest rates, these state-sponsored programs do not reflect the potential of private financing. But private lenders may look closely at these states' experience in deciding whether to enter the market.

## The Future Cost of Long-Term Care

An estimated $56 billion was spent on long-term care in 1987.[23] This was more than 11 percent of all U.S. health care expenditures in that year, and 1.2 percent of the nation's Gross National Product or about $222 per person. Spread over the 7 percent of the population likely to use any long-term care services, average expenditures were about $3,111 per person. But, since the bulk of expenditures (perhaps 90 percent) were concentrated among nursing home residents and the

---

[23]Author's estimate. See chapter II, footnote 9.

chronically disabled elderly in the community, this group—slightly more than 3 percent of the population—may have consumed $6,545 per person that year.[24]

The Congressional Budget Office (CBO) has estimated that long-term care expenditures could increase by 50 percent to 200 percent from 1985 to 2000 (U.S. General Accounting Office, 1988b). The 50 percent increase assumes that the only factor affecting the growth in expenditures is the anticipated increase in the elderly population. Under the assumption that, in addition to the growth in the elderly population, prices continue to rise at the same rate they rose from 1975 to 1984, CBO estimated that spending would double. If the increase in services needed per person based on trends from 1975 to 1984 is included, expenditures are expected to triple by the year 2000.

The doubling to tripling of expenditures is probably an overstatement, given that the technology used in long-term care is so different from that used in acute care. While the increase in the number of people needing assistance is likely to bid up prices, it is not clear that the advances in technology in long-term care will increase the cost and intensity of services at the same rate that they have in other health care sectors. Most of the technological advances in medicine have not diminished the need for technicians, nurses, or physicians. On the contrary, new advances have often led to the need for more health care professionals and often more health care.[25] Most of the technological advances in long-term care, however, have been devices that tend to reduce the need for personal assistance, and in some cases devices that may mean the difference between staying at home or being institutionalized.

## Conclusion

Gaps in, or a lack of, insurance for either health care or long-term care leave millions of Americans at risk for financially catastrophic health care or long-term care expenses. Out-of-pocket health care expenditures relative to income tend to be greater among those under age 65; but for the elderly, long-term care remains the most likely source of financial catastrophe.

---

[24]In 1984, there were 17.1 million chronically disabled Americans of all ages in the community and in institutions.

[25]The development and use of quantitative computerized axial tomography (CAT) scanners, for example, means that less exploratory surgery is performed but more people, including those who are not good candidates for surgery, receive diagnostic CAT scans.

Despite the expansion of Medicare coverage through the Medicare Catastrophic Coverage Act of 1988, Medicaid coverage is likely to remain the primary public source of long-term care financing. Medicaid assistance is most likely to be for nursing home care. In 30 states, assistance with nursing home bills can be obtained once Medicaid-defined assets decline to around $2,000 for single elderly and $3,000 for married elderly couples. In the remaining states, regardless of how far assets are depleted or how expensive the care is, assistance is not available if income exceeds $13,000 (or less in seven states).

Functionally dependent individuals and their families pay the largest portion for long-term care. This financing arrangement and the lack of choice in preparing to meet this contingency are likely to contribute most to emotional outrage, especially on the part of those faced with such a difficult situation. This may lead to increased political pressure for changes in financing this care.

Private financing options do exist, but most have emerged only recently. Private long-term care insurance, in particular, has expanded dramatically since 1987. How rapidly private financing options expand and their impact on Medicaid are of immense public policy concern.

Medicaid provides a critical "safety net" to help ensure that those who need assistance most can obtain it. Medicaid, however, is not a problem-free alternative to self-funding or other insurance mechanisms. Access to, and choice of, nursing home care are impeded for those who must rely on Medicaid.

# V. Ability to Pay for Long-Term Care

## Introduction

The cumulative costs of long-term care can be very expensive. At an average annual cost of $22,000 to $30,000, nursing home costs approach the median income of all families in the United States, which in 1987 was almost $31,000.

Among all chronically disabled elderly living in the community in 1984, yearly expenditures for care averaged $2,780.[1] But expenditures among purchasers of care can vary greatly. For instance, home care for individuals with advanced Alzheimer's disease can exceed $22,000 a year (Neilson and Robinson, 1984). In general, both the risk of needing long-term care and the accumulation of wealth to pay for that care increases with age. However, because few people recognize this risk, savings in anticipation of a need for long-term care are likely to be quite small. In addition, there is both the question of whether people could accumulate sufficient savings to pay for long-term care even if they did recognize the risk and whether such saving is efficient.

The "spousal protection" provisions of the Medicare Catastrophic Coverage Act of 1988, which became effective September 30, 1989, allow more of a couple's income and assets to be protected when one spouse enters a nursing home and seeks Medicaid. States are required to total all nonexempt resources held by either spouse and divide them equally. The spouse remaining in the community is permitted to keep $12,000 to $60,000 in nonexempt assets, depending on the limit set by the state. If this law had been in effect in 1984, potentially less than one-third (30.5 percent) of the couples in this situation could have been on Medicaid within one year instead of the potential 57 percent. A potential 16 percent of all married couples aged 65 or over would have been eligible for Medicaid in six months and about one-half would have been eligible after two years (tables V.1 and V.2).

Most nursing home residents, however, are not married. Most are single women. Among single individuals, nearly 13 percent of the men and nearly 23 percent of the women could have been eligible for Medicaid six months after entering a nursing home. Fifty-three percent of the men could have been on Medicaid in two years, and 50

---

[1] Author's tabulations of the 1984 National Long-Term Care Survey.

## TABLE V.1
## Number and Cumulative Percentage of People Potentially Eligible for Medicaid Assistance during a Nursing Home Stay, by Selected Age, 1984

| Duration | Single People | | | | Married Couples | | | |
|---|---|---|---|---|---|---|---|---|
| | Aged 65–74 | Aged 75 or over | Cumulative percentage aged 65–74 | Cumulative percentage aged 75 or over | Aged 65–74 | Aged 75 or over | Cumulative percentage aged 65–74 | Cumulative percentage aged 75 or over |
| Insufficient Income/Assets | 43,423 | 57,049 | 0.7% | 1.0% | 209,123 | 37,121 | 2.1% | 1.0% |
| During First Week | 0 | 3,926 | 0.7 | 1.0 | 33,513 | 31,567 | 2.5 | 1.9 |
| By First Quarter | 90,245 | 78,023 | 2.3 | 2.3 | 573,468 | 306,391 | 8.3 | 10.2 |
| By Second Quarter | 915,941 | 997,465 | 17.9 | 19.0 | 671,630 | 312,890 | 15.1 | 18.7 |
| By Third Quarter | 692,322 | 786,786 | 29.6 | 32.1 | 641,312 | 331,742 | 21.5 | 27.8 |
| By End of First Year | 399,427 | 472,855 | 36.4 | 40.0 | 712,149 | 267,928 | 28.7 | 35.1 |
| By Second Year, First Quarter | 260,215 | 279,688 | 40.8 | 44.6 | 585,693 | 203,952 | 34.7 | 40.6 |
| By Second Year, Second Quarter | 305,093 | 249,605 | 46.0 | 48.8 | 544,894 | 218,190 | 40.2 | 46.6 |
| By Second Year, Third Quarter | 227,611 | 223,150 | 49.9 | 52.5 | 511,763 | 162,142 | 45.3 | 51.0 |
| By End of Second Year | 187,590 | 240,946 | 53.1 | 56.5 | 389,245 | 133,413 | 49.3 | 54.6 |

| | | | | | | | | |
|---|---|---|---|---|---|---|---|---|
| After Two Years | 2,418,574 | 2,312,733 | 94.2 | 95.1 | 2,087,170 | 806,597 | 70.4 | 76.6 |
| Never without Sufficient Income/Assets | 339,790 | 293,012 | 5.8 | 4.9 | 2,927,778 | 860,919 | 29.6 | 23.4 |
| Total | 5,880,231 | 5,995,237 | 100.0 | 100.0 | 9,887,738 | 3,672,852 | 100.0 | 100.0 |

Source: EBRI simulations of the 1984 Survey of Income and Program Participation, Bureau of the Census, U.S. Department of Commerce.

Note: Assumes that the cost of a nursing home stay is $480 a week and that for couples the provisions of the Medicare Catastrophic Coverage Act of 1988 are in effect (1988 amounts have been deflated to 1984). For single individuals, all assets, including the home, are liquidated. The duration is underestimated since no adjustment is made for the fact that during this time other expenses besides the cost of the nursing home, such as food, mortgage, property taxes, and medical care, must still be met.

## TABLE V.2
## Number and Cumulative Percentage of People Potentially Eligible for Medicaid Assistance during a Nursing Home Stay, by Sex, 1984

| Duration | Single People | | | | Married Couples | |
|---|---|---|---|---|---|---|
| | Males | Females | Cumulative percentage, males | Cumulative percentage, females | Couples | Cumulative percentage |
| Insufficient Income/Assets | 4,002 | 96,470 | 0.2% | 3.9% | 246,241 | 1.8% |
| During First Week | 0 | 3,926 | 0.2 | 3.9 | 65,080 | 2.3 |
| By First Quarter | 21,580 | 146,688 | 1.0 | 5.5 | 879,859 | 8.8 |
| By Second Quarter | 294,873 | 1,618,532 | 12.9 | 22.7 | 984,520 | 16.0 |
| By Third Quarter | 337,217 | 1,141,891 | 26.4 | 34.9 | 973,054 | 23.2 |
| By End of First Year | 241,607 | 630,674 | 36.1 | 41.6 | 980,078 | 30.5 |
| By Second Year, First Quarter | 132,592 | 407,311 | 41.4 | 46.0 | 789,645 | 36.3 |
| By Second Year, Second Quarter | 118,184 | 436,514 | 46.1 | 50.6 | 763,084 | 41.9 |
| By Second Year, Third Quarter | 57,479 | 393,282 | 48.4 | 54.8 | 673,904 | 46.9 |
| By End of Second Year | 114,956 | 313,580 | 53.0 | 58.2 | 522,658 | 50.7 |
| After Two Years | 918,501 | 3,812,807 | 89.9 | 98.8 | 2,893,767 | 72.1 |

|  |  |  |  |  |  |  |
|---|---|---|---|---|---|---|
| Never without Sufficient Income/Assets | 252,360 | 380,442 | 10.1 | 4.1 | 3,788,697 | 27.9 |
| Total | 2,493,350 | 9,382,117 | 100.0 | 100.0 | 13,560,587 | 100.0 |

Source: EBRI simulations of the 1984 Survey of Income and Program Participation, Bureau of the Census, U.S. Department of Commerce.

Note: Assumes that the cost of a nursing home stay is $480 a week and that for couples the provisions of the Medicare Catastrophic Coverage Act of 1988 are in effect (1988 amounts have been deflated to 1984). For single individuals, all assets, including the home, are liquidated. The duration is underestimated since no adjustment is made for the fact that during this time other other expenses besides the cost of the nursing home, such as food, mortgage, property taxes, and medical care, must still be met.

percent of the women could have been on Medicaid within a year-and-one-half.[2]

These simple simulations do not account for other consumption needs of the elderly. The need for long-term care, in particular, is likely to emerge during a time when additional health care supplies and services are consumed. One means of identifying changes in the economic life of older people is to examine a group of these people over time. Longitudinal data enable researchers to examine the same person at different stages of his or her life. Most data bases, however, are cross-sectional rather than longitudinal, questioning people of different ages at the same point in time.

## Economic Status of the Elderly

The economic status of the elderly has improved since 1939, and has improved dramatically since the late 1960s (Smolensky, Danziger, and Gottschalk, 1988; Ross, Danziger, and Smolensky, 1987). Since 1982, a smaller proportion of the elderly have lived in poverty than those under age 65. Today's elderly have much more income and wealth than any previous generation of elderly (Hurd and Shoven, 1985). In 1986, per capita income of elderly people averaged $11,849. In real terms (current 1986 dollars) this is a gain of nearly 40 percent since 1970.[3] In relative terms, the average is more than twice the official poverty threshold for an elderly person (Bureau of the Census, 1985).

The rise in per capita income and the relative decline in the incidence of poverty have fostered the impression that the elderly are quite well off. Although the decline in the prevalence of poverty is an improvement in the economic status of the elderly, focusing on this particular facet gives a limited assessment of their condition. The elderly, as a group, are constantly changing and are made up of heterogeneous subgroups. The dynamic and diverse nature of the elderly population simply cannot be captured in summary statistics.

To understand the improvement in the elderly's economic status, improvements due to the addition of relatively wealthier individuals and the death of relatively poorer individuals must be distinguished from the changes in financial status that occur throughout the period an individual is considered elderly. One study suggests that the appar-

---

[2]For individuals, home equity is assumed to be liquidated and all assets spent.
[3]These figures exclude persons living in group quarters and institutions.

164

ent gains in economic status belie the data. It concludes that for the period 1968 through 1982, the elderly experienced a substantial drop in economic status with the passage of time. It argues that the reason the elderly as a group appear to have improved their economic position over time is that new groups enter old age in considerably better financial position than previous groups (Duncan, Hill, and Rodgers, 1985).

Another study argues that whether the economic status of the elderly has improved over time depends on how demographic and retirement pattern changes are interpreted and included in the analysis. It shows that the decline in the average income of elderly groups as they age is apparent only when one examines data that do not differentiate between demographic and economic changes. It argues that both elderly men and women experience large "one-time" income declines on retirement, and women experience another decline on becoming widows. Controlling for the influences associated with sex, labor force participation, and marital status, the study concluded that the economic well-being of elderly groups generally increased with age over any 10-year period from 1949 through 1979 (Ross, Danziger, and Smolensky, 1987).

With Social Security payments indexed to inflation and an increasing number of elderly retiring with private pension benefits, the income of the elderly population has tended to keep pace with inflation, while the income of the working population has not. In chart V.1, the median income of families headed by people aged 25 to 64 and those headed by people aged 65 or over are converted to an index with a base of 100 in 1970 and plotted against the consumer price index (CPI). The chart compares the relative increases in the median income of elderly and nonelderly families. The lines comparing nonelderly and elderly families can be thought of as expressing the cumulative percentage increase in nominal income since 1970.

Chart V.1 illustrates that the income of the elderly has increased faster than inflation, while the income of nonelderly families has just kept up with the rate of inflation. However, one should not infer from the graph that all elderly persons have increased their incomes during the 1970s and 1980s. The data do not distinguish between the group effect of greater numbers of elderly people retiring with higher levels of income from Social Security and private pensions and that of elderly who are already in retirement and whose income, except for the annual indexing of their Social Security benefit, is fixed.

The data in chart V.1 also do not reveal whether the absolute level of income of elderly and nonelderly families would be considered

165

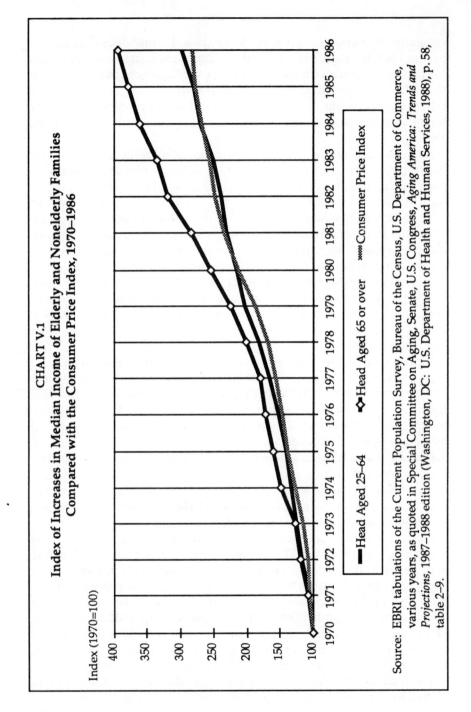

**CHART V.1**

**Index of Increases in Median Income of Elderly and Nonelderly Families Compared with the Consumer Price Index, 1970–1986**

Index (1970=100)

Head Aged 25–64      ◇ Head Aged 65 or over      ∽ Consumer Price Index

Source: EBRI tabulations of the Current Population Survey, Bureau of the Census, U.S. Department of Commerce, various years, as quoted in Special Committee on Aging, Senate, U.S. Congress, *Aging America: Trends and Projections*, 1987–1988 edition (Washington, DC: U.S. Department of Health and Human Services, 1988), p. 58, table 2–9.

adequate. In 1986, household income of the elderly ($19,816) was 58 percent of the average household income of the nonelderly ($34,285). Adjusting for family size by comparing per capita income, the ratio of elderly to nonelderly income increases to 97 percent ($11,285 and $11,594, respectively). Adjusting for taxes, however (before the Tax Reform Act of 1986 took effect), and family size, the ratio of the elderly's to the nonelderly's per capita income increased to nearly 109 percent ($9,574 and $8,783, respectively). As indicated in table V.3, the after-tax income per household member of $9,574 for the elderly was surpassed only by the after-tax income of persons aged 45 through 64.

Increases in retirement income and in the value of accumulated savings have drastically reduced the poverty rate among the elderly. Since 1982, their poverty rate has been less than that of the population at large (chart V.2). In 1987, the poverty rate was 12.2 percent among the elderly and 13.7 percent among the nonelderly. Until 1979, substantial improvements in the poverty rate among the elderly were followed by improvements among all age groups, including children. After 1979, however, the poverty rate among children increased, giving the impression that the decline in the poverty rate among the elderly has been at the expense of children. Detailed assessment of the historical poverty rates of children and the elderly do not support this contention. The two age groups are mutually exclusive (Palmer, Smeeding, and Torrey, 1988).

Poverty rates, however, do vary tremendously by age, sex, and race. Among all adults, the elderly have substantially higher rates of poverty than the nonelderly (12.2 percent versus 10.8 percent in 1987) (chart V.2). Children accounted for the slightly higher poverty figures for the total nonelderly group. Children, who represent more than one-fourth of the U.S. population and who are more than twice as large a group as the elderly, have a substantially higher poverty rate than most adult groups (20.6 percent). In general, poverty is greatest among the oldest age groups, nonwhites, and women. In 1986, among people aged 85 or over, the poverty rate was 17.7 percent; among women in this age group (66.9 percent of the age group), the poverty rate was 19.7 percent.

Elderly minorities, especially blacks and Hispanics, are more likely to live in poverty than elderly whites. Elderly blacks are nearly three times as likely as whites to be poor, and Hispanics more than twice as likely. In 1985, elderly blacks experienced a poverty rate of 31.5 percent compared with 11 percent among whites. Among elderly Hispanic Americans the incidence of poverty was 23.9 percent.

167

TABLE V.3
# Mean and per Capita Household Income, before and after Taxes, 1986

| Ages | Number of Persons in Households (in thousands) | Before-Tax Income | | After-Tax Income | |
|---|---|---|---|---|---|
| | | Mean | Per capita | Mean | Per capita |
| 15–24 | 11,996 | $18,155 | $ 7,865 | $14,894 | $ 6,452 |
| 25–29 | 25,547 | 27,012 | 10,206 | 21,050 | 7,953 |
| 30–34 | 33,393 | 31,342 | 10,184 | 23,927 | 7,775 |
| 35–39 | 33,984 | 35,975 | 10,750 | 27,048 | 8,082 |
| 40–44 | 28,985 | 39,665 | 11,699 | 29,737 | 8,771 |
| 45–49 | 22,177 | 41,833 | 12,993 | 31,033 | 9,639 |
| 50–54 | 18,354 | 40,235 | 13,861 | 29,877 | 10,293 |
| 55–59 | 16,331 | 36,141 | 14,250 | 27,052 | 10,673 |
| 60–64 | 14,135 | 31,267 | 14,211 | 23,921 | 10,872 |
| 65 or over | 33,358 | 19,816 | 11,285 | 16,811 | 9,574 |
| | | | | | |
| All Households | | 32,259 | 11,551 | 24,653 | 8,894 |
| Householder under Age 65 | | 34,285 | 11,594 | 25,930 | 8,783 |
| Householder Aged 65 or over | | 19,816 | 11,285 | 16,811 | 9,574 |
| Ratio of Elderly/Nonelderly | | 57.8% | 97.3% | 64.8% | 109.0% |

Source: Bureau of the Census, U.S. Department of Commerce, "Household After-Tax Income: 1986," *Current Population Reports*, Special Studies, Series P-23, no. 157 (Washington, DC: U.S. Government Printing Office, 1988), pp. 22–25, table 2, and p. 29, table 3.

Elderly women are also twice as likely to be poor as elderly men. In 1986, women represented nearly 58.6 percent of the total elderly population but more than 71.3 percent of the elderly poor. In 1986, the poverty rate among elderly women was 15.4 percent, compared with 8.8 percent among elderly men. Among elderly women living alone (60.8 percent of the women) the poverty rate was 21.6 percent. Nearly 55 percent of elderly black women were living in poverty (Villers Foundation, 1987).

Poverty rates for individuals and families aged 65 or over are defined differently from the poverty rates for people under age 65. The differences are related to the lower U.S. Department of Agriculture "economy" food budget suggested for people aged 65 or older and are based on the notion that the elderly need not consume as much food as the

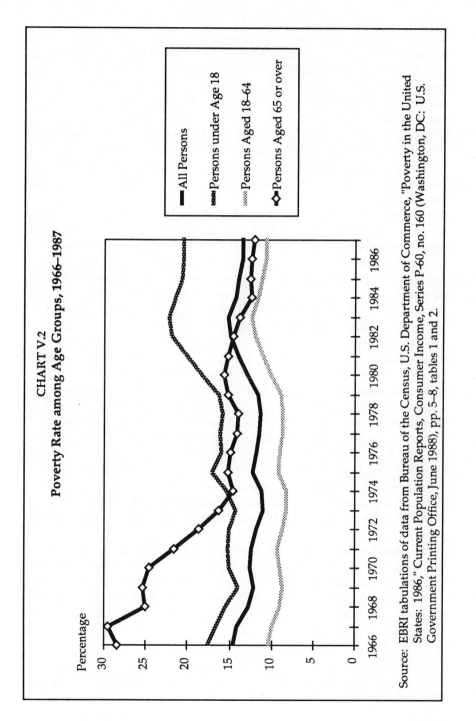

CHART V.2
Poverty Rate among Age Groups, 1966–1987

Percentage

- **All Persons**
- **Persons under Age 18**
- Persons Aged 18–64
- ◇ Persons Aged 65 or over

Source: EBRI tabulations of data from Bureau of the Census, U.S. Department of Commerce, "Poverty in the United States: 1986," Current Population Reports, Consumer Income, Series P-60, no. 160 (Washington, DC: U.S. Government Printing Office, June 1988), pp. 5–8, tables 1 and 2.

nonelderly. The poverty threshold falls by nearly 8 percent when people living alone reach age 65, and by more than 10 percent when either member of a two-person family reaches age 65. In 1987, the threshold for a single adult under age 65 was $5,909, while for a single adult aged 65 or older it was $5,447. That same year, nonelderly couples were considered poor when their income was $7,641 or less. For elderly couples the standard was $6,872. While it may make sense that the elderly have smaller appetites than younger adults, it hardly follows that they also need 8 percent to 10 percent less money for housing, utilities, transportation, and health care (Palmer, Smeeding, and Jencks, 1988).

The elderly are more likely to own their own homes, but may be less likely to be able to maintain them. While they are less likely to own an automobile and thus avoid the costs of maintaining a car, they may need other transportation, such as taxies and buses. The elderly pay more for health care and perhaps more for utilities, to stay warm in the winter and cool in the summer. Whether the elderly need 8 percent to 10 percent less, or whether they need even more money for housing, utilities, transportation, and health care, remains a question.

When the official poverty definition is expanded to include all those whose income is within 125 percent of poverty (the near poor), it becomes clear that the financial position of a significant number of elderly persons is precarious. The percentage of nonelderly with incomes within 125 percent of poverty is 17.9, compared with 20.7 percent for the elderly (table V.4). While nearly 3.5 million elderly lived in poverty in 1986, another 2.3 million lived within 125 percent of the poverty threshold. Near poverty means $6,569 per year in income for single elderly individuals and $8,288 for married elderly couples. To put this in perspective, a regimen of prescription drugs to control high blood pressure for an otherwise relatively healthy 65-year-old can exceed $600 per year, or 10 percent of the near-poverty threshold for single people.[4]

The elderly who are poor or near poor are disproportionately those over age 75 and single women. In 1986, of all elderly people aged 75 or older, 27.1 percent were poor or near poor, compared with 16.8 percent among those aged 65 to 74. About one-half (50.1 percent) of all poor and near poor elderly were aged 75 or older. Nearly two-

---

[4]Unpublished data from 100 chart reviews of hypertension patients at the Family Health Center, University of Maryland, Baltimore, conducted in 1987 by Maria Delgado and Melissa B. Friedland.

## TABLE V.4
## Percentage of the Population with Income below 125 Percent of Poverty, by Age, Sex, and Race, 1986

| Population | Aged 65–74 | | Aged 75–84 | | Aged 85 or over | |
|---|---|---|---|---|---|---|
| | Total (in thousands) | Percentage in poverty | Total (in thousands) | Percentage in poverty | Total (in thousands) | Percentage in poverty |
| All Races | | | | | | |
| Female | 9,624 | 20.3% | 5,237 | 30.7% | 1,536 | 34.5% |
| Male | 7,608 | 12.5 | 3,143 | 19.0 | 759 | 23.1 |
| White | | | | | | |
| Female | 8,581 | 17.8 | 4,756 | 28.3 | 1,407 | 32.5 |
| Male | 6,855 | 10.0 | 2,881 | 15.9 | 692 | 21.3 |
| Black | | | | | | |
| Female | 852 | 43.3 | 432 | 57.5 | 112 | 59.9 |
| Male | 615 | 35.7 | 262 | 44.6 | 59 | 39.8 |
| Other | | | | | | |
| Female | 191 | 26.7 | 50 | 30.8 | 16 | 31.6 |
| Male | 138 | 28.9 | 67 | 33.7 | 8 | 56.5 |

Source: EBRI tabulations of the March 1987 Current Population Survey, Bureau of the Census, U.S. Department of Commerce.

thirds (61.1 percent) of poor elderly, and more than one-half (56.6 percent) of the near poor, were single women (both unmarried and married women not living with their spouses). In all, more than one-half (58.2 percent) of all poor and near-poor elderly in 1986 were unmarried women, and about one-third (32.8 percent) were single women aged 75 or older (chart V.3).

## Today's Elderly

The economic well-being of today's elderly is reflected in the sources of their income and in the nature of their assets.

*Sources of Income*—Differences in poverty between elderly couples and elderly individuals and between individual men and individual women reflect differences in sources of income. The principal sources of family income in 1986 included Social Security (34 percent of all income), earnings (26 percent), income from assets (23 percent), private and public pensions (14 percent), veterans' payments (1 percent), and Supplemental Security Income and other cash assistance programs (0.9 percent). Poor or near-poor elderly are distinguished from higher-income elderly (those with family income at or above 400 percent of poverty) by their significantly greater reliance on Social Security and their low reliance on earnings, assets, or pensions as income sources (Chollet, 1987b). Among the poor and near poor, Social Security constituted more than 75 percent of family income, while pensions contributed 3 percent (table V.5). Conversely, among those with the highest family income, Social Security contributed less than 18 percent while pensions constituted 15 percent. Interest payments and dividends, however, were the single largest source, providing almost 32 percent of income among those with family income at or above four times the poverty rate.

Social Security as a source of retirement income is most important for those with relatively lower retirement income, and pensions are more important for those with higher levels of total retirement income. In 1985, among married couples, Social Security represented 82 percent of income for those with incomes below $10,100 and 18 percent for those with incomes of $30,100 or more. For individuals, Social Security represented 75 percent of income for those with incomes below $4,200, while Social Security represented 22 percent of income for individuals with $13,700 or more in income. Pensions accounted for 5 percent of income for low-income couples and 1 percent for low-income individuals, but accounted for 17 percent of income for high-income couples and 16 percent for high-income individuals.

# CHART V.3
## Proportion of Poor and Near-Poor Elderly, by Marital Status, Sex, and Age, 1984

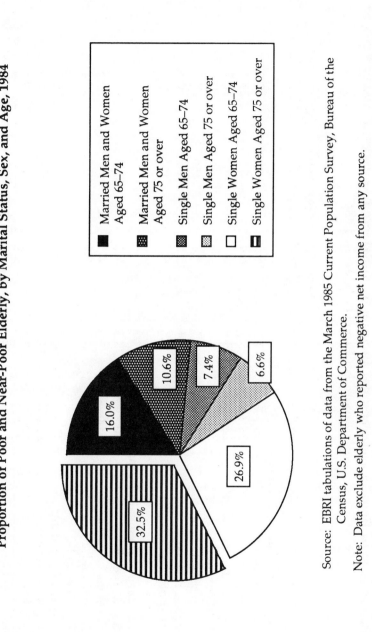

Married Men and Women Aged 65–74

Married Men and Women Aged 75 or over

Single Men Aged 65–74

Single Men Aged 75 or over

Single Women Aged 65–74

Single Women Aged 75 or over

16.0%

10.6%

7.4%

6.6%

32.5%

26.9%

Source: EBRI tabulations of data from the March 1985 Current Population Survey, Bureau of the Census, U.S. Department of Commerce.

Note: Data exclude elderly who reported negative net income from any source.

**TABLE V.5**

**Percentage of Family and Personal Income from Selected Sources, Persons Aged 65 or over, by Poverty Status, 1986**

| Source of Income | Total | Family Income as a Percentage of Poverty Income | | | | |
|---|---|---|---|---|---|---|
| | | 0–99% | 100–124% | 125–199% | 200–399% | 400%+ |
| Percentage of Family Income | | | | | | |
| Social Security | 33.7% | 73.7% | 76.8% | 69.3% | 43.0% | 17.8% |
| Earnings | 26.3 | 5.1 | 6.4 | 8.9 | 21.8 | 33.9 |
| Interest and dividends | 23.4 | 3.9 | 5.0 | 8.9 | 16.7 | 31.7 |
| Pensions and veterans' benefits | 15.2 | 4.3 | 5.8 | 9.6 | 17.5 | 15.9 |
| Public assistance | 0.9 | 12.4 | 5.5 | 2.6 | 0.5 | 0.1 |
| All other | 0.6 | 0.7 | 0.5 | 0.6 | 0.5 | 0.6 |
| Percentage of Personal Income | | | | | | |
| Social Security | 40.7 | 78.3 | 82.6 | 73.4 | 49.8 | 21.5 |
| Earnings | 13.6 | 1.6 | 2.1 | 3.5 | 8.8 | 22.2 |
| Interest and dividends | 26.0 | 3.7 | 5.1 | 10.3 | 20.2 | 36.5 |
| Pensions and veterans' benefits | 17.4 | 4.2 | 5.7 | 10.3 | 20.4 | 19.1 |
| Public assistance | 1.0 | 11.7 | 4.1 | 2.0 | 0.4 | 0.1 |
| All other | 0.5 | 0.5 | 0.5 | 0.5 | 0.3 | 0.6 |

Source:  EBRI tabulations of the March 1987 Current Population Survey, Bureau of the Census, U.S. Department of Commerce.
Note:  Data exclude elderly who reported negative income from any source.

In 1986, Social Security payments provided about three-quarters of the personal income of all the elderly with family incomes within 200 percent of poverty, and nearly one-half of all personal income among elderly persons between 200 percent and 399 percent of poverty (table V.5). By comparison, among the elderly in higher-income families (400 percent of poverty or more), Social Security provided 22 percent of personal income and 17 percent of family income. On average, higher-income elderly derived more than three-fourths of their personal income from earnings (22 percent), assets (37 percent), and employer-provided pensions (19 percent). The poor and near-poor elderly derived a total of 13 percent to 17 percent of their personal income from these sources. About 22 percent of the elderly had income totaling 400 percent of poverty or more.

Studies suggest that the death of a husband substantially increases the likelihood that a widow will become poor.[5] One study found that from 1973 to 1975, the poverty rate for couples in which the husband survived fell by 8 percent to 7 percent, while the poverty rate of surviving widows rose 42 percent. In addition, 37 percent of the widows who were not poor in 1973 were poor two years later (Hurd and Wise, 1987). Poverty, however, is not necessarily a permanent condition. Individuals and families move into and out of poverty. Another study found that among elderly couples in which the husband remained alive during the 10 years surveyed, 21 percent were poor at some time during those years. Among those in which the husband died, the risk of poverty was substantially greater—53 percent were poor at some time during the 10 years (Holden, Burkhauser, and Myers, 1986).

The authors of the first study cited above contend that individuals are more likely to persist in poverty than are couples (Hurd and Wise, 1987). Their analysis of widowhood poverty revealed the possible correlation between lifetime wealth accumulation and mortality. By comparing groups in which the husbands died to those in which the husbands survived, they found that in the years prior to the husband's death, the couples had less wealth than the couples who did not experience the husband's death. Eight years prior to the husband's death, the median wealth was nearly 8 percent less than the median wealth of those couples in which the husband did not die. Four years before, the differential was 10.5 percent, and one year before it was 8.9 percent; but in the year after the husband's death the differential was nearly 54 percent. The authors argue that "it seems unlikely that

---

[5]See, for example, Holden, Burkhauser, and Myers, 1986, or Hurd and Wise, 1987.

wealth differentials of such persistence could be attributed to differences in medical expenses," and that these results "raise the possibility that lifetime health differences are associated with differences in lifetime earnings." It may not be surprising that poor health would have a direct effect on retirement income and wealth, since poor health may have led to early retirement or inability to maintain a job; but without data on health care expenditures it is impossible to determine the degree to which the differential in wealth was due to poor health prior to retirement, chronic illness, death after retirement, or to some combination of these factors.

Income among the elderly is much more equally distributed than among the nonelderly, reflecting the relative importance of Social Security income and other public retirement programs (Fuchs, 1984). Among those included in the Longitudinal Retirement History Survey who were aged 58 to 63 in 1968, the wealthiest 10 percent of the sample had a mean income of $65,363 while the poorest 10 percent had an average income of $1,838. Ten years later, when respondents were aged 68 to 73, the mean income of the wealthiest 10 percent had declined to $52,117 while the average income of the poorest 10 percent had increased to $4,070 (in 1982 dollars) (Fuchs, 1984).

*The Elderly's Assets*—Table V.6 shows the distribution of net wealth by age. Nearly 20 percent have net wealth of $75,000 or more—with the elderly generally holding more net wealth than the nonelderly. However, the percentages with net wealth of $30,000 or more declines in older age groups. Except for those aged 75 or older, nearly one-quarter had net wealth of less than $5,000; for those aged 75 or older, the proportion was closer to one-third.

In 1984, mean net wealth among the elderly was comparable to the population aged 45 to 64. Among the elderly, this average included families with zero or negative net wealth (18 percent) as well as a like number (21 percent) with net wealth of $75,000 or more. By age groups, average net wealth peaked at $55,600 among those aged 55 to 64 in 1984 (table V.7). Among those aged 85 or over, net wealth was less than one-sixth this amount, at $9,100. In all age groups, home equity was the single most important source of wealth. Among the elderly, home equity averaged $33,700, or 67 percent of net wealth. Comparisons of the mean, median, and 75th percentile suggest that large asset values are held by relatively few individuals. Median net wealth among the elderly was $31,200, slightly more than the median among those aged 45 to 64. The top one-quarter of the elderly population had net wealth of $66,000, which was also slightly more than the top one-quarter of the nonelderly population aged 45 or over.

**TABLE V.6**

**Distribution of Net Wealth, by Age, 1984**

| Age Group | Less than $5,000 | $5,000–$9,999 | $10,000–$19,999 | $20,000–$29,999 | $30,000–$49,999 | $50,000–$74,999 | $75,000 or More | Total |
|---|---|---|---|---|---|---|---|---|
| 45–54 | 27.6% | 4.6% | 10.7% | 11.5% | 18.8% | 11.7% | 15.2% | 100.0% |
| 55–64 | 23.4 | 3.8 | 8.5 | 10.0 | 18.6 | 14.5 | 21.2 | 100.0 |
| 65–74 | 24.4 | 3.8 | 9.1 | 9.8 | 16.8 | 14.9 | 21.2 | 100.0 |
| 75 or over | 30.8 | 4.8 | 8.2 | 7.9 | 15.5 | 13.2 | 19.6 | 100.0 |

Source: EBRI tabulations of the 1984 Survey of Income and Program Participation, Bureau of the Census, U.S. Department of Commerce.

Note: Percentages may not add to 100 because of rounding.

## TABLE V.7
# Assets of the Noninstitutionalized Population Aged 45 or over, by Age, 1984

| Age Group | Mean | Median | 75th Percentile |
|---|---|---|---|
| | (in thousands of dollars) | | |
| **45–54** | | | |
| Net wealth | $45.6 | $26.1 | $53.7 |
| Home equity | 42.1 | 36.0 | 65.0 |
| Liquid assets | 9.7 | 1.3 | 8.0 |
| Other illiquid assets | 11.3 | 0.0 | 0.0 |
| Business equity | 5.2 | 0.0 | 0.0 |
| Total debt | 2.0 | 0.2 | 1.1 |
| **55–64** | | | |
| Net wealth | 55.6 | 34.0 | 66.0 |
| Home equity | 45.3 | 38.0 | 67.0 |
| Liquid assets | 18.9 | 3.5 | 16.7 |
| Other illiquid assets | 8.2 | 0.0 | 0.0 |
| Business equity | 4.1 | 0.0 | 0.0 |
| Total debt | 1.1 | 0.0 | 0.5 |
| **65–74** | | | |
| Net wealth | 52.9 | 33.6 | 67.4 |
| Home equity | 37.3 | 30.0 | 60.0 |
| Liquid assets | 20.1 | 4.8 | 22.5 |
| Other illiquid assets | 7.2 | 0.0 | 0.0 |
| Business equity | 1.2 | 0.0 | 0.0 |
| Total debt | 0.4 | 0.0 | 0.1 |
| **75–84** | | | |
| Net wealth | 46.7 | 28.0 | 64.9 |
| Home equity | 28.3 | 15.0 | 45.0 |
| Liquid assets | 19.3 | 4.2 | 23.9 |
| Other illiquid assets | 4.4 | 0.0 | 0.0 |
| Business equity | 1.4 | 0.0 | 0.0 |
| Total debt | 0.2 | 0.0 | 0.0 |

**(continued)**

TABLE V.7 (continued)

| Age Group | Mean | Median | 75th Percentile |
|---|---|---|---|
| 85 or over | | | |
| Net wealth | $ 9.1 | $ 0.0 | $ 5.2 |
| Home equity | 5.7 | 0.0 | 0.0 |
| Liquid assets | 4.8 | 0.0 | 1.2 |
| Other illiquid assets | 0.0 | 0.0 | 0.0 |
| Business equity | 0.0 | 0.0 | 0.0 |
| Total debt | 0.3 | 0.0 | 0.0 |
| Total Population Aged 45–64 | | | |
| Net wealth | 50.6 | 30.0 | 60.0 |
| Home equity | 43.7 | 37.0 | 66.0 |
| Liquid assets | 14.3 | 2.1 | 12.0 |
| Other illiquid assets | 9.7 | 0.0 | 0.0 |
| Business equity | 4.7 | 0.0 | 0.0 |
| Total debt | 1.6 | 0.1 | 0.8 |
| Total Population Aged 65 or over | | | |
| Net wealth | 50.3 | 31.2 | 66.0 |
| Home equity | 33.7 | 25.0 | 52.0 |
| Liquid assets | 19.7 | 4.4 | 22.7 |
| Other illiquid assets | 6.1 | 0.0 | 0.0 |
| Business equity | 1.3 | 0.0 | 0.0 |
| Total debt | 0.3 | 0.0 | 0.0 |

Source: EBRI tabulations of the 1984 Survey of Income and Program Participation, Bureau of the Census, U.S. Department of Commerce.

Marital status and the availability of assets seem to be closely related. Mean net wealth among married elderly couples ($59,100) was more than the mean net wealth of those who were no longer married (table V.8). Most of this difference, however, is found in the holdings of illiquid assets (including nonresidential, nonbusiness real property and life insurance) and home equity. Among single individuals, net wealth was lowest for those who had been divorced ($36,200) and highest for those who had never married ($62,200). For widows, net wealth averaged $51,200; home equity, in particular, was critical since among owners it represented more than 89 percent of their net wealth. Unmarried elderly persons living alone tended to average higher net wealth than elderly persons in the same marital status group living with others (table V.9).

TABLE V.8
# Mean and Median Wealth among Selected Elderly, by Marital Status, 1984

| Type of Wealth | Mean | Median | 75th Percentile |
|---|---|---|---|
| | (in thousands of dollars) | | |
| **Married (n = 12.3 million)** | | | |
| Total net wealth | $59.1 | $41.0 | $71.1 |
| home equity | 47.9 | 42.0 | 65.0 |
| home equity among owners | 58.1 | 50.0 | 70.0 |
| liquid assets | 22.7 | 7.9 | 27.7 |
| illiquid assets | 8.3 | 0.0 | 0.0 |
| business equity | 1.7 | 0.0 | 0.0 |
| **Divorced or Separated (n = 1.3 million)** | | | |
| Total net wealth | 36.2 | 9.9 | 49.3 |
| home equity | 17.1 | 0.0 | 29.0 |
| home equity among owners | 39.5 | 32.0 | 59.3 |
| liquid assets | 15.1 | 1.4 | 15.6 |
| illiquid assets | 3.7 | 0.0 | 0.0 |
| business equity | 0.7 | 0.0 | 0.0 |
| **Widowed (n = 8.0 million)** | | | |
| Total net wealth | 51.2 | 32.6 | 71.2 |
| home equity | 26.5 | 15.0 | 43.0 |
| home equity among owners | 45.6 | 40.0 | 60.0 |
| liquid assets | 18.9 | 4.9 | 23.1 |
| illiquid assets | 5.4 | 0.0 | 0.0 |
| business equity | 0.8 | 0.0 | 0.0 |
| **Never Married (n = 1.4 million)** | | | |
| Total net wealth | 62.2 | 24.9 | 70.0 |
| home equity | 21.8 | 0.0 | 35.3 |
| home equity among owners | 50.8 | 40.0 | 62.5 |
| liquid assets | 33.9 | 7.7 | 34.8 |
| illiquid assets | 4.3 | 0.0 | 0.0 |
| business equity | 2.3 | 0.0 | 0.0 |

Source: EBRI tabulations of the 1984 Survey of Income and Program Participation, Bureau of the Census, U.S. Department of Commerce.

**TABLE V.9**

# Mean and Median Wealth among Selected Single Elderly, by Living Arrangement, 1984

| Type of Wealth | Living with Others | | | Living Alone | | |
|---|---|---|---|---|---|---|
| | Mean | Median | 75th percentile | Mean | Median | 75th percentile |
| | | | (in thousands of dollars) | | | |
| **Divorced or Separated** | | | | | | |
| Total net wealth | $19.3 | $3.6 | $34.9 | $39.8 | $11.8 | $51.3 |
| home equity | 11.8 | 0.0 | 12.3 | 18.2 | 0.0 | 30.0 |
| home equity among owners | 40.1 | 42.5 | 63.1 | 39.4 | 30.0 | 55.0 |
| liquid assets | 7.9 | 0.6 | 6.7 | 16.6 | 1.6 | 20.9 |
| illiquid assets | 0.0 | 0.0 | 0.0 | 4.4 | 0.0 | 0.0 |
| business equity | 0.0 | 0.0 | 0.0 | 0.9 | 0.0 | 0.0 |
| **Widowed** | | | | | | |
| Total net wealth | 39.6 | 15.2 | 55.0 | 55.9 | 40.0 | 75.4 |
| home equity | 20.4 | 0.0 | 35.0 | 29.0 | 20.0 | 45.0 |
| home equity among owners | 46.4 | 40.0 | 60.0 | 45.4 | 39.9 | 59.9 |
| liquid assets | 12.8 | 1.3 | 12.7 | 21.3 | 6.0 | 28.1 |
| illiquid assets | 6.1 | 0.0 | 0.0 | 5.1 | 0.0 | 0.0 |
| business equity | 0.5 | 0.0 | 0.0 | 0.9 | 0.0 | 0.0 |

(continued)

**TABLE V.9 (continued)**

| Type of Wealth | Living with Others | | | Living Alone | | |
|---|---|---|---|---|---|---|
| | Mean | Median | 75th percentile | Mean | Median | 75th percentile |
| | (in thousands of dollars) | | | | | |
| Never Married | | | | | | |
| Total net wealth | 70.9 | 22.6 | 65.9 | 57.0 | 29.3 | 73.0 |
| home equity | 21.2 | 0.0 | 35.0 | 22.2 | 0.0 | 40.0 |
| home equity among owners | 48.0 | 35.0 | 62.0 | 52.6 | 45.0 | 65.0 |
| liquid assets | 39.1 | 7.5 | 32.0 | 30.9 | 8.0 | 35.3 |
| illiquid assets | 6.4 | 0.0 | 0.0 | 3.0 | 0.0 | 0.0 |
| business equity | 4.2 | 0.0 | 0.0 | 1.0 | 0.0 | 0.0 |

Source: EBRI tabulations of the 1984 Survey of Income and Program Participation, Bureau of the Census, U.S. Department of Commerce.

Although married couples averaged substantially higher net wealth than unmarried individuals, variation in wealth among married couples was greater than among unmarried individuals. This variation was concentrated in holdings of liquid assets. At the median and average, liquid assets were a relatively small component of net wealth, but for those with substantial holdings their value was extremely high. The most important component of net wealth—home equity—was more evenly distributed among couples relative to other asset types, and was comparably distributed, although at a lower average, within various groups of unmarried elderly.

Unfortunately, given the relative paucity of wealth data, income is not a very good indicator of the wealth of the elderly. Joint distributions of income and wealth suggest that for less than one-half of the elderly income and wealth are not correlated (Chollet and Friedland, 1988c).[6] While the likelihood of higher net wealth at higher levels of family income is apparent in each group, a significant minority, regardless of marital status, hold either large sums of wealth but receive low incomes or have large annual incomes but no net wealth.

## Tomorrow's Elderly

Each successive group of people entering the ranks of the elderly has been better off than the previous group. It is speculated that this is likely to continue. People reaching age 65 during the next 15 years or so were either babies or not yet born during the Great Depression, were in their prime working years during the growth period of the 1960s, and experienced substantial appreciation in their homes during the inflation of the 1970s. In general, they should have been in a relatively good position to capture the high real interest rates and stock market boom of the late 1970s to mid-1980s (Edmondson, 1987). Demographers have nicknamed those born prior to 1938 the "good-times" generation (Horn, 1978).

Between the good-times generation and the baby boom lies what is referred to in the popular press as the "sandwich generation"—those born between 1938 and 1944. This nickname symbolizes those who are now "sandwiched" between financing their children's education

---

[6]For most elderly, the correlation between income and wealth, although positive, is not very strong (only about 0.5). Never-married elderly persons living alone had the highest correlation at 0.7. In most cases, annualized net wealth (which adjusts for age) reduces the correlation between assets and family income. This reflects the more even distribution of assets among elderly persons of different ages but with similar marital status and living arrangements relative to the distribution of income by age.

and their parents' long-term care (Miller, 1981). However, since this situation is not likely to be unique to this particular generation, the nickname might be best thought of as describing that generation sandwiched between the good-times generation and the baby boom: too old to have been affected by the dramatic surge in the population, too young to reap directly all the advantages of the economic expansion of the 1960s and 1970s, and too small to receive the same kind of special attention marketers and politicians have given to other age groups.

A microsimulation model has been developed to assess the retirement income of future retirees. The Employee Benefit Research Institute/ICF pension and retirement income simulation model (PRISM) was developed by ICF Incorporated in 1979 for the President's Commission on Pension Policy. Under contract to EBRI and others, ICF has enhanced PRISM periodically to reflect changes in federal legislation. The basis of the model is 1979, when the Census Bureau's Current Population Survey (CPS) was matched to Social Security earnings histories. The estimating parameters, however, have been recalculated using the 1984 CPS as a benchmark (Chollet, forthcoming, b). The model simulates many of life's events for workers in 1979. Each worker faces probabilities of unemployment, changing jobs, getting married, having a child, getting divorced, and dying, in conjunction with his or her age. Each year, until the individual reaches age 67, a new array of probabilities are faced. The output of the model is the expected retirement income from Social Security, pensions, and individual retirement accounts (IRAs) for the survivors at age 67.

For each generation retiring through the year 2021, PRISM suggests that both recipiency and the average value of retirement income, in real terms, are likely to increase. Compared with those now retiring, the workers born between 1945 and 1954 are more likely to have employer-sponsored pensions, Social Security, and annuity income from IRAs, but less likely to have income from earnings and Supplemental Security Income (SSI) (table V.10). The decline in earnings reflects the propensity of workers to retire earlier. The projected decline in SSI suggests that fewer retirees will have insufficient Social Security benefits.

Table V.11 presents average annual income by marital status projected for each source of retirement income among those with such income. Among married couples in the first half of the baby boom, real 1985 Social Security income is projected to average $12,800 per year, compared with $9,500 among married couples retiring now. Among single people, the average is projected to be $6,800, compared

TABLE V.10
# Percentage of Retiree Families of Different Generations with Retirement Income at Age 67, from Various Sources

| Income Source | Workers Currently Retiring[a] | Baby Boom Retirees[b] | Percentage-Point Difference |
|---|---|---|---|
| **All Retiree Families** | | | |
| Social Security | 86% | 97% | 11% |
| Employer-sponsored pensions | 48 | 71 | 23 |
| Earnings | 35 | 29 | −6 |
| Supplemental Security Income | 10 | 3 | −7 |
| | | | |
| **Married Couples** | | | |
| Social Security | 94 | 98 | 4 |
| Employer-sponsored pensions | 59 | 83 | 24 |
| Earnings | 44 | 39 | −5 |
| Supplemental Security Income | 2 | | −2 |
| | | | |
| **Single Individuals** | | | |
| Social Security | 77 | 95 | 18 |
| Employer-sponsored pensions | 36 | 60 | 24 |
| Earnings | 25 | 21 | −4 |
| Supplemental Security Income | 21 | 5 | −4 |

Source: Emily S. Andrews and Deborah J. Chollet, "Future Sources of Retirement Income: Whither the Baby Boom?" in Susan M. Wachter, ed., *Social Security and Private Pensions: Providing for Retirement in the Twenty-First Century* (Lexington, MA: D.C. Heath and Company, 1988), p. 77, table 4-1.
[a] Aged 55–64 in 1979.
[b] Aged 25–34 in 1979.

with $4,800 among single workers retiring today. These averages are in 1985 dollars and, therefore, the increases are in real terms; that is, they reflect increases above anticipated inflation. Average real income from employer-sponsored pensions among married baby boom couples is projected to exceed $14,000, double the amount among couples retiring now ($7,100). Among single individuals, average projected pension income for the first half of the baby boom is expected to be $9,600, compared with $5,300 among individuals retiring now. Average IRA annuity values are expected to increase from $500 for couples

185

## TABLE V.11
## Average Income at Age 67 among Recipient Families of Different Generations, from Selected Sources, 1985 Dollars

| Income Source | Average Income of Workers Currently Retiring[a] (in thousands) | Average Income of Baby Boom Retirees[b] (in thousands) | Percentage Increase in Average Income for Future Retirees |
|---|---|---|---|
| Married Couples | | | |
| Social Security | $9.5 | $12.8 | 34.7% |
| Employer-sponsored pensions | | | |
| total | 7.1 | 14.3 | 101.4 |
| defined contribution plans | 4.4 | 11.3 | 156.8 |
| defined benefit plans | 6.5 | 8.7 | 33.8 |
| Single Individuals | | | |
| Social Security | 4.8 | 6.8 | 41.7 |
| Employer-sponsored pensions | | | |
| total | 5.3 | 9.6 | 81.1 |
| defined contribution plans | 3.3 | 8.5 | 157.6 |
| defined benefit plans | 5.1 | 6.5 | 27.5 |

Source: Emily S. Andrews and Deborah J. Chollet, "Future Sources of Retirement Income: Whither the Baby Boom?" in Susan M. Wachter, ed., *Social Security and Private Pensions: Providing for Retirement in the Twenty-First Century* (Lexington, MA: D.C. Heath and Company, 1988), p. 79, table 4-2.

[a]Aged 55–64 in 1979.
[b]Aged 25–34 in 1979.

and $400 for single individuals currently retiring to $3,000 and $2,000, respectively, for the first half of baby boom retirees.

The projected increases in real retirement income among baby boom retirees reflect the assumed real wage growth and the increased labor force participation among women. Higher preretirement wages result in higher postretirement Social Security benefits, and increased labor force participation among women enhances the likelihood that women will receive their own Social Security benefits rather than rely on the 50 percent spousal benefit.

Ironically, wage replacement rates from Social Security benefits and pension income combined are projected to decline slightly relative to current replacement rates (Andrews and Chollet, 1988). For the most part, the projected decline is due to scheduled reductions and the progressivity in the Social Security benefit formula. Lower lifetime earnings provide a lower Social Security benefit than higher lifetime earnings, but provide a higher wage replacement rate. Among married men currently retiring, Social Security benefits and pension income replace 49 percent of preretirement average earnings. For the first half of the baby boom, the replacement rate is projected to fall to 45 percent. For unmarried women, the replacement rate is expected to decline from 77 percent to 53 percent.

The relative importance of pension income is projected to increase as the wage replacement rate for Social Security benefits declines and the wage replacement rate for pension income increases (Andrews and Chollet, 1988). This is reflected in table V.12, which shows the percentage of total retirement income from different sources. Overall, Social Security benefits decline from 46.1 percent of total retirement income to 38 percent, while pension income increases from 22.7 percent to 36.1 percent. The decline in the importance of SSI is telling, dropping from 2.1 percent of retirement income to 0.3 percent.

PRISM's projections of retirement income for the first half of the baby boom suggest that a greater proportion of baby boom retirees will receive pensions, compared with workers now retiring, and that their real pension income and Social Security benefits will be higher. The basis for this is the assumption of economic and real wage growth, since the proportion of employers with pension plans is assumed not to expand. PRISM assumes real wage growth is constrained to the Social Security actuaries' low growth alternative III. The assumed rate of wage growth is about one percentage point higher than inflation (Chollet, forthcoming, b). Although the alternative III assumptions for economic growth are regarded as pessimistic assumptions

187

TABLE V.12
# Percentage of Total Retirement Income at Age 67 among Retiree Families of Different Generations, from Various Sources

| Income Source | Workers Currently Retiring[a] | Baby Boom Retirees[b] | Percentage-Point Difference |
|---|---|---|---|
| **All Retiree Families** | | | |
| Social Security | 46.1% | 39.7% | −6.4% |
| Employer-sponsored pensions | 22.7 | 37.8 | 15.1 |
| Earnings | 28.8 | 22.2 | −6.6 |
| Supplemental Security Income | 2.1 | 0.3 | −1.8 |
| **Married Couples** | | | |
| Social Security | 47.1 | 37.7 | −9.4 |
| Employer-sponsored pensions | 22.7 | 36.6 | 13.9 |
| Earnings | 29.8 | 25.7 | −4.1 |
| Supplemental Security Income | 0.3 | 0.0 | −0.3 |
| **Single Individuals** | | | |
| Social Security | 43.8 | 43.8 | 0.0 |
| Employer-sponsored pensions | 22.7 | 40.2 | 17.5 |
| Earnings | 26.0 | 15.3 | −10.7 |
| Supplemental Security Income | 7.4 | 0.7 | −6.7 |

Source: Emily S. Andrews and Deborah J. Chollet, "Future Sources of Retirement Income: Whither the Baby Boom?" in Susan M. Wachter, ed., *Social Security and Private Pensions: Providing for Retirement in the Twenty-First Century* (Lexington, MA: D.C. Heath and Company, 1988), p. 80, table 4-3.
[a]Aged 55–64 in 1979.
[b]Aged 25–34 in 1979.

by Social Security Administration actuaries, historically these assumptions have tended to be optimistic.

The baby boom did not begin to enter the labor market until after 1961; about one-half had entered the labor market by 1976, and all had entered by 1984. Real gross weekly earnings of all workers in private, nonagricultural employment in the United States declined 9.1 percent from 1970 to 1981. After increasing at an annual rate of 2.6 percent between 1960 and 1973, real wages in manufacturing have since been relatively flat (Marshall, 1986).

Real wage growth reflects gains in productivity; productivity depends on the amount and vintage of capital per employee (machines, tools, equipment, and the amount of modern technology incorporated in them per worker) and the relative abilities of the work force. In terms of employee ability, future groups of retirees will have attained substantially higher levels of education than either current retirees or those likely to retire in the next 10 years. In 1980, more than one-half (57 percent) of those who were aged 65 to 74, and 67 percent of those aged 75 or older, had not completed high school (Bureau of the Census, 1984). Less than 9 percent (9 percent and 7.2 percent, respectively) had attained a college degree or better. Among those aged 25 to 34 in 1980 (essentially the first half of the baby boom), less than 16 percent had not finished high school and 23.3 percent had already completed college or beyond.

The availability of advanced technological machines depends on the economy's ability to develop sources from which employers can borrow at rates lower than the expected rate of return from the production envisioned from the technology. Over the past decade, capital formation has been adversely affected by high real interest rates. The 1987 trade deficit of approximately $175 billion is in part symptomatic of high real interest rates. Moving toward a balance of trade is likely to lower real interest rates, but during the process it is likely that U.S. productivity will decline. Reduced demand for U.S. goods and services is likely to have an adverse effect on real wages and capital formation.

The PRISM projections are not all rosy. Some of the workers and their dependents included in the 1979 model are projected to be poor when they are aged 67. Among workers expected to reach age 67 between the year 2012 and the year 2021, PRISM results suggest that about 18 percent will have retirement incomes below 125 percent of poverty.[7] Single women are most likely to be in this group. PRISM projections indicate that 43 percent of single women will have retirement incomes at 125 percent of poverty or less (Chollet, 1987b). PRISM does not simulate income from all sources; consequently, using retirement income as a proxy for all income would tend to overstate the number of people with less than near-poverty levels of income. How-

---

[7]Income from savings may move some of these individuals above this threshold. In 1988, income from savings represented between 4 percent and 5 percent of total income for those with family income below 125 percent of poverty, while for those with income at 400 percent of poverty or greater, income from savings as a source of retirement income was closer to 37 percent.

ever, income from accumulated assets, which would be the major source of omitted income, tends to be concentrated among those with relatively higher income. In 1984, only about one-third of poor and near-poor elderly reported asset income; among the poor or near poor reporting asset income, the average was about $1,500.

## Economic Vulnerability of the Disabled

An individual's ability to avoid nursing home placement in spite of chronic conditions is in large part dependent on the availability of informal care (from family and friends) and the availability of community-based services. It is also based on income and the ability to liquidate assets to pay for care. Table V.13 suggests that in 1984, among those in the community aged 45 or older with limitations, 27 percent had income within 125 percent of poverty, and 48.8 percent had income within 200 percent of poverty. In contrast, less than one-quarter of the nondisabled population (24.5 percent) had income less than 200 percent of the poverty threshold.

In 1984, an estimated 32 percent of the elderly reported limitations requiring assistance from others. The disabled tend to have less income than the nondisabled, primarily because they tend to be older. Among all 75-year-olds, for example, 23.7 percent had incomes within 125 percent of poverty, and 48.9 percent had incomes within 200 percent of poverty. Those with less income seemed to experience more disability, but only slightly; 29.5 percent had income within 125 percent of poverty, and 54.9 percent had income within 200 percent of poverty. A similar distribution existed among disabled people aged 65 to 74; 24.7 percent had income within 125 percent of poverty, and 46.5 percent had income within 200 percent of poverty.

A comparison of income, net wealth, and age by level of disability in 1984 suggests the importance of assets (savings) in assisting people to remain in the community (table V.14). The substantially less median wealth but similar mean wealth gives the impression that savings were used to remain in the community. Median net wealth and income among the population aged 45 or older who were free from chronic disabilities were twice that of people reporting relatively mild limitations. People with at least one very serious activity in daily living (ADL) limitation (over 1.4 million people) had one-tenth the net wealth of the mildly limited group and were only slightly older. Among the nearly 1 million people with two or three ADL limitations, median wealth was negligible but median family income was in excess of $8,000 a year. Among the population aged 45 or over without any

TABLE V.13
# Limitations of the Noninstitutionalized Population Aged 45 or over, by Poverty Status and Age, 1984

| | Age Group | | | | |
| Poverty Status | 45–54 | 55–64 | 65–74 | 75 or over | Total Aged 45 or over |
|---|---|---|---|---|---|
| **Percentage within Age Group with Any Limitations** | | | | | |
| Below poverty | 21.8% | 32.3% | 41.6% | 59.7% | 37.3% |
| 100%–124% of poverty | 19.9 | 30.7 | 33.8 | 52.7 | 35.4 |
| 125%–199% of poverty | 15.2 | 22.3 | 27.6 | 46.2 | 28.0 |
| 200%–399% of poverty | 7.5 | 15.0 | 21.2 | 41.0 | 17.8 |
| 400%+ of poverty | 4.8 | 7.1 | 14.2 | 39.1 | 9.6 |
| | | | | | |
| All income classes | 8.6 | 15.0 | 23.3 | 45.7 | 19.2 |
| Below 125% of poverty | 27.9 | 25.8 | 24.7 | 29.5 | 27.0 |
| Below 200% of poverty | 45.2 | 45.2 | 46.5 | 54.9 | 48.8 |
| **Percentage of People in Each Age Group without Limitations** | | | | | |
| Below 125% of poverty | 9.6 | 9.8 | 12.2 | 18.9 | 11.1 |
| Below 200% of poverty | 18.7 | 21.7 | 29.6 | 43.8 | 24.5 |
| **Percentage of All People in Each Age Group** | | | | | |
| Below 125% of poverty | 11.2 | 12.1 | 15.1 | 23.7 | 14.2 |
| Below 200% of poverty | 21.0 | 25.2 | 33.6 | 48.9 | 29.1 |

Source: EBRI tabulations of the 1984 Survey of Income and Program Participation, Bureau of the Census, U.S. Department of Commerce.

chronic limitations, the average age was 60, while for those with any chronic limitation it was 70.

## Conclusion

Poor health, disease, accidents, and chronic disabilities are not confined to specific groups of people. These problems are distributed

191

**TABLE V.14**

**Average Age, Income, and Wealth of the U.S. Population Aged 45 or over Living in the Community, by Disability, 1984**

| Limitations | Average Age | Net Wealth | | Income | | Percentage of Population |
| --- | --- | --- | --- | --- | --- | --- |
| | | Mean (in thousands) | Median (in thousands) | Mean (in thousands) | Median (in thousands) | |
| None | 60 | $53.8 | $33.3 | $25.7 | $20.5 | 81.3% |
| IADL[a] Only | 67 | 34.9 | 20.0 | 13.6 | 10.0 | 15.4 |
| At Least One ADL[b] | 70 | 54.3 | 13.2 | 13.4 | 8.9 | 2.0 |
| At Least Two ADLs | 71 | 23.6 | 11.4 | 10.7 | 8.5 | 0.5 |
| At Least Three ADLs | 72 | 31.5 | 7.4 | 13.1 | 8.1 | 0.9 |

Source: EBRI tabulations of the 1984 Survey of Income and Program Participation, Bureau of the Census, U.S. Department of Commerce.

[a]Instrumental activity of daily living (IADL) limitations include having difficulty getting around the house without assistance and needing help to do light housework, prepare meals, or lift more than 10 pounds.

[b]Activity of daily living (ADL) limitations include needing help with personal needs, such as dressing and undressing, eating, or personal hygiene, transferring into and out of bed, and moving around inside the home.

Note: Percentages may not add to 100 because of rounding.

across the population and, for any individual, can occur at any time.[8] Without health insurance, all but a very few people would find financially catastrophic most ambulatory, acute, or long-term care costs associated with serious illness or injury.

Cross-sectional data on income and assets suggest that for those who become disabled during retirement, income may not be sufficient to meet living expenses and the additional expense of community-based long-term care. Those who remain in the community may be spending their savings to do so. One can only speculate that if assistance from family and friends should no longer be enough or if those providing assistance can no longer endure the burden, care in a nursing home would be sought. At that point, assistance from the state might be necessary to pay for nursing home care.

While many of today's elderly may not be able to afford extensive long-term care, some may be able to afford long-term care insurance. Insurance for any of life's contingencies works best when the potential cost is high and the probability of facing that cost is low, as is the case with long-term care. If a large proportion of today's elderly cannot afford long-term care insurance, or are no longer insurable, public policy questions emerge. Should public policy encourage development of private insurance for tomorrow's elderly with a public financing program for today's elderly, or should a social insurance program be developed for all to help us face the costs of long-term care?

---

[8]There is a positive correlation between poor health and low income, since people with low income (and no health insurance) do not partake of preventive health care, and many people with poor health are unable to work (Burtless, 1987).

# PART THREE
# OPTIONS FOR REFORM

# VI. The Potential for Private Long-Term Care Insurance

## Introduction

The question of the feasibility of private long-term care insurance is central to the public policy debate over financing long-term care. The failure of the private market to sell insurance to a large and diverse segment of the population suggests a need to subsidize the purchase of private insurance, establish a public insurance program, or provide public financing for long-term care. Insurance policies are purchased for many of life's contingencies. For example, casualty insurance provides protection against the financial consequences of property damage. Life and disability insurance provide protection from the loss of earnings resulting from worker death or disability. Health insurance provides protection against the cost of acute health care. Insurance protection against the cost of long-term care, however, has not always been available and is not as widespread as other types of insurance.

Nevertheless, the market for private long-term care insurance in the United States is expanding. One estimate suggests that in 1984 about 16 insurers sold approximately 125,000 policies in a few states (ICF Incorporated, 1985b). By June 1989, there were more than 100 insurers and more than 1.3 million policies had been purchased (Meiners, 1984; Advisory Committee on Long Term Care, n.d.; Van Gelder and Johnson, 1989). Prior to June 1987, no employers offered long-term care insurance through an employer-based plan. As of September 1989, at least 35 employers offered or had made arrangements to offer this option.

Insurance purchased today is intended to finance care that will be needed well into the future. Generally, insurance, by its very nature, is not designed to finance a foreseeable short-term need. In 1980, 0.9 percent of all nursing home expenditures, amounting to $200 million, was financed through private insurance. By 1987, private insurance payments for nursing home care had doubled to $400 million but still only represented 0.9 percent of nursing home expenditures. There are no readily available data to measure the impact of this emerging market on the purchase of community- and home-based long-term care.

197

As a practical matter, there was not much of an insurance market for long-term care prior to 1987. Even now, the market for long-term care insurance is minuscule. However, it does exist and, more importantly, it is changing and growing rapidly. Therefore, it is probably premature to fully judge the potential of the long-term care insurance market, especially since in just the last six months of 1988 many more progressive insurance products were introduced. It may be more appropriate to examine the barriers that have been overcome and the remaining weaknesses in the market, with an eye to developing a public policy that would encourage development of a long-term care insurance market.

## Differentiating Insurance from Savings

Using savings, or self-funding, is an efficient method of financing an event whose occurrence and cost are predictable. However, preparing for an event involving known financial consequences is not the same as preparing for an unpredictable event with unknown costs. An attempt to set aside an appropriate amount would generally result in either over- or undersaving. Those who try to set aside a maximum amount would certainly save too much and therefore deprive themselves of other goods and services needed over their lifetime. Since the future need for long-term care is unknown, and since, if needed, its cost is not predictable, self-funding or saving for this contingency is inefficient. Sharing the risk through insurance—either public or private—is much more efficient.

The risks of needing assistance to remain independent at home or of needing nursing home care are always present, but they increase dramatically with age and long after retirement age. While it is possible to have sufficient savings to cover the cost of long-term care, in 1984, only one-quarter of those aged 75 to 84 had net wealth, exclusive of their home, in excess of $32,500. In the same year, one-half of the population aged 75 to 84 had savings, exclusive of their home, of $6,000 or less. For most people it is quite likely that the cost of care would be greater than either the amount saved or the amount that could have been saved.

The cost of long-term care varies. For example, in 1985 nursing home care could have cost more than $22,000 annually. At-home care for those with Alzheimer's disease or related dementias reached an estimated $14,000 the same year (Hu, Huang, and Cartwright, 1986). Four years of care at $50 a day, for a total of $73,000, would certainly exceed the net wealth of most elderly persons.

For those who never need long-term care, any savings specifically for that purpose would be greater than anticipated expenses. Insurance, on the other hand, represents a known cost but would provide financial protection for an event whose cost could be many times greater than the insurance premium. While saving for its own sake may be desirable, and perhaps ought to be encouraged, insuring for the possibility of needing long-term care is more efficient than saving for this contingency.

Economic theory suggests that the well-being of most individuals, and society as a whole, would be improved if people were able to purchase actuarially fair insurance against the risk of expenses when the risk is small and the potential loss is large.[1] However, one article suggests that even if insurance premiums were not actuarially fair, if the preference to avoid risk is sufficiently great, economic well-being may still be improved with insurance.

Since the risk of needing long-term care increases with age, pay-as-you-go premiums would also increase with age. As with life, disability, and acute health care insurance, the odds of filing a claim increase with age. However, unlike the situation with life insurance and to a lesser degree with disability insurance, the importance of long-term care insurance does not diminish with age. Life insurance and disability insurance offer protection against the loss of earnings due to the premature death or disability of a worker. This tends to be relatively more important while a family has young dependents and few assets. After a person retires, this type of insurance is no longer useful (or available). For this reason, some of the long-term care insurance products that have been proposed and developed are a direct response to the diminishing importance of life and disability insurance and the increasing importance of long-term care insurance as people age (Getzen and Hall, 1987).

In many ways, long-term care is another component of health care and therefore may be viewed as a logical extension of acute health care insurance. In fact, nursing home and home health care have been shown to be cost-effective substitutes for some types of hospital care (Select Committee on Aging, 1986a). The difference is that most acute care requires less than a month's treatment. In 1987, the average length of an acute care hospital stay was 6.4 days (National Center for Health Statistics, 1988b). By inference, long-term care is care lasting more than one month.

---

[1]The price of actuarially fair insurance is equivalent to the average cost of the care times the probability that the care will be needed.

### Current Long-Term Care Insurance Products

As of January 1989, at least 105 insurance companies were selling long-term care insurance (Van Gelder and Johnson, 1989). While there are common elements among them, policies vary considerably, depending on when they were first issued. Over time, many of the restrictive clauses of the early policies have been modified or removed. Typically, individual plans introduced in 1988 paid daily indemnity (fixed) dollar benefits for care received in a skilled, intermediate, or custodial nursing home (Van Gelder and Johnson, 1989). Often, however, the nursing facility must be licensed by the state. Home health care benefits must usually be provided by state-licensed, Medicare-certified, or voluntarily accredited agencies. For most outstanding older policies, prior hospitalization is often required before policyholders are eligible for benefits. The typical policy covers Alzheimer's disease and is guaranteed renewable. Policies are usually sold to people between ages 50 and 79, with premium levels based on the insured's age at the time of enrollment. These premiums remain essentially the same during the policyholder's life unless the premiums for everyone in the same group or class are increased. According to calculations by the Health Insurance Association of America (HIAA), the average premium is about $300 a year at age 50 and $2,100 a year at age 79.

Long-term care policies generally exclude coverage for conditions that existed within a specified time prior to, and immediately following, the purchase of the policy. In a 1984 study of 16 policies, one-half had preexisting condition periods of six months, and one-quarter had preexisting condition periods of up to one year (Meiners, 1984). However, more recent surveys suggest that preexisting condition periods are increasingly likely to be six months. In 1987, the U.S. General Accounting Office (GAO) analyzed 33 policies offered by 25 insurers in 1986 and found that of the 32 policies that had preexisting condition clauses, two-thirds had a six-month exclusionary period (U.S. General Accounting Office, 1987a). HIAA's survey found that in 1988, 21 of 29 HIAA member company policies required a six-month preexisting condition period (Van Gelder and Johnson, 1989).

Policies often require prior institutionalization before policyholders are eligible for either nursing home or home health care benefits. In the most recent HIAA study, 25 of 29 HIAA member company policies required a prior hospital stay before the insured became eligible for nursing home benefits. In these policies, the insured had between 14 and 90 days to enter a nursing home after leaving the hospital. In general, the requirement also applied to home health care benefits:

to be eligible for home health benefits, the insured generally had to have been in a hospital or nursing facility. The 1987 GAO study found that 29 of the 33 policies it examined required prior hospitalization to receive long-term care benefits. Of 28 policies with prior hospitalization requirements, 12 required that nursing home institutionalization be within 14 days of discharge from the hospital, and 13 required nursing home institutionalization within 30 days.

Benefit amounts can vary among policies offered by different insurance companies and even those offered by the same company. Each of the 29 policies included in the 1988 HIAA survey provided a fixed level of benefits, often on a fixed dollar-per-day basis. In most of the policies, the insured chooses the indemnity amount desired and pays a premium based on the desired payment level and his or her age at the time of purchase. The indemnity amount for the policies studied ranged between $10 and $120 per day.

Insurance company policies often limit the length of time the insured is eligible to receive long-term care benefits. While a few place a dollar amount on the maximum benefit received, most set a time limit after which insurance payments will end. Often the maximums (either the dollar level or the length of time for which care is covered) differ depending on whether the insured is in a nursing home or is receiving home health care. The 1988 HIAA survey found that 28 of the 29 policies it studied limited the length of the coverage period. Six of the policies had separate lifetime maximum coverage periods for nursing home and home health care. For these six policies, the median limit for nursing home care was four years, and the median limit for home health care was two years. The remaining policies either set a combined lifetime maximum benefit period for both nursing home and home health care or set separate maximum benefit periods for each of the two services (in this case, if the policyholder is discharged for a certain period, he or she is again eligible for another benefit period).

Unlike typical health insurance policies, deductible periods for long-term care insurance are for a specified time. Health insurance policy deductibles commonly require the insured to pay for a certain amount of care out-of-pocket before health insurance benefits begin. Instead of a predetermined level of expenditures, most long-term care policies offer a choice of deductible periods ranging from none or "first day coverage" to 100 days; the longer the deductible period chosen by the insured, the lower the premium.

Coverage of Alzheimer's disease and related mental and nervous disorders is also expanding. A 1984 study found that of 16 policies that covered certain aspects of long-term care, nearly one-half excluded all mental and nervous disorders (Meiners, 1984). In December 1988, the National Association of Insurance Commissioners amended its model regulations to require all policies to state explicitly whether they include coverage for Alzheimer's disease and related dementias. HIAA found that all 29 of the policies it reviewed in 1988 covered Alzheimer's disease, suggesting that coverage of this disease and related dementias is increasing.

Other increasingly common provisions of long-term care insurance policies include renewability and inflation-adjustment clauses. Renewability provisions guarantee that the policy cannot be canceled unless the policyholder stops paying the premium. Two-thirds of the policies in HIAA's 1988 survey sample were guaranteed renewable, which indicates an increase over HIAA's 1986 survey, when only one-half of the policies contained a guaranteed-renewable clause (Van Gelder and Johnson, 1989).

There is concern that long-term care insurance policies that promise to provide fixed indemnity payments for future services will be unable to provide adequate financial coverage for long-term care. As a result, some insurance companies are beginning to offer an "inflation adjustment" option, which increases the indemnity amount of the benefit over time. While some policies studied by HIAA in 1988 will pay benefits that are increased a certain percentage every specified number of years, other policies anticipate higher future costs and set the future indemnity amounts accordingly. HIAA found that most of the 29 policies it surveyed in 1988 offered some protection against inflation.

A new approach to long-term care insurance integrates long-term care coverage with life insurance coverage. According to the 1988 HIAA study, at least nine companies introduced long-term care coverage as part of individual life insurance policies, and many experts predict more companies will pursue this method of insuring against long-term care expenses. Coverage is made available through a rider to the life insurance policy. If the policyholder requires long-term care, the life insurance policy provides that a set percentage of the death benefit will cover some of the expenses. The value of the death benefit (usually 2 percent per month) is reduced as the rider continues to cover some of the policyholder's long-term care expenses (Van Gelder and Johnson, 1989).

## Problems Inhibiting the Development of the Market

The design of long-term care policies has been influenced by a variety of factors. Weak market demand and relatively little tax and regulatory influence have left policy design to insurers without much input from consumers or legislators. Without clear market signals, and with poor data, insurers have struggled to find products that are attractive yet do not jeopardize the companies' financial health. This has resulted in the marketing of fixed-dollar rather than service benefits. The cost of these policies, relative to their benefit, and their strict claims requirements have led to criticism of many of the policies on the market (Consumers Union, 1988; Firman, Weissert, and Wilson, 1988). These criticisms tend to center around the requirement of a prior hospitalization or receipt of services at a skilled nursing facility prior to covering benefits received at an unskilled facility. Such requirements would disqualify most long-term care claimants.

Many of the limitations criticized have been removed or modified in policies introduced since the latter half of 1988. Within the constraint against incurring too much potential liability, responsible insurance companies have begun to respond to consumer preferences and to the criticism of consumer groups. However, many market barriers must be overcome before private long-term care insurance offers real protection to a broad spectrum of the population.

## Identifying the Demand for Long-Term Care Insurance

A market exchange requires that there be people who are both *willing* and *able* to purchase a product at a price at which firms are *willing* and *able* to produce it. In most markets the bias is in favor of the consumer. While consumer demand will encourage supply, it is much more difficult (and expensive) for producers to create a market demand. An emerging supply of a product in advance of demand puts the onus on advertisers not only to demonstrate why individuals should buy their particular product but also why they should buy such a product at all. It is critical that the demand for long-term care insurance become more vigorous so that market discipline will encourage insurers to sell policies consumers want and discourage unfavorable policy designs.

Convincing consumers of the risk and financial consequences of long-term care has been a fundamental barrier to the development of long-term care insurance (Meiners, 1983). In general, people are not aware of the financial risk associated with long-term care (Rice, 1987). Some deny the possibility of becoming dependent on others. Others incorrectly assume that needed care will be covered either through their current health care insurance or through Medicare, employer-provided health insurance, or some other policy that supplements

Medicare. In 1984, an American Association of Retired Persons' survey found that among its members (a relatively well-informed group) who thought they might need to spend time in a nursing home, almost 80 percent thought that Medicare would pay for most of the cost of a nursing home stay lasting a month or longer (Rice, 1987). An October 1987 survey found that 49 percent of 1,000 random respondents of all ages, and 49 percent of those aged 65 or over, either did not know about or incorrectly described Medicare coverage of nursing home care (R L Associates, 1987). Furthermore, many may have presumed, in large part correctly, that they would receive assistance from the state (primarily through Medicaid).[2]

Encouraging people to understand and accept the risks they face and to voluntarily purchase insurance has been difficult with other types of insurance as well. For example, some kinds of casualty insurance are now required under certain circumstances because few people purchased it voluntarily (Kunreuther, 1978). Lenders will not usually provide a mortgage without the borrower obtaining fire insurance, and most states now require the purchase of automobile liability insurance to maintain motor vehicle registration. Furthermore, relatively few people purchase health insurance that is not employer sponsored.

How people think about low-probability events with large financial consequences has been the subject of fairly extensive research by psychologists (Slovic, Fischhoff, and Lichtenstein, 1976). Flood insurance has been especially intriguing since it is inexpensive yet rarely purchased, even by those in relatively high-risk areas. One study funded by the National Science Foundation concluded that most homeowners in high-risk areas had not even considered how they would recover from a flood or earthquake and had considered such events as being so unlikely that they ignored the possible consequences (Kunreuther, 1978). The idea of purchasing insurance tended to have meaning only after there was evidence, such as repeated flooding, that they would have reaped a return from "investing" in a policy. Despite the existence of low-cost flood insurance, flood victims who were without insurance have exerted intense pressure on the government to provide assistance following a catastrophe.

---

[2]The extent to which the existence of Medicaid discourages the purchase of private insurance is under investigation in eight states. These states, with grants from the Robert Wood Johnson Foundation, are looking for ways to encourage the purchase of private long-term care insurance (Robert Wood Johnson Foundation, 1989).

Gathering the information necessary to decide to purchase long-term care insurance requires that individuals recognize the need at least to ask how they would meet the financial consequences of long-term care. If they assume that long-term care is already covered, then the decision to investigate additional options would not be rational. Even if they recognize the financial risk of long-term care, their determination of whether long-term care insurance makes sense (assuming they are aware of its existence) would require knowing the strengths and limitations of Medicaid. At this point in the development of the market, however, even the purchase of long-term care insurance bears its own set of risks. There is a risk that the benefits purchased will be inadequate and that they will not be paid if a claim needs to be made. For most other types of insurance, these issues are negligible, but because long-term care insurance may be purchased long in advance of the need for its use, inflation and insurer solvency are very real concerns.

Public policy can go a long way toward encouraging the demand side and shaping the supply side of the long-term care market. For example, the Medicare Catastrophic Coverage Act of 1988 (MCCA) requires the Secretary of Health and Human Services to notify Medicare recipients annually of what Medicare does and *does not* cover. In addition, the fact that the MCCA does not extend coverage for the primary cause of catastrophic expenses for most Medicare recipients (i.e., long-term care) has not gone unnoticed by some elderly and the press. This, too, should encourage more people to think about how their own long-term care will be financed and should begin to encourage the demand for long-term care insurance.

The tax code can also be used to call attention to the importance of long-term care insurance. A tax credit or deduction for the purchase of long-term care insurance would make consumers aware of its existence and might make people ask why it is necessary. However, persuading individuals of moderate income to purchase long-term care insurance will depend on how the tax incentive is structured. Encouraging relatively younger workers, in particular, to purchase long-term care insurance would be a more effective way to expand the market than appealing primarily to older people, who are more likely to be retired, since only relatively higher-income retirees will be able to take advantage of the tax incentive.

If consumer demand and competition among insurers do not ensure that all polices are adequate in terms of their benefits, public policy can intervene by establishing minimum standards with respect to benefits and the terms under which they must be provided, by using tax incentives or by direct regulation.[3] Public policy can also protect consumers from the consequences of insurer insolvency by establishing financial standards, requiring specific levels of reinsurance (insurance bought by insurance companies), or establishing a public reinsurance program, similar to the Pension Benefit Guaranty Corporation, which insures private pension plans.

*Medicaid: Altering the Demand for Insurance*—Many have suggested that Medicaid discourages demand for long-term care insurance (Knickman, 1988; Pauly, 1989). As a safety net, Medicaid stands as the insurer of last resort. In a general sense, especially in states with medically needy programs or "spend-down" provisions, Medicaid can be thought of as nursing home insurance with a very large deductible (most nonexempt assets) and a very large copayment (virtually all available monthly income). While the "cost" of seeking assistance from Medicaid also includes its institutional bias and limited access to nursing homes, most people cannot be expected to know this. On the other hand, some contend that, because surveys have found that few elderly persons are aware of Medicaid coverage, the program is not likely to be a deterrent to the purchase of private insurance (Rivlin and Wiener, 1988).

With assistance from the Robert Wood Johnson Foundation, at least eight states have begun studies on what they can do to facilitate the development of the private insurance market. Most of their attention is expected to focus on the costs and benefits of easing Medicaid eligibility for those who purchase sufficient qualified long-term care insurance (Meiners, 1988a). Such changes in the Medicaid program could be advocated if, because of the private insurance market, total Medicaid expenditures declined. Medicaid does not currently allow states to receive federal funds for these expenditures. Consequently, unless states are willing to finance the entire cost of care for new Medicaid recipients, each state would have to petition the Health Care Financing Administration to allow these changes or petition Congress to change federal Medicaid law.[4]

**Measuring Risk and Expected Cost**

In addition to low demand, a significant obstacle faced by insurers in developing long-term care insurance policies has been their inabil-

---

[3]States are responsible for regulating insurance sold within their borders. Most states have already passed legislation and continue to revise regulations that address many of the consumer protection concerns.

[4]Legislation was introduced during the first session of the 101st Congress to allow states to undertake these demonstration projects.

ity to accurately project long-term care costs and usage. Data are needed to enable insurers to understand the risk factors associated with the need for long-term care, the related course of care and its cost, and the impact of insurance on the use of services. Because of a lack of appropriate data, the expected cost of long-term care is not known, and the development of both risk assessment to minimize adverse selection and uniform measures to assess the need for long-term care has been inhibited. Moreover, the lack of appropriate data has limited full assessment of effective care, which could help in the development of case-managed programs.

The lack of appropriate data, in conjunction with insurers' experience with other health care costs, may have contributed a great deal to the development of fixed indemnity long-term care insurance plans. Without appropriate data, almost any other approach could have left insurance companies in a financially vulnerable position. The lack of data is likely to change because the government, in response to growing concern about long-term care, has increased the number of survey questions asked in official data collections (U.S. Department of Health and Human Services, 1987). Furthermore, insurance companies should soon be able to draw from their own marketing and claims data.

## Unanticipated Increases in the Cost of Long-Term Care

For both consumer and insurer, unanticipated increases in the cost of long-term care is a troublesome problem. Part of the financial risk associated with needing long-term care is, of course, cost. Since risk increases with age, the relevant cost is related not so much to the immediate period (the next year or two) but to a point well beyond. For consumers, true protection comes from a service benefit insurance policy that covers the cost of the service. However, because insurers lack relevant data and are not much better than consumers at predicting future cost, they have been disinclined to sell policies covering the cost of long-term care services. Since inflation is an uncertain risk for both insurer and insured, without sweeping changes in the delivery system, service benefit policies are unlikely to develop rapidly.[5] Consequently, individuals are likely to be either over- or underinsured.

---

[5]Service benefit policies do exist, but they usually have total dollar limits. That is, they either pay for the daily cost of a nursing home stay *up to some daily limit*, have a fixed lifetime benefit, or both. Under the former arrangement, the total number of days covered does not decrease, but as the cost of care increases beyond the daily limit a smaller percentage of the daily cost is covered. Under the latter arrangement, although each day covered is paid in full, as the cost of a nursing home stay increases the total number of days covered decreases.

Several different approaches have been taken to offset the risk of inflation. The most common approach has been to offer a wide range of daily benefits. This enables the consumer to choose the level of benefits that most closely fits his or her expectations about the cost of long-term care and to choose the amount of inflationary risk to insure against. That is, if current nursing home costs are $60 a day but are expected to double within the insured's lifetime, he or she may wish to purchase a policy that will pay $120 a day. Of course, despite the anticipated cost of $120 per day, the insured has the option of risking the expected inflation by purchasing a policy that pays less than $120 a day.[6]

More recently, policies have begun to offer options that either let the insured adjust their expectations of inflation or purchase policies in which the benefits are automatically increased in response to inflation. These changes reduce the risk of unanticipated inflation somewhat but not completely, since these options are based on past inflation but do not necessarily accommodate future inflation. That is, benefits can be increased either by some fixed percentage of past inflation or after past inflation has passed a specified threshold. Other policies simply increase benefits by some fixed percentage, regardless of the actual rate of past inflation or changes in anticipated future inflation.

Integrating the financing with the delivery of long-term care or assembling a comprehensive system of managed care with negotiated prices may ultimately be the way to mitigate the risk of inflation associated with unanticipated increases in the cost of care. Although unanticipated inflation jeopardizes a policy's real benefit, this does not mean that the insurance has no value. Whatever the insurance benefit level, the proportion of care paid directly out-of-pocket will be less. Unfortunately, extremely rapid unanticipated price increases, for all practical purposes, could leave policyholders in the same relative financial position they would have been in without having purchased the insurance. That is, if the true cost of care is several times the benefit level purchased, the policy in conjunction with insufficient income is not likely to alter a person's options or the financial consequences of entering a nursing home.

**Adverse Selection**

Insurance enables individuals to pool the cost of an unexpected event. For example, if everyone had a 0.1 percent chance of incurring

---

[6]On the other hand, dollar limits may, at the margin, serve to ration care so that the insurance benefits are wisely spent.

a $100 loss, 10 people could join together and pool the risk by contributing $10 to a fund that would be used to pay the unlucky person in the group who incurs the $100 loss. For $10, everyone would be insured against the potential loss of $100. If, however, the risk is variable and individuals know their own risk but others do not, this arrangement would break down due to the potential for adverse selection; that is, just those with the greatest risk would be more likely to purchase the insurance. Selection bias would lead to higher prices, making the price of the insurance no longer actuarially fair to those with low risk or to those who do not know their risk. In this example, contributions of $10 would no longer cover the expected risk of the group if, out of 20 people, 10 have a greater-than-average risk and 10 have a less-than-average risk, but only the 10 with the higher risk participate. In this case, an insurer could either raise the price as suggested by the risk faced by the group or prohibit the high-risk individuals from entering the pool. Raising the price relative to how risk-adverse the group is could leave the low-risk group uninsured, since they might not want to purchase insurance that is no longer actuarially fair to them. Prohibiting high-risk individuals from entering the group would tend to increase the cost of administering the insurance and therefore would also lead to increases in the price of the policy—tending to force out the lower-risk people.

Marketing individual long-term care insurance policies to relatively older people necessitates that insurers worry about adverse selection. Although the risk is not yet predictable, there is concern that individuals who believe they are likely to need assistance will be more inclined to purchase insurance. For insurers, assessing that risk is both difficult and costly. Only an imprecise set of factors can begin to predict who is likely to need and subsequently use formal long-term care services. Insurers, however, are financially at risk if their risk assessment techniques prove to be inaccurate. Marketing policies to younger people removes some of the speculative aspects of adverse selection.[7] Both the financial risk imposed by insuring people who know their risk is greater than average, and the cost of trying to detect them can be

_____
[7]Bruce Boyd of TIAA-CREF points out that there is an inverse relationship between administrative costs incurred to determine adverse selection and actual claims. Lower expenses for medical underwriting may result in more claims, and more effort to reduce adverse selection will raise administrative costs but reduce claims (personal communication with author). The relationship, however, is not necessarily dollar for dollar. Kim Ballard of The Prudential also notes that if just a few younger people are aware of long-term care insurance, insurers would still need to worry that those who sought the policy did so because their odds for claiming benefits were greater than average.

nearly eliminated by selling policies to individuals who are currently working.

### Insurance-Induced Demand, or "Moral Hazard"

Moral hazard refers to the effect insurance may have on the insured's incentives. For example, the outbreak of fire is not likely to be intentional; but, because of the existence of insurance, the probability of a fire occurring is increased due to increased carelessness or, in extreme cases, due to arson. The existence of health insurance is not likely to make people less careful with their health, but once ill, it is likely to alter the choice of practitioners and services used (because the price of care to the insured has been reduced) and therefore the cost of care (Arrow, 1963; Pauly, 1968; Arrow, 1968; Bishop, 1981). For long-term care insurance, the question of insurance-induced changes in behavior centers around the concern that insured individuals would be more inclined to overstate their disability or to substitute paid assistance for assistance from family or friends.

The potential for overstating a disability or replacing informal services with formally paid services puts insurers at risk for not having appropriately priced the expected cost of long-term care. This risk has generally discouraged the development of service-based benefits. Acute health care insurance has not been immune from insurance-induced demand for care. Moral hazard is one of the many contributing factors to the growing consumption of health care services.[8] The response to the rising cost of health care by employers, the insurance industry, and public payers of health care has been to redesign health insurance plans by moving away from first dollar coverage (instituting coinsurance and deductibles), placing a greater emphasis on managed care (health maintenance organizations and utilization review), and examining reimbursement alternatives (prospective payment or preferred provider arrangements). Lessons learned from these changes in health insurance should provide suggestions for the development of long-term care insurance that is service based.

---

[8]Of the many factors contributing to the rising share of health care attributable to Gross National Product (including moral hazard, population growth and aging, inflation, defensive medicine, and medical uncertainty), advances in technologies are probably the most important (Schwartz, 1987). For a literature review and another view of the role of health insurance in explaining the rise in medical expenditures, see Manning et al., 1987.

## Tax Law Issues

The tax code does not explicitly recognize long-term care. Therefore, there has been ambiguity concerning the tax treatment of premiums paid for long-term care insurance, the benefits received by policy-holders, and, until April 1989, the long-term care insurance reserves held by insurers. Tax treatment not only affects the price of insurance but, perhaps more importantly, it affects the ability of employment-based plans to spur market development. Some insurance products sold on an individual basis (accident, health, life, and disability insurance, for example) are also provided as an employee benefit. Employer-sponsored benefit programs account for a large percentage of the accident, health, life, and disability insurance policies sold and are an essential component of the development of the markets for these policies.

Paraphrasing the Internal Revenue Code of 1986 (IRC), expenses for medical care are defined under section 213(d) as amounts paid for the diagnosis, cure, mitigation, treatment, or prevention of disease; for the purpose of affecting any structure or function of the body; for transportation primarily for and essential to medical care; or for insurance (including Medicare Part B premiums). It is not clear whether assistance to function on a daily basis or to remain independent in spite of chronic disabilities would be included. The question raised is how to distinguish between medical and nonmedical services when both are necessary for individuals to remain independent in their own homes.

Section 213(d) also enables amounts paid for certain lodging away from home to be treated as payment for medical care as long as the lodging is not lavish or extravagant and the stay away from home is primarily for and essential to medical care, which is specified to require: (a) that care is provided by a physician in a licensed hospital (or in a medical care facility that is related to, or the equivalent of, a licensed hospital), and (b) there is no significant element of personal pleasure, recreation, or vacation in the travel away from home. The IRC limits allowable expenditures to $50 for each night for each individual.

Even more ambiguous than the portion of long-term care that may not be considered medical care for income tax purposes is how the IRC would treat long-term care insurance. If the definition of medical care does not exclude long-term care or is amended to explicitly include it, then long-term care expenses, including long-term care insurance premiums that exceed 7.5 percent of adjusted gross income,

211

would be deductible from an individual's federal income tax. Furthermore, if the definition of medical care under section 213(d) includes long-term care, long-term care insurance purchased by an employer on behalf of an employee would not have to be included in the employee's gross income.[9] Moreover, if the definition of medical care includes long-term care (whether individually purchased or paid for by an employer), the benefits received when a claim is filed would not be included as taxable income.

While the earnings on reserves held for life insurance policies are not treated as taxable income to either the policyholder or the insurer, the tax treatment of earnings for similar reserves held for long-term care policies is not clear. IRC sections 801(a) and 816(b) include in their definition of life insurance companies those companies that issue noncancelable health and accident insurance contracts and whose life insurance reserves plus unearned premiums and unpaid losses make up more than 50 percent of their total reserves. IRC section 804(a) excludes from policyholders' taxable income their share of the reserves' investment yield.

Revenue ruling 89-43, issued on April 10, 1989, clarified that the reserves held for long-term care insurance are not subject to taxation. However, the ruling did not go so far as to define long-term care insurance as accident or health insurance. The longer interest on reserves is able to compound without taxation the lower premiums charged can be. One estimate suggests that favorable tax treatment could reduce premiums by 11 percent for policies sold to people aged 65 and by 33 percent for policies sold to people aged 55 (Technical Work Group on Private Financing of Long-Term Care for the Elderly, 1986). Since most insurers were operating on the assumption that reserves would be treated as clarified in the revenue ruling, prices are not expected to change. Insurers, however, have probably heaved a tremendous sigh of relief.

One article suggests that insurance is more likely to be developed and sold for: (1) events for which services to be purchased are not very different when the price is subsidized by insurance; (2) events for which risk is very random; and (3) events for which people prefer to avoid the financial consequences (Pauly, 1968). For long-term care, perhaps only the second condition holds. The first condition is unpre-

---

[9]As prescribed by section 105(b) of the IRC.

dictable, and people are only beginning to recognize and respond to the financial consequences of long-term care. Presumably the increased demand for long-term care insurance has resulted in part from the fact that more people have learned about its delivery and financing. The controversy over and the debate and passage of the Medicare Catastrophic Coverage Act of 1988 provided an opportunity to educate people and to make them aware that, despite both improvements in Medicare coverage and increased Medicare premiums, requiring long-term care remains the most financially catastrophic health-related event the elderly face.

Very little is known about how people would respond if insurance reduced the out-of-pocket cost of nursing home care, home health care, or adult day care. Most families do everything they can to avoid placing a family member in a nursing home. Chapter III provided some limited evidence that families do not substantially alter their assistance when publicly financed community-based services are provided. In Canada, where health care is provided by each province, the coverage of long-term care has led to a tendency to substitute formal long-term care for hospital care rather than for informal family assistance. In demonstration projects in the United States in which community-based services were provided, families did not alter the amount of time they spent as caregivers. Whether, over time, attitudes about familial obligation would change is difficult to predict.[10]

Despite the preferences of most people to avoid entering a nursing home, Social Security Administration actuaries have assumed that nursing home insurance with no limit on the years of coverage and paying the full cost of care would have resulted in a 50 percent increase in nursing home days in 1986 (assuming the supply of beds also increased) (Technical Work Group on Private Financing of Long-Term Care for the Elderly, 1986). Cutting the maximum number of years covered to six and imposing a 90-day elimination (waiting) period, the increased use of nursing home days relative to the amount that would have been used in the absence of the insurance fell to 22 percent.

---

[10]Evidence of a change in attitudes toward familial obligation due to the introduction and continuation of Social Security is very difficult to interpret. The frequency of children providing financial assistance to their parents has declined since the program's inception. However, it should be kept in mind that more of our parents are living longer and there are fewer children per surviving parent. Therefore, while the frequency of assistance may be declining, thanks to Social Security and other improvements in sources of retirement income, total lifetime expenditures by children on behalf of their parents may not be declining.

# Controlling Expenditures and Protecting Consumers

More than 27 demonstration projects conducted and studied over the past 20 years have been devoted to the question of whether home- or community-based care can be a cost-effective substitute for nursing home care. These projects have shown that in most cases home- or community-based care is not a cost-effective substitute for nursing home care. The reason is that, although the risk of institutionalization is quite low, some individuals needed nursing home care regardless of how much home health care was available. While not everyone needed nursing home care, many needed home health care services. As a consequence, since the reduction in institutionalizations was small and the need for home health care was so great, home health care costs exceeded the savings from the reductions in institutionalized days (Weissert, 1988; Kane, 1988).

The most extensive and rigorous demonstration project directed at this question was the National Long-Term Care Channeling Demonstration, known as the "channeling" demonstration, which operated at 10 sites basically from June 1982 to March 1985. Each site was in a different state. Five sites tested a "basic case management model," while the other five tested a "financial control" approach to case management (Carcagno and Kemper, 1988). In both models, each client received a comprehensive assessment of his or her needs. A care plan was developed and services were arranged for its implementation. The plan was monitored to ensure that services were provided or modified as needed, and the client's needs were reassessed on a regular basis (Phillips, Kemper, and Applebaum, 1988). The fundamental difference between the two approaches was that in the financial model case managers were given much more discretion and authority to purchase services not currently available in the community to meet client needs. Their one constraint was that specified costs per person and costs per program could not be exceeded.

There were few real differences in the outcomes between the two case management approaches. There was no measurable difference in mortality rates, nursing home use, or hospital use. There was, however, a difference in the number of days that clients were bedridden. Although clients in the basic model were no different from the control group (untreated group) in terms of measured levels of limitations, after six months they had fewer days in which they were restricted to bed. Clients in the financial model were significantly more disabled than the control group at both 6 and 12 months.

The biggest difference, however, was in the cost of the two approaches.

The startup costs for the financial control model were greater than those of the basic model but the ongoing costs were lower. The combined costs were higher in the financial control model. Initial costs per client averaged $204 in the five basic model sites and $206 in the five financial control models. Initial administrative costs were $330 per client in the basic model and $340 in the financial control model. Monthly costs per client in the basic model averaged $92, while for the clients in the financial model they averaged $86 (Thornton, Will, and Davies, 1986).

While there were no measurable differences in mortality rates or nursing home or hospital use between the group in the case management program (regardless of the model) and the control group (those not receiving case management), there were differences in the quality of both the clients' lives and those of their families. Not surprisingly, clients in both models had fewer unmet needs and were more confident and satisfied with care arrangements one year later than those not receiving any assistance from the demonstration project. Among those receiving case management, there was higher "global" life satisfaction at six months, and in the financial model this difference was still significant after one year. However, no measurable differences were found in other psychological aspects of well-being such as contentment, self-perceived health, and social interaction. Family caregivers were happier with case management, although this difference was not statistically significant at 12 months for the basic model (Carcagno and Kemper, 1988). In the basic model, the amount of care provided by families was the same as the amount provided by the control group families. Only in the financial model was there some evidence of reduced efforts by family or friends. Most of the withdrawal of informal assistance was on the part of friends.

While in-home care and community-based services might not substitute for nursing home care, case management offers the possibility of making the delivery of long-term care more equitable, rational, and efficient. Integrated into a long-term care insurance policy, it may enable insurers to control expenditures or share the risk of unexpected expenditures with the case management enterprise.[11] Unfortunately,

---

[11]Insurance industry executives suggest that they would be inhibited from establishing a case-managed service benefit by the potential litigation and ensuing "bad will" that could result if a beneficiary felt that he or she were entitled to some service that the case manager denied. However, case management is increasingly becoming incorporated into acute care health insurance programs.

to date little is known about how to establish effective case management strategies (Kane and Kane, 1987).

The term "case management" could refer to almost any form of arrangement that coordinates long-term care services. Services have already been developed to provide information and to refer people to sources of assistance. This type of service is particularly helpful for adult children who do not live near their parents, as it can identify community services and provide some assurance about the level of competence of the services purchased. Referral services may be able to do much more, and together with the myriad of volunteer organizations, quasi-public agencies, and the efforts of entrepreneurial endeavors, new enterprises are likely to emerge that may be able to assess client and family needs and to assist them in coordinating care.

In an extreme case, a case management enterprise could participate in assuming the insurance risk. The social health maintenance organization (S/HMO) and the life care community (or continuing care community), discussed in chapter II, represent mechanisms for integrating the delivery and financing of long-term care. S/HMOs have not only integrated insurance with the delivery of long-term care, they have removed the barriers between acute and long-term care. Life care communities do not cover acute care, nor do they explicitly manage long-term care, but the structure of the life care community lends itself to managing this care (Bishop, 1988).

Case management is too often regarded as a device to reduce health care expenditures; therefore, for purposes of long-term care, it ought to be viewed of as "case coordination" or "care management." Essentially, it is carried out by a multidisciplinary team (physician, nurse, social worker, and pharmacist). This team, perhaps led by the nurse or social worker, can assess a situation, evaluate options, and assist functionally dependent persons and their families in coordinating care or altering physical structures so that those who are functionally dependent can maintain their independence in a dignified manner. As client advocates, perhaps working with insurers to provide benefits that are not included in the contract, case management teams may be an important tool in protecting consumers and effectively spending beneficiaries' dollars.

A managed care system has the potential, but without appropriate data systems and research it may be less effective than anticipated. Preferred provider organizations (PPOs) and health maintenance organizations (HMOs) are quite illustrative of both the limitations and the potential of case management. In both cases, these alternative health care delivery systems were promoted as solutions to managing employer health care expenditures. Although somewhat effective, they have not yet proven to be as effective as promised (Friedland, 1987b). Most PPO plans were sold to employers on the basis of the discount offered by physicians and hospitals that had agreements with the PPOs. Providers were initially chosen as preferred by PPOs because of their willingness to discount their prices—not because they were more effective at delivering care. Only recently, and long after their introduction into the market, have PPOs been able to collect the data necessary to choose efficient providers based on more appropriate criteria than the discount. Similarly, HMOs must provide the same standard of care as other providers and must purchase the same inputs (physicians, nurses, receptionists, supplies, office space, etc.) as traditional physician offices. Therefore, an HMO's ability to control health care expenditures has been derived primarily from the types of patients attracted (usually younger and, therefore, healthier people), economies associated with the purchase of equipment and supplies because of their size, their ability to control access to care, and because of hospital discounts. In general, HMOs have tended to lower the cost of health insurance but have not changed the rate at which its cost is increasing (Newhouse et al., 1985).

## Consumer Protection

Given the variations that already exist in policy design and the difficulty of comparing products, ensuring that market demand will protect consumers is likely to require regulation to standardize policy terminology and marketing techniques (Select Committee on Aging, 1987c; U.S. General Accounting Office, 1987a and 1989). Insurance is regulated by each state, usually through an insurance commissioner. In December 1986, the National Association of Insurance Commissioners (NAIC) drafted model regulations for state legislatures to use as guides for writing their states' laws on long-term care insurance. The purpose of these regulations is to promote the public interest, to publicize the availability of long-term care insurance policies, to ensure flexibility and innovation, and to protect consumers from deceptive sales or enrollment practices. Substantial amendments to the original model act, incorporated in June 1987 and December 1988, provide even more stringent guidelines (Advisory Committee on Long Term Care, 1988). As of July 1989, 28 states or territories had incorporated some version of the NAIC model act, and nine states had incorporated the model act in more stringent legislation. The remaining 19 jurisdictions have not yet amended their insurance laws to deal explicitly with the emerging market for long-term care insurance.[12]

The NAIC model act specifies that no long-term care insurance can be canceled, made nonrenewable, or otherwise terminated on the grounds of a policyholder's age or deterioration in mental or physical health. Policies cannot establish new waiting periods when an existing policy is replaced by a policy offered by the same company. Nor can a policy cover only skilled nursing care or provide significantly more coverage in a skilled facility than in facilities providing lower levels of care. The model defines and places limits on waiting periods associated with preexisting conditions. Furthermore, it prohibits long-term care insurance policies from requiring prior institutionalization either in a hospital or in a high-skilled facility before paying benefits. In addition, any advertisement stating that a policy covers home health care or a home benefit cannot condition receipt of these benefits on prior institutionalization. If a policy does condition coverage of noninstitutional care on prior receipt of institutional care, the model act limits the required amount of institutionalization to 30 days.

Under the model act, consumers have the right to examine a policy and return it for a full refund of the premiums paid. These rights must be stated prominently on the policy's first page. Direct mail response solicitations must give consumers 30 days, and other consumers must be given 10 days, after receiving the policy to return it with no questions asked. Policy applications must also include an outline that describes the policy's principal benefits and coverage; a statement of principal exclusions, reductions, and limitations; a statement of the renewal provisions; and any reservations in the policy regarding changes in premiums. Group policies must provide covered individuals with a way to continue coverage after they leave the "group" or if the "group" no longer continues to participate in the insurance program.

Standardization of terms and clear outlines of coverage, along with well-informed agents and a much better-informed consumer, can go a long way toward creating strong enough market demand to discourage abuses such as misleading statements and the use of "fear tactics." However, the potential for abuse is tremendous. Sales abuses practiced by some salespeople selling Medicare supplemental insurance, or Medigap policies, are not likely to be tolerated in the sale of long-term care insurance. To the extent that abuses are apparent, federal legislation is likely to be passed more quickly than legislation

---

[12]In addition to the 50 states, insurance is regulated through governing bodies in the District of Columbia, Guam, the Virgin Islands, American Samoa, and Puerto Rico.

regulating the sale of Medigap policies. This was clearly part of the concern that prompted the NAIC to take a proactive posture in developing model regulations. The U.S. General Accounting Office has already recommended that Congress pass legislation similar to the Baucus-Pepper supplemental Medicare insurance reform measures (Select Committee on Aging, 1987c; U.S. General Accounting Office, 1989).

Perhaps the most important consumer protection issue is whether the policy or insurance company will still exist by the time policyholders claim benefits. The best policies are guaranteed renewable, which means that as long as premiums are paid, insurance companies will not drop coverage because of a policyholder's deteriorating health or advancing age. However, despite this guarantee, insurers reserve the right to cancel a policy or a group (class) of policies if reserves are insufficient to meet potential liabilities. Furthermore, consumers have no recourse if an insurance company goes bankrupt.

## Developing a Group Market

Companies that sell long-term care insurance policies to groups or organizations such as associations, or to individuals by virtue of their employment, should be able to reduce the cost of insurance. First, the costs associated with maintaining a sales force to sell policies on a one-on-one basis (administrative, commissions, salaries) are immediately reduced. Second, depending on the group, the cost of systematically evaluating to ensure that those at greatest risk are not the only individuals buying the policy can be eliminated.[13]

### When a Group Is Not a Group

Data are not yet sufficient to estimate the expected long-term care costs for a particular group formed on the basis of a specific association, such as a firm's employees. Consequently, the pricing and structure of group long-term care insurance policies look like that of individual policies marketed to specific groups. Currently, the major difference between policies marketed to groups and those marketed to individuals is the lower premiums for group policies. But an employment-based product offers some additional advantages to both the consumer and the insurer. Since active employees are less likely to need long-term care assistance, both because of their age and because

---

[13]Encouraging the participation needed to eliminate individual underwriting may require employers to pay a portion of the long-term care insurance premium.

they are capable of working, adverse selection is less likely to be a problem and the chances of insuring a sufficient level of low-risk population increases as more of the group participates. This ensures lower premiums and should eliminate the need for individual screening of insurance applicants.

If participation is high, selling to a relatively young group also gives an insurer more time to adjust premiums to the risk that is being insured. As insurers obtain more information from their claims data, they will be better able to understand the factors that need to be used to determine policy pricing. As pricing estimates become more accurate, premiums can be increased or decreased to accurately reflect cost. If policyholders include a diverse population of young and old, then in some sense the younger members of the group can subsidize the *risk* to the insurance company for the uncertain costs of long-term care and therefore reduce the premiums for everyone. That is, the younger group provides a buffer for the insurer if the premiums charged to the older group turn out to be incorrectly calculated, thereby reducing some of the insurer's risk.

### Long-Term Care Insurance as an Employee Benefit

Like employer-provided health insurance, employer-sponsored long-term care insurance offers the potential to increase the share of privately financed long-term care. Group long-term care insurance could provide more coverage than an individual policy at the same cost. Employment-based groups are younger and healthier populations, and if there is sufficient participation, they minimize the need for and cost of screening for adverse selection. Marketing and administrative costs should be substantially less than those incurred in the sale of individually marketed policies. Insurance executives suggest that the differential could be 20 percent to 30 percent.

Employer interest in long-term care has resulted in a few major employers offering long-term care insurance. Prior to June 1987, perhaps no employer offered a long-term care insurance plan, but by September 1989, at least 35 employers offered plans or were planning to do so. A partial list is provided in table VI.1. Some programs were initiated only for retirees, but most are now sold to active workers and retirees, their spouses, and their respective parents. In virtually all of these programs, the entire premium is paid by the employee. The employer pays part of the administrative and marketing costs. Despite the lack of premium subsidy, employee interest has been somewhat surprising. Although a majority of employees are not enrolled,

220

a disproportionate share of enrollees are in their late thirties to mid-forties.

Most of the plans are designed to prefund the cost of the rising risk. In that way, they are like whole or universal life insurance, with premiums based on the lifetime risk of needing long-term care and priced according to the purchaser's age at the time of initial purchase.[14] Premiums remain basically the same while the policy is held.[15] Relative to the risk of needing long-term care, this fixed premium is high in the early years but low in later years.

Table VI.1 identifies some of the features of employment-based policies that were offered by employers in 1988. Typically, employment-based policies offer employees a choice of benefits ranging from $50 to $200 for each day spent in a nursing home, with daily home health care benefits of one-half the nursing home benefit. Deductibles, which are usually expressed as the *period of time* that must elapse before benefits are paid, are usually from three to four months, and benefit periods are usually limited to between four and six years. None of the plans automatically and fully adjust benefits for inflation, but a few offer participants the option of increasing benefits every two years, and others increase benefits by some fixed amount automatically. A three-year, $100-a-day nursing home benefit (with a $50-a-day home health care benefit) after a 60-day waiting period can cost about $10 a month for those who purchase the policy at around age 30. Purchasing the policy at age 40 can raise the premium 56 percent, and purchasing it at age 50 is likely to nearly triple the premium over the cost at age 30.

*Using Flexible Benefit Plans*—Flexible benefit, or cafeteria plans, may offer a unique opportunity to finance long-term care insurance. Flexible benefit plans allow employees to choose among benefits, often paying for them with pretax earnings. The value of benefits is excluded from employees' taxable income if they are employer paid. If long-term care insurance qualifies under tax law as a benefit option, its inclusion in flexible benefit plans would give people flexibility to make choices based on their personal situations. Employees no longer interested in day care for children, for example, could switch to long-term care insurance.

---

[14]Purchasing long-term care insurance this way not only keeps the premiums level but may also alter preferences for protection by encouraging individuals to get into the habit of planning for long-term care as one of life's contingencies.
[15]Premiums can be modified by age class, however.

**TABLE VI.1**
# Group Long-Term Care Insurance Products

| Companies | Carrier | Premiums | Participation | Benefits | Maximums |
|---|---|---|---|---|---|
| Aetna Life and Casualty Co. | Aetna | After-tax payroll deduction and pension deduction or direct-billed. Entry-age level premiums. | Number of eligibles: 41,000 retirees; participation rate: 7.2% actives, 15% retirees. | Custodial care in nursing home and/or private home care. Home care is 50% of daily benefit amount. Three options: $50, $75, or $100/day. | $1 million. |
| American Express Co. | Travelers[a] | Employees pay Travelers directly or payroll deduction; entry-age priced. High-option monthly level premiums: 30 = $10, 40 = $16, 50 = $32, 60 = $72, 70 = $208, 80 = $408. Low-option premiums are one-half these amounts. | Number of eligibles: 20,000; participation rate: 7.5% | Covers nursing home care, custodial care, home health care, and adult day care in non-residential care facilities. Choice of two benefit plans: high option— $100/day for nursing home care and $50/day for home health care; low option—one-half these amounts. | $75,000 or $150,000. |
| Army and Air Force Exchange Service of Dallas | Aetna | After-tax. | Number of eligibles: 23,000 actives, 10,000 retirees; participation rate: 6% actives, 15% retirees. | Covers home health care, nursing home care, and custodial care; $40, $60, $80, or $100/day for nursing home care, and $20, $30, $40, or $50/day for home health care. | $73,000, $109,500, $146,000, or $182,500. |

| Eligibles | Waiting Period | Prior Facility Use Required | Inflation Adjustment | Features |
|---|---|---|---|---|
| Employees/ spouses and retirees/ spouses; parents not covered. | 90-day waiting period before benefits paid. | No, and no prior nursing home care. Must need help with 2 of 5 ADLs to receive benefits. | No. Covered individuals may increase plan option. | Portable on individual basis; 90-day premium waiver period; extended term provision; return of contributions provision—return of premiums if active premium-paying employee dies before using benefit; retirees and portables (those who terminated employment) reduced by 10% each year. |
| Employees/ spouses at any age; parents, parents-in-law, and retirees and their spouses under 80 years old. | 90-day waiting period of covered services before benefits paid; only one qualifying waiting period per lifetime. | No prior hospital or nursing home care. | No. Covered individuals may increase benefit amount. | Portable; access to Eldercare Resource Referral Service; premiums waived after 120 days of nursing home care; no death benefit. |
| Employees/ spouses, parents, parents-in-law, and retirees and their spouses. | 90-day waiting period before benefits paid. | No, and no prior nursing home care. Must need help with 2 of 5 ADLs to receive benefits. | Yes. | Portable; no death benefit. |

**(continued)**

**TABLE VI.1 (continued)**

| Companies | Carrier | Premiums | Participation | Benefits | Maximums |
|---|---|---|---|---|---|
| Bell Atlantic Corporation | Mutual of Omaha | Entry-age priced. Monthly level premiums: 30 = $12, 50 = $32, 65 = $100. | Number of eligibles: 27,000 actives, 38,000 retirees; participation rate: NA. | 80% of costs up to $100/day for nursing home care and $50/day for home health, hospice, custodial, or adult day care. | Five-year benefit. |
| CNA Insurance | CNA | After-tax. | Number of eligibles: 14,500; participation rate: 23%. | Covers any level of care in a facility. Three levels of coverage: $60, $80, or $100/day. | |
| First Interstate Bancorp. | Travelers[a] | Payroll deduction or direct billing; entry-age priced. High-option monthly level premiums: 30 = $14.16, 40 = $23.64, 50 = $40.44, 60 = $87.16, 70 = $227.48, 80 = $441. Low-option premiums are one-half these amounts. | Number of eligibles: 20,000; participation rate: NA. | Covers home health care, nursing home care, and adult day care; two levels of coverage: $50 or $100/day for nursing home care and $25 or $50/day for home health care. | $75,000 or $150,000. |
| Ford Motor Co.—United Auto Workers[b] | Managed by the Jefferson County Department for Human Services under contract with the Blue Cross and Blue Shield Associations of Michigan and Kentucky. | Financed by employers. | Number of eligibles: 5,000 actives and recent retirees; participation rate: 100%. | Costs of custodial care in an institution and in the home; may include respite care coverage; for costs of non-medical custodial care for severely handicapped employees and retirees so they can live at home. | Two years or approximately $16,000 for each eligible participant. |

| Eligibles | Waiting Period | Prior Facility Use Required | Inflation Adjustment | Features |
|---|---|---|---|---|
| Employees at any age; spouses, parents, parents-in-law, and retirees and their spouses under 80 years old. | 90-day waiting period. | No. | No. Covered individuals under age 65 may purchase a $20 daily benefit increase every 5 years. | Portable; guaranteed renewable; percentage of premium returned (25%), less benefits paid, if the covered individual dies or coverage is terminated after at least one year. |
| Employees/ spouses and retirees under 80 years old. | 90-day waiting period before benefits paid. | | No. However, a rider is offered which allows covered individuals to increase coverage a minimum of $20/day every five years during open enrollment. | Portable; no death benefit. |
| Employees/ spouses at any age; parents, parents-in-law, and retirees and their spouses under 80 years old. | 90-day waiting period of covered services before benefits paid; only one qualifying waiting period per lifetime. | No, and no prior nursing home care. | No. | Portable; access to Eldercare Resource Referral Service; if stop paying premiums after 10 years, receive 30% daily benefit amount and, each additional year of payment, an additional 3% increase in daily benefit amount, up to 75% after 25 years; no death benefit. |
| Hourly workers, their dependents, and some retirees at Ford's truck and vehicle assembly plants in Louisville, KY. | | | NA. | Two-year pilot program; program will be evaluated in 1991 to determine whether it should be continued. |

(continued)

**TABLE VI.1 (continued)**

| Companies | Carrier | Premiums | Participation | Benefits | Maximums |
|---|---|---|---|---|---|
| General Foods Corporation | Aetna | After-tax. | Number of eligibles: 8,000 actives, spouses, and parents; participation rate: NA. | Covers home health care, nursing home care, and custodial care; $40, $60, $80, or $100/day for nursing home care, and $20, $30, $40, or $50/day for home health care. | $73,000–$182,500; increases $36,500 for each additional $20/day of coverage. |
| Harnischfeger Industries | Travelers[a] | Payroll deduction or direct billing; entry-age priced. High-option monthly level premiums: 30 = $14.16, 40 = $23.64, 50 = $40.44, 60 = $87.16, 70 = $227.48, 80 = $441. Low-option premiums are one-half these amounts. | Number of eligibles: 10,000; participation rate: NA. | Covers home health care, nursing home care, and adult day care; three levels of coverage: $50, $70, or $100/day for nursing home care; $25, $35 or $50/day for home health care. | $75,000, $105,000, or $150,000. |
| John Hancock Mutual Life Insurance Co. | John Hancock | Pretax option through flex plan; entry-age priced. Monthly level premiums: 42 = $12.30, 60 = $45.40, 70 = $106. | Number of eligibles: 15,000; participation rate: 8%. | 80% of costs up to $80/day for nursing home care and $60/day for home health care. No choice in options. | Four years. |
| Levitz Furniture | CNA | After-tax. | Number of eligibles: 4,500; participation rate: NA. | Covers nursing home care and home health care; three levels of coverage: $60, $80, or $100/day for nursing home care; $30, $40, or $50/day for home health care. | $120,000, $160,000, or $200,000. |

| Eligibles | Waiting Period | Prior Facility Use Required | Inflation Adjustment | Features |
|---|---|---|---|---|
| Employees/ spouses and parents, parents-in-law. | 90-day waiting period before benefits paid. | No, and no prior nursing home care. Must need help with 2 of 5 ADLs to receive benefits. | Yes. | Portable; return of contributions provision—return of premiums if active premium-paying employee dies before using benefit; retirees and portables (those who terminated employment) reduced by 10% each year. |
| Employees/ spouses at any age; parents, parents-in-law, and retirees and their spouses under 80 years old. | 90-day waiting period of covered services before benefits paid; only one qualifying waiting period per lifetime. | No, and no prior nursing home care. | No. Covered individuals may increase benefit amount. | Portable; access to Eldercare Resource Referral Service; premiums waived after 120 days of nursing home care; if stop paying premiums after 10 years, receive 30% daily benefit amount and, each additional year of payment, an additional 3% increase in daily benefit amount, up to 75% after 25 years; no death benefit. |
| Employees with six months of employment; spouses and retirees under 80 years old; parents not covered. | 90-day waiting period before benefits paid. | | Yes, every 3 years benefit reassessed in terms of inflation; employees may increase coverage for higher premiums. | Portable; no premium refund option; no death benefit. |
| Employees/ spouses under 80 years old; retirees not covered. | 90-day waiting period before benefits paid. | | No. However, a rider is offered which allows covered individuals to increase coverage a minimum of $20/day every 5 years. | Portable; no death benefit. |

**(continued)**

227

## TABLE VI.1 (continued)

| Companies | Carrier | Premiums | Participation | Benefits | Maximums |
|---|---|---|---|---|---|
| Ohio State Teachers Retirement System | Aetna | After-tax pension deduction or direct-billed; entry-age priced. $10 option monthly level premiums: 50 = $3.16, 60 = $6.39, 70 = $13.75. | Number of eligibles: 67,000; participation rate: 15%. | Custodial care in nursing home and/or private home care. Home care is 50% of daily benefit amount. Ranges from $10 to $100/day in increments of $10. | $18,250–$182,500; increases $18,250 for each additional $10/day of coverage. |
| Procter and Gamble | Aetna | After-tax payroll deduction or direct-billed; entry-age priced. Monthly level premiums: 20–24 = $4.20, 40 = $13.20, 60 = $55.10. | Number of eligibles: 27,000; participation rate: 10.9%. | Custodial care in nursing home and/or private home care; home care is 50% of daily benefit amount; $60/day for nursing home care; $30/day for home care. | $109,500. |
| Professional Staff of Congress—City University of New York (PSC-CUNY) | John Hancock | After-tax. | Number of eligibles: 10,200 employees, 2,000 retirees; participation rate: NA. | 80% of costs up to coverage maximum; three levels of coverage: $60, $80, or $100/day for nursing home care; $45, $60, or $75/day for home health care. | $87,600, $116,800, or $146,000. |

228

| Eligibles | Waiting Period | Prior Facility Use Required | Inflation Adjustment | Features |
|---|---|---|---|---|
| Retirees/ spouses, parents, and parents-in-law. | 90-day waiting period before benefits paid. | No, and no prior nursing home care. Must need help with 2 of 5 ADLs to receive benefits. | Yes. Covered individuals may purchase $10/day in additional coverage without medical underwriting in years ending in 0 and 5; additional purchases in other years are allowed subject to medical underwriting. | Portable on individual basis; 90-day premium waiver period; no death benefit. |
| Employees/ spouses, parents and parents-in-law. | 90-day waiting period before benefits paid. | No, and no prior nursing home care. Must need help with 2 of 5 ADLs to receive benefits. | No. | Portable on individual basis; 90-day premium waiver period; extended term provision; return of contributions provision—return of premiums if active premium-paying employee dies before using benefit; retirees and portables (those who terminated employment) reduced by 10% each year. |
| Employees/ spouses, parents, parents-in-law, and retirees/ spouses. | 90-day waiting period before benefits paid. | | Yes, every 3 years benefit reassessed in terms of inflation; employees or members may increase coverage for higher premiums. | Portable; no death benefit. |

(continued)

## TABLE VI.1 (continued)

| Companies | Carrier | Premiums | Participation | Benefits | Maximums |
|---|---|---|---|---|---|
| South Carolina Retirement Systems | Aetna | After-tax. | Number of eligibles: 127,000 actives and spouses; participation rate: NA. | Covers home health care, nursing home care, and adult day care; 8 levels of coverage: $30–$100/day for nursing home care, $15–$50/day for home health care. | $54,750–$182,500; increases $18,250 for each additional $10/day of coverage. |
| State of Alaska | Aetna | Entry-age priced. Monthly level premiums: 55–59 = $26.80, 60–64 = $48.25, 65–69 = $80.45, 70–74 = $128.70. | Number of eligibles: 9,300 retirees; participation rate: 32%. | Reimburses usual, reasonable, and customary up to a fixed maximum: nursing home—$125/day in-state and $75/day out-of-state; home health—$75/day in-state and $40/day out-of-state. Coverage provided for actual expenses incurred under written, covered program of care prescribed by a physician for medically necessary care and for treatment received in a nursing care facility or home convalescent unit. Treatment must also include one of the following: home health aides, licensed practical nursing, occupational therapy, physical therapy, or speech therapy. | Overall maximum $200,000, includes $50,000 home health. |

| Eligibles | Waiting Period | Prior Facility Use Required | Inflation Adjustment | Features |
|---|---|---|---|---|
| Employees and spouses; parents not covered. | 90-day waiting period before benefits paid. | No, and no prior nursing home care. Must need help with 2 of 5 ADLs to receive benefits. | Yes. Covered individuals may increase coverage $10/day during open enrollment. | Portable; return of contributions provision—return of premiums if active premium-paying employee dies before using benefit; retirees and portables (those who terminated employment) reduced by 10% each year. |
| Retirees and spouses; parents not covered. | 90-day waiting period before benefits paid. | No, and no prior nursing home care. | No. | Different benefit levels for care delivered in and out of state; no death benefit. |

(continued)

**TABLE VI.1 (continued)**

| Companies | Carrier | Premiums | Participation | Benefits | Maximums |
|---|---|---|---|---|---|
| State of Maryland | Travelers[a] | Payroll deduction or direct billing; entry-age priced. Low- and high-option monthly level premiums: 30 = $5, $7; 40 = $9, $12.60; 50 = $17, $23.80; 60 = $39.50, $55.30; 70 = $112.25, $157.15; 80 = $220, $308. | Number of eligibles: 60,000; participation rate: 5%. | Three levels of coverage: $50, $60, or $70/day for nursing home care; $25, $30, or $35/day for home health care. | $75,000, $90,000, or $105,000. |

Source: Employee Benefit Research Institute.

[a]These four policies are based on the initial The Travelers product. As of June 1, 1989, The Travelers announced the introduction of its second generation product that will be available with effective dates beginning January 1, 1990. This new product includes case management and offers many additional benefits and options.

[b]Both General Motors Corporation and Chrysler Corporation have initiated employer-paid pilot programs as a result of 1987 contract agreements with the United Auto Workers.

Note: Insurers have signed agreements with at least 18 other employers, but information on these plans has not been made available.

Except for 401(k) arrangements, the tax code explicitly prohibits flexible benefit plans from providing deferred compensation. The tax law question regarding flexible benefit plan financing of long-term care insurance is whether this insurance is, like a pension plan, deferred compensation. The John Hancock Mutual Life Insurance Company was probably the first employer to offer long-term care insurance to its employees through its flexible benefit plan funded through participants' pretax earnings.

*Inhibiting Factors*—There are several barriers to the development of long-term care as an employee benefit.

First, it is unlikely that long-term care insurance will be added to employee compensation without modifying the current benefit structure. As a practical matter, it is difficult to redesign compensation packages. Unless there are dramatic changes in business conditions, changes in employee compensation packages are usually made gradually. Even the recent movement in health insurance away from first dollar coverage that has occurred in response to rapid increases in health care costs has tended to occur carefully and usually in conjunction with the addition of new benefits such as employee savings accounts or health reimbursement accounts.

| Eligibles | Waiting Period | Prior Facility Use Required | Inflation Adjustment | Features |
|---|---|---|---|---|
| Employees/ spouses at any age; parents, parents-in-law, and retirees and their spouses under 80 years old. | 90-day waiting period of covered services before benefits paid; only one qualifying waiting period per lifetime. | No prior hospital or nursing home care. | No. Covered individuals may increase benefit amount. | Portable; access to Eldercare Resource Referral Service; premiums waived after 120 days of nursing home care; ability to change benefit amount; no death benefit. |

Second, employers are not likely to rush to offer new benefits when there is so much uncertainty about the costs and liabilities involved. Employers may already feel "burned" by their experience with post-retirement medical benefits. Well-meaning employers who presumed that they were offering to pay for health insurance after retirement *if they could afford it* have learned from a series of court cases that they may indeed have to provide the benefits even though their financial conditions may change. Moreover, they may not even be able to alter the structure of their promises (such as adding a copayment, for example) despite the substantial increases in the cost of health care (Chollet and Friedland, 1988a). This situation is exacerbated by employers' frustration over their inability to control health care expenditures for either active employees or retirees. Consequently, they are likely to avoid providing new employee benefits, especially if the cost of the benefits is unpredictable or there is a potential liability that they cannot anticipate.

Third, long-term care is clearly not on the same footing as other employee benefits. A dollar in compensation used to purchase an employee benefit that is recognized in the tax code is worth more than a dollar to the employee because it is not considered taxable income.

Since it is not clear how long-term care insurance would be treated in the tax code, a dollar used by an employer to purchase long-term care insurance may have to be reported by the employee as a dollar of taxable income.[16] Employee contributions toward the premium would not necessarily count as tax-deductible medical expenses (Utz, 1988). Benefits received when a claim is filed may also have to be included as taxable income.

In addition, there is no straightforward way for employers to establish a trust fund to finance either long-term care or long-term care insurance at retirement. Normally, a trust fund established for active workers' medical benefits can avoid taxation if the contributions to the trust do not exceed more than 35 percent of the prior year's plan expenses. Reserves of this magnitude may be sufficient for health plans, since the plans essentially are established and priced to provide coverage for that year. But they are unlikely to be sufficient if an employer is funding a benefit over the working life of the employee that will be purchased during retirement.[17]

Prior to 1984, funding in anticipation of paying for a retiree's medical benefits could be done on a tax-preferred basis through a special trust under IRC section 501(c)(9) called a voluntary employee beneficiary association (VEBA). The Deficit Reduction Act of 1984 (DEFRA) severely limited employers' ability to prefund postretirement medical benefits on a tax-preferred basis. This change, however, did not affect many employers, since virtually all of them were financing these benefits on a current-cost basis rather than funding accruing liability by setting aside funds during employees' active work careers. EBRI estimates that in 1988 the accrued unfunded liability for retiree health benefits for active workers and retirees was $169 billion for private employers (Chollet, 1989).

Historically, employers have not been required to disclose unfunded liabilities for postretirement health plans on corporate balance sheets; the existence of an unfunded plan could be relegated to a footnote. However, in February 1989, the Financial Accounting Standards Board proposed a rule that would require employers to determine and report the amount of this unfunded liability on their corporate income statements (by 1992) and balance sheets (by 1997). The net effect of this proposed ruling is that the liability would be taken into account if and when the corporation borrows money; therefore, the cost of issu-

---

[16]The dollar paid by the employer is still deductible as a normal business expense.
[17]There are other limitations, especially for the funding of postretirement medical benefits. For more information, see Chollet and Friedland, 1988a.

ing stocks or bonds and of borrowing from a bank is likely to increase. Furthermore, even if employers want to prefund, they cannot do so on a tax-preferred basis because of DEFRA restrictions.

One way employers may be able to prefund postretirement health benefits on a tax-preferred basis is by saving through their pension funds. IRC section 401(h) enables employers to contribute to a special fund for benefits other than pensions. However, these contributions cannot be more than 25 percent of the total contribution to the pension fund and might not be permitted if the pension plan has reached the full funding limit.[18] The limitations may cause contributions to be insufficient to prefund needed postretirement benefits.

In addition to the fact that tax code restrictions strongly discourage employers from using VEBAs to fund retiree health insurance liability of any type, these trusts may be poorly suited to the kind of long-term care insurance benefit employers may wish to provide. VEBAs are not structured as employee-owned capital accumulation accounts. Employer contributions to a VEBA are not associated with particular employees, and workers who terminate employment before retirement cannot withdraw funds from them. Although employer contributions to either an IRC section 401(h) trust (designed as subsidiary to the pension benefit) or an IRC section 105(h) trust (a medical expenditure account) are made on behalf of specific workers, these trusts are not intended for employee capital accumulation either. These trusts may best be used by employers to fund a defined service benefit, which employers may wish to avoid in designing a long-term care plan for retirees.[19]

Despite tax code ambiguities, employment-based long-term care policies have been developed, marketed, and sold. While this suggests that tax policy may not be a deterrent, it certainly has not encouraged policy development and marketing. The number of employers provid-

---

[18]A March 23, 1989, Internal Revenue Service (IRS) private letter ruling suggests that contributions to 401(h) trusts are permitted even if the pension plan's full funding limit has been reached. However, budget legislation moving through Congress at the time of this writing would reverse this ruling.

[19]At least one employer has used section 105(h) based on an IRS letter ruling to establish a tax-exempt "medical expenditure account" to finance health insurance benefits for current workers and retirees. While 105(h) plans have not been used widely or at all to fund accrued liability for future benefits, employee benefit consultants have suggested that these plans may be useful for that purpose since unused balances can be rolled over to subsequent years—a feature that obviously is critical to capital accumulation. However, 105(h) accounts may be poorly suited for funding benefits that may not be paid for a substantial number of years, since employer contributions cannot be deducted as a business expense until distributions are made from the account in payment of participants' health care bills.

ing access to long-term care insurance is still relatively small. When asked about factors inhibiting the provision of long-term care insurance, 52 percent of the responding 139 member firms of the Washington Business Group on Health said that cost was an important barrier. Slightly more than one-third of the respondents cited as inhibiting factors fear of government mandates for employer contributions, lack of employee interest, and the concern that employee pressure would eventually result in employer contributions. Less than one-third of the respondents (30 percent) felt that unfavorable tax treatment was inhibiting the development of long-term care insurance (Washington Business Group on Health, 1987).

Employers have little incentive to offer long-term care insurance as an employee benefit for a number of reasons, including: the disadvantages of this type of insurance compared with other benefits such as pension plans, 401(k)-type cash or deferred compensation arrangements, and accident and health plans; anxiety over entering into financial obligations with unpredictable costs; and the difficulty inherent in changing nonwage compensation packages. Employees are not likely to encourage change in employer positions since the majority probably do not recognize that protecting income during retirement requires planning for long-term care. With minimal employee interest and employer hesitation, additional tax advantages for providing long-term care insurance may be necessary to increase the number of employers providing this insurance.

*Issues of Funding, Vesting, and Portability*—Providing favorable tax treatment to encourage long-term care insurance is likely to raise questions about how to structure the benefit so that employees retain the value in their plan after leaving an employer (portability) and obtain an unrevocable right or "entitlement" to accrued benefits (vesting). Congress may want assurance that plans receiving preferential tax treatment do not discriminate in favor of highly paid employees and that the insurers will be financially capable of fulfilling their promises. Clarification of the tax code alone is unlikely to lead to product development that accommodates these concerns.

Portability of long-term care insurance benefits may be particularly difficult to achieve, especially given the way long-term care insurance policies have been developing. Currently, plans incorporate prefunding into the policy. When contributions to the plan cease, unless the recipient is receiving benefits, these plans no longer have any value. However, plans do offer the option of converting to an individual policy when an employee either leaves an employer or an employer decides to abandon plan sponsorship. Except for an additional admin-

236

istrative charge (currently around 2 percent of the premium) paid to the insurance company, all other terms of the policy remain the same. This enables policyholders to maintain coverage.

Still, the value of the premiums paid to prefund future benefits is not maintained unless the premium continues to be paid. While the policy is portable, the value of the prefunded portion of the policy usually is not.[20] If an employee went to work for another firm that also offered access to long-term care insurance or paid for long-term care insurance, there probably would not be a way to incorporate the prefunded value of the former policy into the new policy. Portability of this sort would require that the former insurance plan return the entire premium plus earnings on that premium and that the new insurance plan be willing to accept this payment in exchange for a policy with the same premium that would have been charged if the employee had first purchased this policy from the new insurer.

## Conclusion

We are all at risk of needing long-term care. Fortunately, most of us will not need very extensive assistance; however, some of us will. Rather than trying to save for this uncertain and potentially expensive need, pooling financial risk through insurance would be efficient. Saving for this contingency is not.

In a four-year period starting in 1985 and accelerating after 1987, the market for long-term care insurance expanded dramatically. However, it is still relatively small—at most, 4 percent of the elderly held policies in September 1989. Furthermore, private insurance is still an insignificant source of long-term care financing—less than 1 percent. Nevertheless, development of this market offers the potential for providing individuals with financing options that have not previously existed as well as the possibility of altering the financing and delivery of long-term care.

So many factors have inhibited market development that it is somewhat surprising that the market exists at all. Especially significant has been the lack of consumer interest, which has put the onus on insurers not only to convince consumers why they should purchase their particular version of long-term care insurance but why they should consider buying this sort of insurance at all. Weak consumer demand has also left much of the development of insurance products

---

[20]Recent policy designs have included provisions to refund part of the premiums paid.

to insurers. Insurers' inability to accurately project expected costs and utilization without strong market signals or the encouragement of tax and regulatory policy has led to the development of a fixed dollar rather than a service benefit.

Many of the initial policies were laden with so many liability-limiting provisions that consumer groups questioned their value. Insurance policies introduced since the middle of 1988, however, have improved dramatically. Many no longer require prior hospitalization before benefits can be claimed. Alzheimer's disease and related dementias are more likely to be covered, home health care or care in a nursing facility is less likely to require prior care in a higher-level or skilled nursing facility, and many policies now include provisions to adjust benefits to inflation.

Despite the many recent improvements in long-term care insurance policies, some fundamental problems remain. First, there is no guarantee that the insurance benefit will be sufficient to guarantee access to needed care 20 to 40 years after the policy is purchased. Second, there is no guarantee that the insurer or the policy will still exist when benefits are needed. Third, there seems to be no easy way to ensure portability or to exchange the prefunded portion of one insurance policy for a new one.

Private long-term care insurance provides millions of people with the potential to pool the financial risk of needing assistance. This potential would be maximized if employers offered access to long-term care insurance and encouraged employees to buy it. However, even if employers do become an important distribution mechanism for long-term care insurance, as with other voluntary employee benefits, universal coverage is not likely.

# VII. The Importance of Long-Term Care to Employers

## Introduction

Employers amass economic resources of land, labor, and machinery and mold them into goods and services. The distribution of the goods and services is affected by the financial return to landowners, lenders of capital, and the labor used in production. Changes in the size and distribution of the labor force have a direct effect on production. This affects employers and employment as employers compete for the best workers and employees seek the best employment opportunities.

The symbiotic relationship between employers and employees is evident in the financing of public programs such as Medicare, Medicaid, and Social Security. These programs are structured to be financed on a pay-as-you-go basis from payroll, income, sales, and property taxes. One consequence of pay-as-you-go financing is that, holding all else constant, the more beneficiaries relative to the number of workers, the greater the potential tax burden on employees and employers. Therefore, the financial well-being of these publicly financed programs is of the utmost importance to employers and employees—not only because they are financing the programs but also because they are potential beneficiaries.

For most aspects of economic security, except long-term care, there exists a public-private partnership, with employers playing a significant role in the relationship. From this perspective, it seems natural that employers would be drawn into the public policy debate over the financing and delivery of long-term care and would evaluate the feasibility of employment-based long-term care insurance. Most employee benefits began out of concern for the welfare of employees and corporate goodwill and image but eventually emerged as management tools to attract and retain quality employees, to foster a productive working environment, or to encourage early retirement (Graebner, 1980; Kamerman and Kahn, 1987).

The changing age distribution of the population and the corresponding changes in the labor force may lead employers to assist in providing either long-term care or long-term care insurance. Employers have already begun to offer "elder care" benefits to accommodate active employees who are also caregivers to a spouse or parent. Some employers provide assistance to retirees or to retiree clubs (Levin,

239

1988). As of September 1989, at least 35 employers either provided or were about to provide access to long-term care insurance. Most of these plans are open to employees and their spouses, parents of employees and their spouses, and retirees. Surveys of employers and discussions with benefit consultants and employee benefit managers suggest a reserved but sincere interest in evaluating the feasibility of either assisting caregivers or providing access to long-term care insurance. As more employers learn about the financing and delivery of long-term care, it is expected that increasing numbers will address the issue.

The establishment of employer-sponsored long-term care insurance programs as a traditional employee benefit is not likely to be quick or spontaneous. Employers are not likely simply to add another benefit, especially if liability is not predictable or controllable. Changes in employee compensation are more likely to occur in an awkward and incremental fashion. The intensity of employee demand will be critical, as will the public policy response to financing long-term care. Employers and employees currently share in the cost of long-term care financing and are certain to share in it even if the financing is changed. But, in the long run, the relative magnitude and distribution of the cost will be affected by the actions employers, employees, and legislators take in the short term.

## An Overview of Employee Benefits

Employers are extremely important to the economic security of employees and their dependents and retirees. Employers provide access to group health insurance for 65 percent of the U.S. population. Ninety percent of full-time workers in medium-sized and large establishments[1] have employer-provided health insurance. In 1988, 45 percent of full-time participants in an employer-provided health plan had coverage that continued after retirement, even if retirement was before age 65, when Medicare benefits begin. In addition, in the same year about 80 percent of full-time workers in medium-sized and large establishments had a pension plan (Bureau of Labor Statistics, 1989a). In 1986, 49 percent of all full-time employees were covered by pension plans (Piacentini and Cerino, forthcoming).

Employer-based pension plans are an important source of income security for retirees. In 1986, 40 percent of the population aged 65 or over reported income from private or public pensions. Among the

---

[1]Private nonfarm establishments that employ 100 workers or more.

elderly who reported pension income from a private employer plan, 7 percent received at least one-half of their total income from one or more plans, and among those with family income of at least twice the federal poverty income level, 43 percent reported pension income (see chapter V). Among elderly couples and individuals reporting private pension income in 1986, 50 percent received 20 percent or more of their total income from one or more private pensions.

For retirees formerly employed by public employers, pensions are an even more important source of income. In 1986, 78 percent of elderly couples and individuals reporting public pension income derived 20 percent or more of their total income from public pensions, and 36 percent reported one-half or more of their total income came from public pensions (Grad, 1988). The increased importance of government employee pensions as a source of retirement income for government retirees is probably due to the fact that, until recently, most government employees were not required to contribute to Social Security.

Employer-sponsored health insurance benefits for retirees have also become an important and fairly common employee benefit. In 1988, 45 percent of private-sector workers in medium-sized and large establishments in the United States had health insurance plans that continued benefits after retirement (Bureau of Labor Statistics, 1989a). Until recently, many employers may have initiated retiree health benefits rather casually, as a presumed low-cost alternative to enhanced pension benefits (Chollet and Friedland, 1988b). However, health care inflation has made retiree health plans a very valuable supplement to retirement income. For low-income retirees, the value of their retiree health benefits (automatically indexed to the rising cost of health care) can exceed the amount of their pension benefit over time (Doran, MacBain, and Reimert, 1987).

Among the current elderly population, 28.6 percent, or 7.3 million retirees, supplement Medicare with health insurance benefits from a past employer (Chollet, 1989). This figure excludes elderly persons who have retiree health coverage as dependents. Although retiree health insurance benefits are more common among pension recipients, a significant number of elderly persons without pension income also report health insurance benefits from a past employer.

Employer and worker contributions to pension plans represent an important form of private saving. Although workers may substitute pension saving for individual saving, studies indicate that private pensions probably increase net saving among workers (Ippolito, 1986;

241

Korczyk, 1984; Friedland, 1983).[2] Individual retirement savings opportunities—even those accorded tax advantages comparable to pension contributions—are apparently less effective than pensions in encouraging widespread saving among workers. For tax year 1987, fewer than 13 percent of workers reported any contribution to an individual retirement account (IRA), compared with more than 58 percent of ERISA-mandated eligible workers who participated in an employer pension plan (Piacentini, 1989). Among workers not participating in an employer pension plan (potentially displacing discretionary saving), 11 percent reported an IRA contribution. Although this lower IRA contribution rate reflects the lower income of workers without pension plans, the differential between employer pension participation and the rate of IRA contributions among workers is consistent with estimates indicating that employer pensions force saving.

The success of employer pension and savings plans in facilitating retirement saving and employers' roles in financing health care among workers and retirees suggest that employment-based plans can serve as noteworthy models for plans designed to finance the expected expenses of long-term care or long-term care insurance over employees' working years. The structure of such plans for long-term care, however, is likely to be critical to its acceptability to employers and employees. Employers are unlikely to consider adopting any plan that has unpredictable costs and liabilities, and employees are unlikely to appreciate employers' efforts on their behalf if they themselves do not recognize the risks of not incorporating this contingency into their retirement planning.

## A Convergence of Pressures

### Pressures from Outside the Firm

*The Changing Labor Force*—Firms that traditionally have relied on new entrants into the work force have already faced rising labor costs. Workers under age 24 were born between 1964 and 1972, the beginning of the "baby bust." Fast-food outlets and grocery stores have been increasing wages to attract entry level workers (Bernstein,

---

[2]That is, while an additional dollar in pension funding might lead individuals to reduce savings, for the majority of people the reduction in private savings would be less than the addition to the pension fund. On net, total savings from both pension funds and other forms of saving are increased.

1987). Projections by the U.S. Department of Labor (DOL) indicate that between now and the year 2000, the labor force will grow at a slower rate than at any time since the Great Depression (Johnston et al., 1987). Between 1986 and the year 2000, the number of men in the labor force aged 16 to 25 is projected to remain constant. DOL's moderate projections estimate a range of growth of ±0.05 percent (table VII.1). Overall, the labor force is projected to grow 1.2 percent per year, less than one-half the average growth rate during the 1970s.

The National Institute on Aging macroeconomic-demographic model (MDM) is a large computer simulation model that simultaneously estimates demographic change and economic growth to produce macroeconomic projections between 1980 and the year 2055. The model simulates how demographic change will affect U.S. economic growth. The economic growth, in turn, determines employment and earnings. Table VII.2 presents projected employment by age and sex as well as some aggregate labor market variables between 1980 and the year 2055. Prior to the year 2010, annual rates of growth in employment are projected to be greatest among women aged 25 to 64; after the year 2010, employment is expected to grow fastest among men aged 65 or over. Earnings are expected to grow at a slower rate after the year 2010, while the total number of hours worked will decline at a faster rate than prior to the year 2010.

The MDM projections are remarkably similar to more recent DOL projections through the year 2000. MDM projects that in that year the labor force will number 132.5 million people, or 6.3 million fewer than the more recent DOL projections. However, the MDM projections show similar growth rates—1.14 percent per year between 1980 and the year 2000 (compared with DOL's 1.2 percent). Between the year 2000 and the year 2010, MDM projects that the annual labor force growth rate will be 0.69 percent. During the time when the baby boom generation is retiring (between the year 2010 and the year 2030), the labor force is expected to grow 0.15 percent annually (table VII.2).

The decline in the growth of entry level workers and the eventual overall decline in employment growth are likely to raise the cost of labor. In fact, MDM projects that total compensation as a share of Gross National Product (GNP) will increase dramatically between now and the year 2055. The average annual GNP growth rate is projected to be 1.12 percent, while between 1980 and the year 2055, total compensation is expected to increase 1.84 percent per year. The rising share of compensation is reflected in the declining unemployment rate, which during this period is projected to decline from 7.7 percent to slightly more than 4 percent.

243

## TABLE VII.1
## Civilian Labor Force, by Sex, Age, Race, and Hispanic Origin: 1986 and Moderate Growth Projections through the Year 2000

| Group | Number (in millions) | | Percentage Change | Percentage Distribution | Growth Rate |
|---|---|---|---|---|---|
| | 1986 | Projected, 2000 | 1986–2000 | Projected, 2000 | 1986–2000 |
| Total, Aged 16 or over | 117.8 | 138.8 | 17.8% | 100.0% | 1.2% |
| Men, Aged 16 or over | 65.4 | 73.1 | 11.8 | 52.7 | 0.8 |
| 16–24 | 12.3 | 11.5 | -6.1 | 8.3 | -0.4 |
| 25–54 | 44.4 | 53.0 | 19.4 | 38.2 | 1.3 |
| 55 or over | 8.8 | 8.6 | -1.8 | 6.2 | -0.1 |
| Women, Aged 16 or over | 52.4 | 65.6 | 25.2 | 47.3 | 1.6 |
| 16–24 | 11.1 | 11.1 | 0.1 | 8.0 | c |
| 25–54 | 35.2 | 47.8 | 35.8 | 34.4 | 2.2 |
| 55 or over | 6.1 | 6.8 | 10.1 | 4.9 | 0.7 |
| White, Aged 16 or over | 101.8 | 116.7 | 14.6 | 84.1 | 1.0 |
| Black, Aged 16 or over | 12.7 | 16.3 | 28.8 | 11.8 | 1.8 |
| Asian and Other,[a] Aged 16 or over | 3.4 | 5.7 | 71.2 | 4.1 | 3.9 |
| Hispanic,[b] Aged 16 or over | 8.1 | 14.1 | 74.4 | 10.2 | 4.1 |

Source: Howard N. Fullerton Jr., "Labor Force Projections: 1986 to 2000," *Monthly Labor Review* (September 1987), p. 20, table 1.
[a]Includes American Indians, native Alaskans, Asians, and Pacific Islanders. The historic data are derived by subtracting "Black" from the "Black and other" group projections.
[b]Persons of Hispanic origin may be of any race. Labor force data for Hispanics are not available before 1976.
[c]The rate is −0.05 percent to 0.05 percent.

## TABLE VII.2
## Projected Employment by Age, Sex, and Aggregate Labor Market, 1980–2055

| Years | Men (in millions) | | | | Women (in millions) | | | | Aggregate Labor Market | | | | |
|---|---|---|---|---|---|---|---|---|---|---|---|---|---|
| | Aged 16–24 | Aged 25–64 | Aged 65 or over | Sub-total | Aged 16–24 | Aged 25–64 | Aged 65 or over | Sub-total | Employment (in millions) | Labor force (in millions) | Hours worked per worker | Compensation rate (1972 dollars) | Average annual compensation (1972 dollars) |
| 1980 | 12.1 | 44.4 | 1.9 | 58.4 | 9.7 | 28.2 | 1.1 | 39.0 | 97.4 | 105.5 | 1,508 | $5.51 | $8,312 |
| 1990 | 10.8 | 53.0 | 2.1 | 65.9 | 9.3 | 36.2 | 1.4 | 47.0 | 112.9 | 119.1 | 1,509 | 6.25 | 9,434 |
| 2000 | 11.1 | 55.9 | 1.8 | 68.8 | 10.8 | 45.1 | 1.1 | 57.0 | 125.8 | 132.5 | 1,471 | 7.47 | 10,998 |
| 2010 | 12.5 | 56.7 | 2.1 | 71.3 | 12.2 | 50.6 | 0.9 | 63.6 | 134.9 | 142.0 | 1,426 | 8.62 | 12,287 |
| 2020 | 11.8 | 56.4 | 2.9 | 71.0 | 11.5 | 52.9 | 1.1 | 65.6 | 136.7 | 143.4 | 1,397 | 9.59 | 13,398 |
| 2030 | 12.8 | 55.4 | 3.4 | 71.8 | 12.6 | 53.9 | 1.3 | 67.8 | 139.6 | 146.3 | 1,369 | 10.82 | 14,806 |
| 2040 | 12.8 | 57.0 | 3.4 | 73.2 | 12.6 | 57.2 | 1.2 | 71.1 | 144.3 | 150.8 | 1,344 | 12.79 | 17,185 |
| 2050 | 13.0 | 57.1 | 3.7 | 73.9 | 12.8 | 58.0 | 1.3 | 72.2 | 146.1 | 152.3 | 1,309 | 15.37 | 20,123 |
| 2055 | 13.4 | 57.3 | 3.9 | 74.5 | 13.2 | 58.2 | 1.4 | 72.8 | 147.3 | 153.5 | 1,291 | 16.86 | 21,763 |
| | | | | | | Rates of Growth | | | | | | | |
| 1980–2010 | 0.11% | 0.82% | 0.33% | 0.67% | 0.77% | 1.97% | −0.67% | 1.64% | 1.09% | 1.00% | −1.19% | 1.50% | 1.31% |
| 2010–2055 | 0.15 | 0.02 | 1.39 | 0.10 | 0.18 | 0.31 | 0.99 | 0.30 | 0.20 | 0.17 | −0.22 | 1.49 | 1.26 |
| 1980–2055 | 0.14 | 0.34 | 0.96 | 0.33 | 0.41 | 0.97 | 0.32 | 0.84 | 0.55 | 0.50 | −0.21 | 1.50 | 1.29 |

Source: Projections based on National Institute on Aging, National Institutes of Health, Public Health Service, U.S. Department of Health and Human Services, *Macroeconomic Demographic Model* (Washington, DC: U.S. Government Printing Office, 1984), tables 10-8 and 10-9.

The rising cost of labor is likely to encourage employers to alter their mix of capital (plant and equipment) and labor. The demand for specific products and available technology will affect the degree to which employers will be able to substitute machines for people. However, replacing employees with machines could raise the per person cost of labor, even if the total cost of labor is reduced, if lesser-skilled employees are replaced with fewer higher-skilled employees. If the demand for employees to maintain the more complicated machinery grows relatively faster than the supply of employees, then per person labor costs will be bid up either directly (through wages) or indirectly (through higher training costs).

*Changes within the Labor Force*—Two of the most pervasive labor force trends have been the propensity toward earlier retirement and the growing proportion of women in the labor market. The implication of these trends is profound. Together, they point directly to the need to examine how employee compensation is attracting and retaining women. Since labor force growth is declining, it will be increasingly necessary to retain workers aged 55 or older. The participation of women in the labor force began to grow at a small, relatively constant rate before the turn of the century and began to increase dramatically during World War II. The labor force participation rate among women aged 25 to 44 grew 40 percentage points, from 29.9 percent in 1940 to 73.3 percent in 1985 (chart VII.1).

Not surprisingly, the fastest growth in the labor force participation of women has been among married women. But of particular note is the fact that among married women the fastest increase in the labor force participation rate has been among mothers. From 1960 to 1986, the labor force participation rate of women aged 20 to 24 increased by 33.1 percentage points for women who were married; 16.4 percentage points for women who were separated, divorced, or widowed; and 1.6 percentage points for women who were single. Similarly, for women aged 25 to 34, the labor force participation rate increased most for married women (38.7 percentage points), followed by separated, divorced, or widowed women (22.9 percentage points), and single women (1.2 percentage points) (Bureau of the Census, 1986c).

A growing proportion of the labor force consists of workers with children. Between 1960 and 1987, the proportion of married women in the labor force with a child under age 6 more than tripled (Bureau of the Census, 1987b). In 1987, about 66.9 percent of mothers with children under age 18 were in the work force (Bureau of the Census, 1987b). Furthermore, between 1970 and 1988, the proportion of children under age 18 who lived with one parent doubled from 12 percent

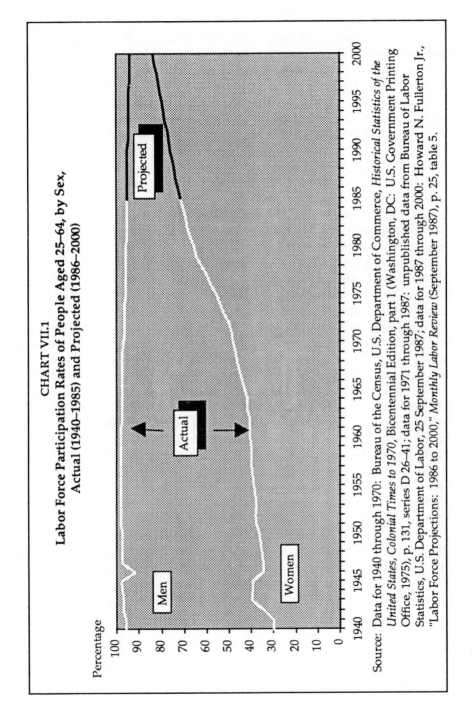

CHART VII.1
Labor Force Participation Rates of People Aged 25–64, by Sex,
Actual (1940–1985) and Projected (1986–2000)

Source: Data for 1940 through 1970: Bureau of the Census, U.S. Department of Commerce, *Historical Statistics of the United States, Colonial Times to 1970*, Bicentennial Edition, part 1 (Washington, DC: U.S. Government Printing Office, 1975), p. 131, series D 26–41; data for 1971 through 1987: unpublished data from Bureau of Labor Statistics, U.S. Department of Labor, 25 September 1987; data for 1987 through 2000: Howard N. Fullerton Jr., "Labor Force Projections: 1986 to 2000," *Monthly Labor Review* (September 1987), p. 25, table 5.

to 24 percent (Bureau of the Census, 1989a). Most of these families (90 percent) were headed by a woman (Saltford and Heck, 1989).

With more working mothers and single-parent households, day care for preschool children and care for "latch-key" children has continued to be a troublesome issue. Since the baby boomers are still in their childbearing years, the need for quality, affordable day care for children is not likely to diminish in the short run. During the 1988 presidential campaign, both candidates proposed plans for addressing child care, and in recent years Congress has seriously considered legislation mandating that employers enable new parents or employees with a sick child or elderly parents to take unpaid leave without losing either benefits or their jobs (Saltford, 1988).

Increasingly, employees will be preoccupied with arranging for the day care of a dependent, but for a growing number and proportion of workers the dependent will be a chronically ill parent or spouse rather than a child, and for some it will be both a parent and a child. Currently, close to one-quarter of all employees may be caregivers, and perhaps three-quarters of these are responsible for an adult.[3] Among caregivers who worked while providing assistance, 20 percent had cut back on their hours, 29 percent rearranged work schedules, and slightly less than 20 percent took time off without pay (Select Committee on Aging, 1987b). The trend toward delaying childbearing will, in the short run, increase the possibility of employees finding themselves forced to provide care to both a child and a dependent adult. However, the full impact of this trend will appear when these children have grown and entered the labor force. Then it will be even more likely that they will have parents to care for while they are employed. Children born to a 30-year-old parent today will be 50 years old when their parents are in their eighties.

Despite the strong trend in increased labor force participation of women, successive groups of employees are retiring earlier (Andrews, 1986). In 1970, 83 percent of all men aged 55 to 64 were in the labor force, but by 1986 this rate had dropped to 67.3 percent. The participation rate for women aged 55 to 64 also declined during this period, but only slightly, from 43 percent to 42.3 percent. Relatively few people aged 65 or over were working in 1986—only 16 percent of men

---

[3]In a survey of employees working at one site of The Travelers Insurance Company, 28 percent of the respondents indicated they had caregiving responsibilities—primarily (81 percent of the time) a parent or a spouse's parent (The Travelers Companies, 1985). In a survey of IBM employees, 30 percent were found to be taking care of elderly relatives (Saltford and Heck, 1989).

and 7.4 percent of women. A decade-and-a-half earlier (1970), 26.8 percent of men and 9.7 percent of women aged 65 or older were in the labor force (Bureau of Labor Statistics, 1985 and 1987c).

Employers are likely to be affected by these changes in the labor force in several different ways. First, as purchasers of labor, the slower rate of growth in the labor force is likely to exert upward pressure on the cost of labor. Second, the changing work force—older, with a larger percentage of women—is likely to lead to increased pressure for new employee benefits. Unless employee compensation is restructured, the addition of new benefits will further increase the cost of labor. Third, employers with unfunded postretirement medical benefits may find their labor costs relative to revenues or profits increasing as the ratio of retirees to active workers increases. Fourth, as taxpayers, employers will continue to help pay for Social Security, Medicare, and Medicaid. Barring reductions in benefits and depending on productivity, the growing number of beneficiaries and recipients relative to the base of financial support could lead to tax increases.

Employer responses to these changes are likely to differ, in large part depending on the products they produce, available technology and capital, and management philosophy. But nearly all employers can expect to be affected. Employer interest in providing elder care benefits or access to long-term care insurance might be encouraged initially by concern about productivity. Undoubtedly, corporate executives will seriously consider the argument that employee productivity and morale are adversely affected when they themselves are struggling desperately to provide care to a dependent spouse, parent, or other relative. Small changes in benefits such as flexible hours, referral services, and counseling services may go a long way toward mitigating losses in productivity. Other employers may restructure benefits because it is in their corporate culture to be innovative and progressive leaders in terms of responsiveness to employees (Kamerman and Kahn, 1987). Others may find their way to change because of union negotiation, while others may respond to competition and feel that they must act to attract and retain better employees. Regardless of how the process is initiated, key employees in senior executive positions have begun to learn more about how long-term care is currently financed and delivered.

Over time, employees, too, may be increasingly willing to change the structure of their compensation to include long-term care insurance. Assuming there is continued economic growth, the relative decline in the growth of the labor force and the move toward higher-skilled labor will result in increases in real wages for some segments of the labor force. Concern has been raised that the sheer number of people in the labor force who were born during the baby boom would tend to reduce wages, but simulation results from one study suggest that the wages of men born during the baby boom will increase but those of women will not (Levine and Mitchell, 1988). This study expects that between 1985 and the year 2020, despite the aging of the work force, wages will increase 4.4 percent to 7.8 percent (depending on the simulation and the age groups examined); however, while the rate of wage increase for men is expected to increase from 8.6 percent to 12.2 percent, the simulations for women suggest declines ranging from 7.8 percent to 10.3 percent. The Social Security Administration expects real wages (wage increases beyond inflation) to rise between 0.9 percent and 1.7 percent annually until the turn of the century and to remain steady at a 1.4 percent annual rate of growth until the year 2010. The MDM projections suggest average annual real wage increases of 1.5 percent between 1980 and the year 2055 and average annual real increases in yearly compensation of 1.29 percent.[4]

*Changing Attitudes and Expectations*—Employers, employees, and retirees contribute to the financing of Social Security, Medicare, and Medicaid. Payroll taxes imposed on employers and employees finance current Social Security recipients and Medicare Part A benefits. Federal income taxes finance three-quarters of Medicare Part B and the federal portion of Medicaid expenditures. The state portion of Medicaid funding comes from general revenues, especially from property, sales, and income taxes.

Consequently, in addition to the changing age structure of the population (i.e., a growing ratio of beneficiaries to active workers), the financial health of these three programs can directly affect the cost per worker or taxpayer. Unless the average retirement age or productivity increases, public programs financed by active workers on a pay-as-you-go basis will continually require either greater contributions from employers and active employees, contributions from beneficiaries, or a combination of both. Moreover, improvements in public plans may not necessarily mean that employers will be able to change their benefits in response. This was evident in the "maintenance of effort" provisions of the Medicare Catastrophic Coverage Act of 1988 (MCCA), which required that employers providing postretirement health benefits to Medicare recipients provide retirees with cash or new

---

[4]Annual compensation is expected to increase at a slower rate because of an expected decline in the total number of hours worked.

benefits to the extent that the new Medicare benefits replaced existing provisions in their health plans.[5]

In addition, there has been a steady progression toward a substantial public program that would cover long-term care. The effort that eventually culminated the enactment of MCCA was initiated by Health and Human Services Secretary Otis Bowen's attempt to introduce an administration proposal for legislation that would cover long-term care. The proposal was deflected by President Reagan's request for a year-long commission study, and a compromise eventually emerged that expanded Medicare coverage of acute care but did not include long-term care. The late Rep. Claude Pepper (D-FL) tried to amend the bill to include coverage of chronic home health care but was asked to remove the amendment to ensure the bill's passage in exchange for a vote by the full House of Representatives on his proposal as a separate bill.[6]

Public reaction to MCCA has been vocal and negative. This may be due primarily to the increased monthly premium ($4) and to the anticipated supplemental premium ($22.50 per $150 in federal income tax liability), but it may also be due to the expectation that a premium of this magnitude would increase benefits in ways visible to beneficiaries. If it were to go into effect in January 1991, the prescription drug benefit would be a noticeable improvement in benefits. What is probably most noticeable to beneficiaries is that long-term care is not covered.

There seems to be public recognition that long-term care is an important issue for the country. In a survey for the Health Insurance Association of America conducted by the University of Maryland Center on Aging, nearly 47 percent of the public recognized long-term care for the elderly and the disabled as extremely important (Meiners, 1989). While only 2.5 percent of the respondents claimed to have had personal experience with such care, 29.9 percent of those responding acknowledged that someone in their family had needed long-term care in the past five years. In this survey, 76.5 percent did not expect the government to pay for long-term care; 35 percent were in favor of

[5]The law specifies that the new benefits must be in excess of 50 percent of the value of the provisions they replace. Technically this provision is only in effect for the first two years of the new law, but prior to the movement toward repeal of the law, it had been expected that the law would be amended to make this requirement permanent.

[6]In June 1989, the bill was defeated by a vote of 169-243. Many who opposed the bill claimed their opposition was due to the fact that it had not gone through normal committee consideration before reaching the House floor.

a government program for everyone; 60 percent were in favor of a government program for the needy; and 72 percent were in favor of government support to help people buy long-term care insurance. Overall, 66.4 percent of the respondents were in favor of an arrangement in which the government would provide one-third and private sources two-thirds of the funding. An additional 10.5 percent were in favor of a 50-50 funding arrangement.

However, in a survey done by R L Associates (1987) for the American Association of Retired Persons and the Villers Foundation (now Families USA), 47 percent of the respondents replied that someone in their family had needed long-term care at some time in the past, and an additional 14 percent of the respondents had friends who had to find or provide long-term care for a spouse or parent. Of the respondents, 60 percent felt strongly, and 27 percent agreed somewhat, that the absence of a long-term care program is a national family crisis. In terms of responsibility, 86 percent felt that it may be time to consider some kind of government action or insurance program, such as Social Security or Medicare, to help with long-term care. Sixty-one percent felt that a federal government program should be an entitlement program rather than one available only to the poor; 27 percent thought it should serve only the poor.

### Pressures from Within the Firm

Declining fertility rates combined with longer life expectancies have increased the number of elderly people relative to the nonelderly. In 1900, 4 percent of the population was aged 65 or over; in 1988, the elderly represented more than 12 percent of the population. As the number of elderly people grows relative to the number of nonelderly, the financing of public programs such as Social Security, Medicare, and Medicaid becomes an increasingly important public policy issue. Social Security benefits have already been reduced and taxes increased by the 1977 and 1983 Social Security Amendments, which help maintain the program's financial integrity through at least the year 2030. Medicare is projected to experience financial difficulties by 1995, and Medicaid, despite the growing number of people likely to need assistance, is expected to continue to contain program expenditures by restricting access to health care.

The insolvency of the Medicare program and actions by states to contain Medicaid expenditures will precede the retirement of the baby boom generation that is now between the ages 26 and 45. Population projections indicate that in the year 2030 the number of elderly persons will increase by 140 percent, and increase the proportion of elderly to 21 percent and the proportion that is aged 85 or over to 5 percent.

Declining fertility rates will also slow the growth rate of the labor force and thus the number of potential taxpayers and consumers. Projections to the year 2000 place the annual growth rate at around 1.2 percent—less than one-half the average growth rate during the 1970s. Projections of annual growth rates beyond the year 2000 are even smaller (0.27 percent through the year 2055). Relatively tighter labor markets are likely to raise the cost of labor to employers. Employer responses to these increases are likely to vary, depending partly on the products produced, but for most employers the cost of production is likely to rise.

Tighter labor markets could also result in lowered minimum hiring standards. Concern about the quality of future workers has already prompted some larger employers to focus attention and money on the public school system. More than 64 percent of 130 major corporations recently surveyed ranked primary and secondary education as their major concern, an increase from 42 percent two years earlier (The Conference Board, 1988). Even if wages are not driven up, training costs (including remedial education) may raise the unit cost of labor.

As the composition of the labor force changes, employers are likely to experience new pressures from employees to consider a different mix of employee benefits. Two aspects of this change include the larger number of working mothers and the increasing number of adults with a chronically ill parent or family member. Most of the growth in the labor market has been among women in general, and women with young children in particular. Since women born during the baby boom are still in their childbearing years, the demand for day care is likely to increase in the short run.

Declining fertility rates not only reduce the growth in new employees and new taxpayers but also mean that there will be fewer adults to assist parents and family members with chronic disabilities. Longer life expectancies without commensurate reductions in disability means that more people will need long-term care. Increasing numbers of employees will become caregivers. Recognition that Medicare, supplemental Medicare insurance (Medigap), and other forms of health insurance do not cover long-term care and that coordinating this care is confusing, stressful, and time consuming may also encourage the formation of new employee benefits.

As members of the baby boom generation advance to senior positions in their firms while providing long-term health care at home, employers are more likely to evaluate the actual and potential needs

253

of their employees as caregivers. A growing share of employees may be willing to see their compensation restructured to include some form of long-term care insurance or elder care benefits. The absence of this development, however, is likely to intensify pressure either to establish or expand public programs or to mandate employer-provided assistance.

*Rising Health Care Costs*—Any enthusiasm over the prospects for restructuring employee compensation to address long-term care must be tempered by the state of crisis felt by employers over their health care plans. Managing health care costs has once again become of primary concern to employers. The issue of managing health care costs has become quite emotional since many employers went through significant changes in their health plans to initiate cost management strategies following the 1982 recession. During that period, many firms saw profits decline appreciably while health care costs increased. Since then, the rate of growth of health care expenditures in nominal or current dollar terms has subsided, but in real terms, that is, adjusted for the general rise in prices, it has not (Friedland, 1987b) (chart VII.2). From 1970 to 1987, employer health care expenditures increased 6.9 percent per year in real terms.[7]

As large payers of health care expenses (employers, insurers, and public payers) have moved to control expenditures, health care providers have found it increasingly difficult to finance uncompensated care. Providers' responses, in turn, have resulted in making it even more difficult for those without health insurance to obtain care. Since the percentage of the population without health insurance has not declined despite the economic recovery, legislators have increasingly looked to legislative solutions to assist those without health insurance. Since 1982, more than 15 percent of the population has been found to be without any source of health insurance. In 1986, an estimated 17 percent of the nonelderly population, or 37 million Americans, were without any source of health insurance (Chollet, 1988b).

*Postretirement Medical Benefits*—Employers have become increasingly concerned about their postretirement health plans. Since neither vesting nor funding standards for retiree health benefits are specified in law, very few employers have funded the accruing liability for retiree health benefits, either for active workers or retirees. Employers who did fund plans were limited by the Deficit Reduction Act of 1984, which placed stringent ceilings on tax-qualified contributions to retir-

---

[7]For more on the role and response of employers in the changing health care market, see McArdle (1987) and Employee Benefit Research Institute (1989).

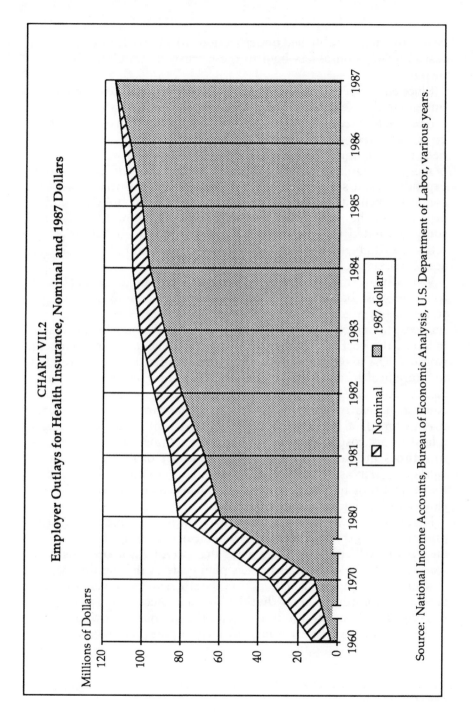

CHART VII.2

Employer Outlays for Health Insurance, Nominal and 1987 Dollars

Millions of Dollars

Source: National Income Accounts, Bureau of Economic Analysis, U.S. Department of Labor, various years.

ee health trusts established under section 501(c)(9) of the tax code and taxed earnings on assets held in these trusts as unrelated business income.

Since employer policy toward retiree health benefits has been largely unregulated by federal law, employers have generally believed themselves free to alter or terminate health benefits for both current workers and retirees already receiving benefits. However, over the last decade, when employers have attempted to terminate plans as part of mergers, acquisitions, or bankruptcy reorganizations, or to contain expenditures, a series of court cases have upheld retirees' rights to continued benefits based on the wording of plan documents and the depiction of the plan to workers and retirees (Schmidt, 1989). One study estimated that in 1988, the value of unfunded liabilities for retiree health benefits was $91 billion for retirees and $188 billion for active workers (Chollet, 1989).

Virtually all employers finance postretirement medical benefits on a current-cost basis rather than funding the accruing liability by setting aside funds during employees' active work lives. While current-cost financing does not change the cost of the benefits provided, it forces the cost of benefits for current beneficiaries onto current workers. The magnitude of the unfunded liability is directly related to future health care costs and the number of retirees. Financing on a current-cost basis becomes more or less expensive depending on a company's relative growth. For instance, the current cost of postretirement medical benefits per active employee will be relatively small if health care costs do not increase and the number of active workers to retirees increases. However, if the number of retirees to active workers is increasing—the situation for many employers—the cost of the postretirement plan per employee will also increase. Rising health care costs further accelerate plan costs.[8]

Regardless of whether a plan is financed on a current basis or is prefunded, longer life expectancies will mean that retiree health insurance plans will cost more. For plans that prefund, the propensity of workers to retire earlier also raises plan costs as the funding period is shortened and the benefit period lengthened. However, the real issue for employers today is that the Financial Accounting Standards Board has declared its intent to require that accountants who adhere to the profession's standards identify on a corporation's balance sheet

---

[8]From 1985 to 1986, employer costs for health insurance increased four times faster than general prices.

the accruing unfunded liability associated with postretirement medical benefits. The addition of a liability without a corresponding asset is likely to affect the corporation's ability to raise capital. To the extent that undisclosed estimates of a firm's unfunded liabilities have not been anticipated in stock prices, the first reports could dramatically affect stock prices. This additional information could also raise the interest rate a corporation would have to pay for money raised either by issuing bonds or by borrowing from a bank.

*Employees and Long-Term Care*—Trying to keep a family member out of an institution is likely to adversely affect employees and consequently employers. If employees use sick leave, come in late, leave early, extend lunch hours, or need to make personal telephone calls because they are trying to juggle two or three hats at once—employee, parent, and caretaker or care coordinator—their work probably suffers. Productivity can also be impaired when an employee refuses to accept a promotion, reduces his or her hours, or quits because he or she is caring for someone who is chronically ill. Studies suggest that from 12 percent to 30 percent of caretakers have quit their jobs to become full-time caregivers (Brody et al., 1987).

Providing long-term care for aging family members affects women particularly. More than 70 percent of informal caregivers are women.[9] Women who leave the work force to raise their children typically lower their earning potential (Fuchs, 1983). Consequently, as daughters or daughters-in-law, they may have fewer disincentives to leave the labor market again to care for an elderly parent (because their wages are likely to be lower than their husbands'). Women tend to marry men older than themselves and because of their longer life expectancy will continue to compose a disproportionate share of the single elderly. As younger spouses, women are more likely to become caregivers to their ailing husbands. In addition, as spouses and as widows, women are more likely to bear the financial burden of uncovered expenses incurred with their husbands' illnesses.[10] In 1988, among people aged 65 to 74 living in the community, the ratio of women to men was 1.3 to 1; among those aged 75 to 84, the ratio was 1.7 to 1; and among people aged 85 or older, the ratio of women to men was 2.6 to 2 (Bureau of the Census, 1988d).

---

[9]EBRI tabulations of the 1982 National Long-Term Care Survey.

[10]Using longitudinal data, it has been estimated that widows have a 30 percent greater likelihood of becoming impoverished than they would have if their husbands had not died (Holden, Burkhauser, and Myers, 1986, table 3).

Women who reduce their work hours, change jobs, or leave the labor force to become caregivers may be less likely during their retirement years to be in a position to finance health care needs that are not covered by Medicare or other health insurance. Any diminution of financial independence is exacerbated by the fact that women are more likely to need long-term care, since they tend to report lower health status and more chronic conditions than men the same age (Verbrugge, 1982).

As more employees begin to recognize the need for current financing and delivery of long-term care, they may be increasingly willing to restructure their employee compensation package to include the purchase of long-term care insurance. On the other hand, their recognition could lead to additional political pressure to expand Medicare and Medicaid. At this point, it is too soon to know. Extensive education and debate are necessary before a national consensus emerges. Unfortunately, for most people, that education is a result of first-hand experience.

## Issues for Restructuring Employee Benefits

Decline in productivity, concern for employees, and employees' growing awareness of the limits of Medicare coverage (as well as the coverage of other health insurance policies) could encourage employers to restructure employee benefits to include information and counseling, time off to care for a dependent, and alternative delivery or financing options such as adult day care or long-term care insurance. Conferences and workshops for human resource specialists are increasingly addressing long-term care insurance and elder care issues.

Employers seem increasingly aware of how dependent care can affect productivity, absenteeism, labor turnover, and morale. However, relatively few large firms have taken formal action to counter these potential problems. In a survey of personnel executives in 1988, 71 percent recognized the potential loss associated with caregiving demands; however, not more than 5 percent of 1,000 large corporations had instituted formal benefit changes (Saltford and Heck, 1989).

A few relatively large employers have taken bold and innovative steps toward direct involvement in the delivery and financing of long-term care. Most of these firms have moved toward formalizing elder care benefits such as flexible hours or time off. Others have added sources of assistance through their employee assistance programs. IBM, for example, has established a nationwide referral network that provides employees in any of its locations with help in finding assistance for their parents, who may well live on the other side of the country.

As stated earlier, more than 35 employers as of September 1989 provided access to long-term care insurance programs for their retirees, their active workers, or both. The plans offered to active workers were also available to their spouses and to the workers' and spouses' parents. In most of these plans the parents could purchase the insurance regardless of whether or not the employee participated. For the employer, these plans incur the expenses of soliciting and evaluating bids from insurers; informing and educating employees through brochures, leaflets, and meetings; and administering the payroll deductions for the purchase of the insurance. Premiums are paid by employees or their dependents who are eligible to purchase the insurance. Financial risk associated with the insurance plan seems to be held at arm's length from the employer.

The approach taken thus far may not fully accommodate other concerns such as employee retention. As currently structured, once an employee has gained access to a group insurance policy, participation is no longer contingent on his or her employment. The employer has done a great service by educating consumers and giving them the opportunity to purchase a policy at 20 percent to 30 percent less than the same policy sold individually, but the employee can continue to purchase the same policy upon leaving the employer.[11]

The Task Force on Long-Term Health Care Policies issued a series of 41 recommendations that would encourage development of the private insurance market (Task Force on Long-Term Health Care Policies, 1987). The report explicitly recognized the need to promote the availability of long-term care insurance through employment. It recommended that, at the very least, tax laws should not discourage employers from making long-term care insurance available to employees through cafeteria plans and flexible spending accounts. It also recommended that individuals be permitted to use vested pension and retirement savings (including IRAs, Keogh plans, annuities, and stock bonus and employee stock ownership plans) to purchase long-term care insurance either before or after retirement and avoid taxation on the transfer.

This proposal may not be feasible for defined benefit pension plans because the present value of the defined benefit is based on current,

---

[11]There may be a handling charge associated with the individual billing, but it is not likely to be more than 2 percent of the premium.

not projected, salary. Consequently, the value of the defined benefit pension plan over most workers' careers may be too small to pay long-term care insurance premiums. Another difficulty would be how long-term care insurance would be treated in terms of joint and survivor annuity elections. Furthermore, there is the question of what would happen in the case of divorce settlements that include a pension.

The proposal assumes that individuals will be motivated by the relative advantages provided by long-term care coverage; namely, that withdrawn funds used to purchase long-term care insurance and any benefits paid by the plan are tax exempt. The relative tax advantage, however, may not be a compelling argument for workers to invest in long-term care insurance, given the illiquidity and risk of the investment in conjunction with recently reduced marginal tax rates.

Some observers have recommended setting up special trusts or expanding existing funding vehicles to pay for long-term care or long-term care insurance. The Task Force on Long-Term Health Care Policies recommended removal of the restrictions on funding postretirement medical benefits on a tax-preferred basis that were imposed in the Deficit Reduction Act of 1984. During the 100th Congress, Sen. Dave Durenberger (R-MN) introduced a bill to amend the tax code to provide "uniform Federal tax treatment for employer-provided health care benefits for retired employees." The bill would have established a new retiree health care trust for the payment of benefits provided to former employees (or their spouses) after they have reached age 70. Rep. Rod Chandler (R-WA) introduced a similar bill to amend the tax code to, among other things, expand the postretirement health and long-term care benefits that may be provided through a pension plan. Essentially, this approach would have relied on existing trusts, such as those available through Internal Revenue Code (IRC) section 401(h) and cash or deferred arrangements under IRC section 401(k), to enable an employer to pay for medical and long-term care benefits.

Restructuring employee benefits to include consideration of long-term care or long-term care insurance may require the development of criteria to evaluate the different proposals. For instance, it seems reasonable that the value of a long-term care insurance plan plus the asset value of a reduced pension benefit be at least equivalent to the value of the pension benefit that would have resulted if long-term care insurance had not been purchased. That is, purchase of long-term care insurance should not result in reduced total asset value at retirement. This may be difficult to achieve if the benefits paid by the insurance plan are unindexed and if the long-term care insurance plan provides current coverage as well as an accumulation to finance future coverage. Whether the reduction in future retirement well-being is significant will depend on the amount of the premium associated with current coverage.

Another criterion might be that adequate retirement income should not be reduced for retirees who never need long-term care. While all retirees need adequate income, not all will be functionally dependent. But what constitutes adequate income is a subjective matter. Nevertheless, any proposal to reduce disposable retirement income must recognize some standard for income adequacy. In addition, workers who reduce their pensions in exchange for long-term care insurance must not lose asset value because they fail to make annual contributions to the plan. That is, either the insurance must be portable or the prefunded portion of the long-term care insurance must be returned to the employee. An important strength of the pension system—and particularly of defined contribution pensions—is that a change in employment does not diminish the value of the accumulated asset even if no additional contributions are made.

Finally, long-term care insurance and a reduced pension must be adequate to ensure access to long-term care. Long-term care insurance that does not pay for the services needed does not, by itself, guarantee access to long-term care. Rapid price increases of long-term care services, in conjunction with insufficient retirement income, may limit an individual's ability to afford the care for which insurance was purchased and retirement income reduced.

## Conclusion

The baby boom has had a tremendous effect on our society. The entry of baby boomers into the labor force, in conjunction with the increased labor force participation of women, has tended to hold down real wages (Andrews and Davis, 1988). Public entitlement programs, financed on a pay-as-you-go basis, have expanded. These programs will eventually face increased claims on the entitlements financed by a growing number of beneficiaries relative to the growing number of potential taxpayers. Longer life expectancies due to declining mortality, but without commensurate reductions in chronic disabilities, are likely to increase the duration of Social Security benefit payments and to increase the probability of a greater use of health care services. Medicaid, too, seems destined to incur a growing portion of these expenditures or be forced to reduce access to care.

Regardless of what employers do, they are likely to be affected by the declining growth of entry-age workers over the next 18 years. In particular, the cost of labor is likely to rise. As the baby boom generation begins to retire, the labor market could become tighter, raising the cost of labor. Upward pressure on wages, however, might not result in an increase in wages for all workers, depending on the distribution of workers responding to the shifts in employment opportunities (Andrews and Davis, 1988). Tighter labor markets could, however, mean that minimum hiring standards are lowered. Concern about the quality of future workers has already prompted some larger employers to focus attention and money on the public school system. More than 64 percent of the 130 major corporations surveyed by the Conference Board ranked primary and secondary education as their major concern, an increase from 42 percent two years earlier (Conference Board, 1988). Even if wages are not driven up, training costs (including remedial education) might raise the unit cost of labor.

The cost of labor could also rise as a result of family problems that hinder productivity. More employees are likely to be desperately coping with a chronically disabled family member. Recognition that Medicare, Medigap, or other forms of health insurance, including employer-provided health insurance, do not cover long-term care, and that coordinating this care is confusing, stressful, and time consuming, may lead to the development of new employee benefits.

Although the shift in the age and composition of the work force will occur over a 50-year period, employers and the public sector have already started to respond to some of the anticipated and initial pressures. Social Security benefits have been reduced for future retirees while taxes were raised, newly expanded Medicare benefits are to be financed entirely by beneficiaries, and some employers have established elder care and long-term care insurance benefits.

The emergence of employment-based long-term care insurance offers tremendous potential for enhancing the economic security of millions of Americans. Legislators have an opportunity to affect the scope and depth of these policies as they are developing rather than after the fact. While the IRS decides whether questions about the tax code are points merely needing clarification or requiring changes in the law, legislation could go beyond clarification and explicitly encourage employers to provide long-term care or long-term care insurance. However, for the most part, employer interest in elder care and long-term care insurance remains tentative at best.

Employment-based group long-term care insurance offers the potential to provide broad-based financing for long-term care. Group-based long-term care insurance, like group health insurance, would be less expensive than the same coverage sold outside the group due to lower marketing and administrative costs. Costs would also be lower because insurers would have a greater opportunity to minimize the effects of adverse selection by selling policies to people unlikely to need the coverage immediately. Moreover, the demand for insurance coverage is likely to grow as more people become aware of the protection it provides. The broader the distribution of insurance coverage, the more likely it is that expansion of the private market will alter public program expenditures.

As more members of the baby boom advance in their firms and begin to provide long-term health care, employers are likely to evaluate their employees' actual and potential long-term care needs. A growing share of employees may be willing to see their compensation restructured to include some form of long-term care insurance or elder care benefit. If employers and employees decide to include long-term care insurance as part of compensation, there is a chance that an equitable public-private partnership could emerge in the area of financing and delivery of long-term care. If employers and employees decide not to finance long-term care insurance as an employee benefit designed to enhance retirement income security, there is an even stronger likelihood that employers and employees will be financing a public program aimed at providing long-term care.

# VIII. Altering the Public-Private Partnership

## Introduction

During the last 10 years, public debate over long-term care has shifted from issues concerning the delivery of care to the question of who should pay. Ten years ago, service and delivery options, availability of care, and quality of care were almost always central to the public policy debate, while any discussion of financing focused on what benefits ought to be covered and on what terms. The debate has also shifted increasingly toward a private-sector solution because of heightened awareness of the emerging long-term care cost burden, the acceptance of increasingly tight fiscal constraints (Lawlor and Pollak, 1985), and overall improvements in the elderly's financial position (Wiener et al., 1986; Rivlin and Wiener, 1988).

Economic and political perceptions brought about by the federal budget deficit may be responsible for this shift in emphasis, but so too may be the recognition that delivery flows from financing. The revenue necessary to finance a public program, or the revenue forgone as a result of tax-favored private financing, can be substantial. Financing, however, is really a means to an end—the delivery of long-term care. Ultimately, it is the availability and effectiveness of long-term care that counts. Furor over financing, however, could impede the formulation of adequate goals from which to appropriately evaluate policy alternatives.

Different perspectives and agendas will lead to different considerations, making the goals for long-term care quite varied. There may be a consensus that our long-term care delivery system ought to provide, fairly and equitably, the most effective, least costly set of services and equipment that promote functional independence and rehabilitation while recognizing the efforts and capacities of family members, the availability of community services, and the dignity of functionally dependent people (Callahan and Wallack, 1981; Pollak, 1986; Somers, 1985; Kane and Kane, 1987; Rivlin and Wiener, 1988). But even reaching a consensus on this primary goal will not necessarily lead to a consensus on how to evaluate the merits of different financing options. Reaching such a consensus will require agreement on such diverse questions as what is fair and equitable, what is effective long-term care, and what is functional dependence. Establishing standards

265

requires an understanding of available community resources and a decision as to what constitutes an acceptable role for the family.

## Financing Long-Term Care: Sorting Public from Private Dollars

Long-term care is currently funded through a combination of public and private financing. In 1987, long-term care expenditures probably exceeded $56.4 billion, with slightly more than one-half (52 percent) financed through public sources, and slightly less than one-half financed through private sources (see chapter IV). Nearly one-half (49 percent) of all nursing home expenditures, which probably accounted for 72 percent of all long-term care expenditures, were financed directly from federal, state, and local public programs. However, more than one-half of nursing home residents received public assistance. Furthermore, more than three-quarters (78.3 percent) of what is classified in the National Health Care Expenditures data as "other personal health care," which includes home health care, is also financed directly through public programs.

Most public expenditures for long-term care are made by Medicaid, but the role of Medicare is more substantial than is usually recognized. Although the size of the expenditure is difficult to estimate, Medicare pays for long-term care delivered in a hospital when poorly delivered long-term care, either at home or in a nursing facility, requires acute care intervention (Vladeck, 1985b). In addition, Medicare prospective payments to hospitals for acute care include expenses associated with delays in getting a hospital patient into a nursing home or arranging appropriate home care. While Medicare prospective hospital payments may encourage earlier discharges, the difficulties in locating a nursing home bed or arranging for sufficient in-home care diminish some of the force of this incentive.

While the mix of public and private dollars may be close to even, distribution of the financing burden is not. Most private expenditures for long-term care are derived directly from those who need the care. On the other hand, most public expenditures for financing long-term care are derived from general revenues. Federal expenditures are primarily financed through income taxes, while at the state and local levels expenditures are financed through a combination of income, sales, and property taxes. The public policy discussion seems to focus on two different aspects of this financing—the emotional issues stemming from the fairness of private financing and the rising cost of publicly financed health care, especially in light of the changing age distribution of the population. Despite this dichotomy of concerns, most public action has focused on limiting public program expenditures at the expense of those who need long-term care. From 1983 to 1987, total expenditures for nursing home care increased 38.1 percent, private expenditures increased 41.1 percent, and public expenditures increased 34.5 percent.

Subtle but vital components of the public policy debate on long-term care are the issues of access and quality. Efficient and effective care means that care is delivered without compromising either the quantity or the quality of care desired by society. As suggested in chapter III, current care delivery (including access and quality) is a direct consequence of the way long-term care has been financed. Public policy decision makers must determine what type of long-term care is to be considered. Should it be only nursing home care or the full range of services needed to maintain independence? Another way of framing this question is: what is it that we want to buy? We may, for example, through tax policy, want to encourage private insurance that covers nursing home care, or we may wish to finance nonrecuperative or chronic nursing home care through the Medicare program, but in either case, do we want to buy or subsidize this care as it is now delivered?

Technological change in the delivery of long-term care is bound to be influenced by the availability of financing. However, we have a relatively limited understanding of what is effective long-term care. We do know that care received at home is preferred to care received in an institution and that the quality of nursing home care responds to different types of caregiving interventions. We also know that case management offers the means to coordinate care and to rationalize and control expenditures, and that assessment and intervention can alter the course of care of functionally impaired people slated for admission to nursing homes (Kane and Kane, 1987; Farfel, 1988). But we know little about how to structure reimbursement mechanisms to foster better care, let alone how to organize the delivery of such care. The scientific basis for evaluating effective care through medicine and gerontology is just emerging. This basis is critical to the development of rational public policy. Ultimately, the challenge for public policy is to promote a financing system that encourages the effective delivery of care. But since this goal is still elusive, the challenge is to encourage the development of effective care, to avoid discouraging advances in technology, and to enable continuous incorporation of more effective care into the delivery system.

The main focus of the emerging public policy discussion has been how to distribute long-term care costs. Most of this debate centers on whether financing ought to be primarily public or private. Implicit in this debate has been the recognition that long-term care is an insurable event. Whether insurance ought to be primarily public or private is the central issue. Movements for reform in either direction have been complicated by different and sometimes competing goals. Consequently, public policy toward long-term care financing is likely to include both public and private funding, possibly leading to an uneasy partnership between the public and private sectors.

## The Case for Private Financing

The case for expanding private financing options is based on the argument that the private insurance market can more efficiently distribute resources and satisfy people's diverse needs. The private insurance market, it is asserted, has been slow to emerge due to inhibiting market barriers. Public intervention is necessary but only to assist in removing some of the impediments. Conducting an educational campaign to encourage demand for long-term care insurance, clarifying or altering tax laws or other laws governing the market, establishing a reinsurance program for private insurance, or collecting data that would assist in the pricing and development of a private market are a few of the types of government activities often suggested that could assist in market development.

It is usually suggested that the market has been slow to develop because the public underestimates and therefore undervalues the financial consequences and risks of needing long-term care. A government campaign to educate citizens about what Medicare does and does not cover, as well as how Medicaid works, and tax incentives that would advertise the desirability of purchasing long-term care insurance are examples of the types of government activities most often suggested that could make consumers aware of the need for long-term care insurance.[1] Insurers have been slow to develop products because of the lack of demand and the uncertainty of how insurance laws and tax laws would apply. The products that have been developed include many provisions that limit benefits in a manner

---

[1] The Medicare Catastrophic Coverage Act of 1988 requires that the Secretary of Health and Human Services annually inform Medicare beneficiaries of what Medicare does and does not cover. In compliance with the law, the first notification was mailed out at the end of January 1989.

that enables insurers to anticipate financial liabilities without appropriate data.

It has been suggested that public policy that eliminates these supply and demand barriers could lead to market expansion, enabling consumers to choose an insurance product that best matches their needs, tastes, and preferences. The expansion of private insurance to middle-income Americans, in particular, could reduce the number from this income group who need Medicaid, enabling a larger percentage of the Medicaid budget to be spent on others in poverty. The preference for a largely private insurance market over a public social insurance program approach also stems from the belief that the private market better serves consumer preferences, offers less potential for waste, and is more likely to be sensitive to consumer demand. Competition among insurers and among providers would help to force insurance companies to design and price policies according to consumer demand.

By comparison, a public program is not considered likely to encourage the same variety and choice that might emerge in a private market. Depending on how a public program is established, it might not be subject to market discipline but rather to congressional action and, therefore, to the demands of special interest groups. In addition, financing a larger share of long-term care through the private sector would reduce the government's explicit financial obligations and consequently some of the tension associated with the budget process that puts groups such as the elderly and the nonelderly into direct competition.

### The Case for Public Financing

The case for expanding public financing of long-term care is frequently made by citing the failure of a large percentage of Americans to purchase adequate insurance protection. As highlighted in chapter VI, economic theory suggests many reasons why *individual* private insurance that provides real protection (i.e., inflation-adjusted service benefits) is unlikely to be held by most citizens. The market is plagued by a variety of structural and plan design problems, including the potential for adverse selection (the propensity of those who are more inclined to use the benefit to purchase the insurance). This disproportionately increases the cost of insurance. Other problems include uncertainty over the use of long-term care services due to the existence of insurance (moral hazard), the rising risk with age of needing long-term care, increasing and unpredictable long-term care costs, a lack of reliable actuarial data for pricing policies, and ambiguity in the tax code and in state insurance regulations.

269

As of January 1989, a relatively small percentage of the population had purchased long-term care insurance—perhaps 4 percent of the elderly and a negligible percentage of the nonelderly. However, as suggested in chapter VI, despite all the barriers against it, a market has emerged and is growing at a phenomenal rate. Ironically, some contend that as private financing options grow and more middle- and high-income individuals purchase policies, the emerging gap between those most likely to receive assistance from the state (mostly through Medicaid) and those who can afford long-term care insurance coverage could encourage the establishment of a publicly financed program.[2]

Accepting the idea that private insurance will expand neither far enough nor fast enough leads to the question of whether to provide insurance through a public program. This concept has meant expanding or improving Medicaid or creating a new social insurance program. The case for making long-term care benefit entitlements subject to a means test (as exists in Medicaid) is based on the fact that the program would target limited public resources to persons with greatest financial need. Also supporting this approach are those who argue that public policy should not protect the assets of the wealthy. However, for those with health insurance who happen to have a fatal heart attack, this asset protection argument is rarely made. That is, we do not expect heart attack victims to sell their homes. On the other hand, Medicaid already finances the bulk of publicly financed long-term care. Easing Medicaid eligibility requirements to improve the social "safety net" could be viewed as a logical extension of current public policy.

The case for expanding the public sector through a social insurance or Medicare-like approach is usually made with the acknowledgement that long-term care is insurable, and is advanced on more altruistic grounds. Social insurance can provide universal coverage to all who qualify (the disabled or the elderly), the costs can be shared by all taxpayers through income taxes or by workers (and to some degree employers) through payroll taxes, administrative economies can be realized, and any cost problems associated with adverse selection could be avoided by universal coverage of the population (Davis and Rowland, 1986). Furthermore, concern over government involvement in preserving private assets could be mitigated by requiring income-

---

[2]This point originated in a speech by Stanley S. Wallack at the Fourth Annual Private Long-Term Care Insurance Conference, Washington, DC, March 1–2, 1988.

related premiums and/or deductibles and asset-related estate and gift taxes. Establishing a universal entitlement program lessens the differences in access to and quality of care between private paying patients and those receiving Medicaid (Rivlin and Wiener, 1988). Unlike private insurance, a social insurance approach can be used to meet other objectives, such as redistributing income, and can be financed in a variety of ways, including on a pay-as-you-go basis.

## Modifying Public Policy to Facilitate Private Financing

Most public policy options to facilitate private financing of long-term care have centered around use of the tax code to encourage product development. Alternatively, the government could intervene directly by becoming an insurer or a long-term care provider. It could build nursing facilities or adult day care facilities to compete with proprietary facilities. It could sponsor the development of case management systems utilizing, for example, Area Agencies on Aging—a structure that already is integrated with local community-based services throughout the United States. In addition, the government already owns and operates a fairly extensive long-term care delivery system through the Veterans Administration (VA). It is feasible that the VA system could be expanded or allowed to compete with private providers.

Historically, however, public policy has tended to encourage government intervention in either the production or purchase of goods and services that the market fails to provide. One analyst contends that, despite the advantages of relying on the market to allocate resources or even to provide information to regulators, there is a deep-seated bias in our political system in favor of intervening through direct determination of products by regulation and other forms of centralized bureaucracy. For example, there has been a strong commitment to public education rather than to individual subsidies to ensure uniform access to private education. Another example is the overwhelming bias favoring the use of direct regulation rather than tax incentives to encourage pollution control. Despite the information collection and resource allocation advantages of the market and previous failed attempts by the government to intervene in areas where the market exists, this bias seems to remain (Schultze, 1977). Perhaps this bias is the basis for Alan Blinder's "Murphy's Law of Economic Policy." He argues quite convincingly that economists are less influential in public policy areas in which they are, for the most part, in agreement, but are highly influential in public policy areas in which they know the least and disagree the most (Blinder, 1987).

As discussed in chapter VI, there has been a great deal of ambiguity in the tax code with respect to long-term care insurance. This has tended to discourage the development of private financing approaches. There are basic questions concerning the tax treatment of long-term care insurance premiums, long-term care benefits, and, prior to April 1989, the tax treatment of long-term care insurance reserves. While these ambiguities in the tax code are not the only factors inhibiting employer interest in long-term care insurance, they have contributed to it. In addition to clarifying current tax treatment, public policy discussions have also suggested additional tax preferences to encourage the development of the private market for public purposes.

### Using the Tax Code to Meet Social Goals

Congress has frequently used the tax code to promote or attain specific social and economic goals. Allowing the deduction of interest for a home mortgage, for example, was an explicit attempt in the 1950s to encourage, subsidize, and support home ownership. In the debate over using tax policy to facilitate private financing of long-term care, the following questions must be answered.

- Do we want to use tax policy to encourage individuals to save specifically for long-term care or long-term care insurance?
- Do we want to use tax policy to encourage employers to provide access to long-term care insurance?
- Do we want to use tax policy to influence the characteristics and provisions of long-term care insurance?
- Do we want to use tax policy to reward, encourage, or adjust for the informal and formal support provided by families to functionally dependent relatives?

An affirmative answer to any of these questions raises other questions: How do we best use the tax code to facilitate our goal or goals? How do we determine who bears the tax burden and who benefits from the special tax treatment?

Every provision in the tax code that is not used by all taxpayers constitutes a subsidy of those who do take advantage of the provision by those who do not. Because some people use a provision and others do not, tax revenues are less than they otherwise would have been. To raise a specific amount of revenue, the tax burden on everyone else must be increased. The difference between the amount of tax revenues collected and the amount that would have been collected if special provisions in the tax code were not exercised is referred to as a tax

272

expenditure. The questions from a public policy perspective are: who bears the burden of the tax expenditure (that is, the exclusion, exemption, deduction, or credit), and how does the burden compare to the social benefit? In terms of long-term care, to what degree would a special tax provision enable a broad spectrum of individuals of different financial means to finance their long-term care and how would the provision alter public expenditures relative to what they would have been in the absence of the provision? This is an issue for which data are limited.

### Specific Public Policy Options to Encourage Private Financing

Public policy options that would use the tax code to encourage private financing of long-term care include:

- Establishing special savings accounts, the earnings of which would be tax deferred and the contributions to which would be subject to either a tax credit or a tax deduction;
- Providing a tax credit or tax deduction for the purchase of qualified long-term care insurance;
- Enabling workers and retirees to convert retirement income into long-term care insurance without paying taxes on the retirement income; and
- Enabling employers to establish a trust fund, the earnings of which would not be subject to taxation and the contributions to which could be based on the expected cost of long-term care or long-term care insurance after a current worker retires.

It has been suggested that by establishing a special savings account similar to an individual retirement account (IRA), individuals could take responsibility for their own long-term care needs. The advantage of such an approach is that it would encourage saving and maximize individual freedom and preferences. The disadvantage is that it would not guarantee access to either long-term care or long-term care insurance. Furthermore, if accounts were opened only by those most able to afford long-term care, public expenditures for this care would not be reduced, but tax revenues would be.

Experience with IRAs has shown that even prior to the restrictions imposed in the Tax Reform Act of 1986, participation was not widespread. EBRI tabulations of the May 1983 EBRI/U.S. Department of Health and Human Services Current Population Survey pension supplement indicated that in 1982 only 17 percent of workers had IRAs. Internal Revenue Service data indicate that in 1986, 15.2 percent of all returns claimed an IRA deduction. Participation among those with adjusted gross income (AGI) of less than $20,000 was 4.1 percent, while among those with AGI in excess of $100,000 participation was 46.1 percent (Shiley and Kalish, 1987-1988).

Given that most long-term care financing proposals based on this concept would limit withdrawals to specific circumstances, it is hard to imagine that the reduced liquidity of such an account would foster wider participation, especially if many people in their working years fail to assess the risk of needing long-term care.[3] Furthermore, saving for long-term care is inefficient and, for many persons, infeasible. Assuming rates of return in an IRA at 1 percent greater than inflation, an individual at age 40 saving for an anticipated nursing home stay of three years at age 80 would need to save (in current dollars) an additional $1,677 per year. If this person relegated this saving to just their working years and retired at age 67, then additional savings would have to be $2,124 a year. If retirement was planned for age 58, then additional savings for long-term care would have to be nearly $4,000 a year.

Providing a tax credit or deduction for long-term care insurance would directly subsidize the cost of an insurance policy. But while this may make a policy affordable for some, the real value of the tax incentive is the public awareness created by attracting taxpayers to a line item credit or deduction. However, if the prices of policies are too high relative to family budgets, it is not likely that the credit or deduction will encourage the purchase of insurance among lower-income individuals. The greater the participation rate among higher-income individuals relative to those with lower income, the greater the subsidy from all taxpayers to those most able to afford long-term care insurance.

Enabling employers to institute a trust fund to finance long-term care or long-term care insurance for retirees would require a definition of employee rights and employer obligations. Employers will not want to establish a fund that incurs a potentially large and unpredictable financial liability, nor will they willingly fund a trust that is not protected from becoming a target for a corporate takeover. Furthermore, unless the promised benefit is simply cash and access to a long-term care insurance policy, the proposition suggested is not sufficiently different from simply expanding the current pension law to include another pension fund, the contributions and distributions of which are not subject to current law limitations. One of the advan-

---

[3]As to the additional savings argument, whether individuals merely shifted current savings to IRAs or net savings were actually increased is still a matter of controversy.

tages of this approach is that it would call to employees' attention the need to consider long-term care as a threat to their income security.

Allowing workers and retirees to convert retirement income into long-term care insurance would offer some of the same advantages as setting up a special account. It would make planning for this contingency explicit. However, if vested pension benefits could be used prior to retirement, there is a danger that retirement income could be reduced. How will individuals making transfers from retirement income at age 45 know whether they will be able to afford the reduction in retirement income associated with the transfer (plus the forgone compounded interest) when they retire? Furthermore, unless the insurance policy is tied directly to inflation, it is likely that the value of the employee's retirement income plus the insurance policy will be less than the value of the retirement income in the absence of the policy purchase.

*Alternative Ways to Conceptualize Employment-Based Long-Term Care Insurance*—There are two ways to prefund long-term care insurance over an employee's working years.[4] The primary distinction between them is whether capital accumulation to purchase the benefit in retirement is separate from the insurance plan ("outside funded") or occurs within the insurance plan ("inside funded"). Long-term care insurance policies sold to employers to date have been essentially inside-funded arrangements. Although the probability of needing such coverage is low for young employees, the coverage does have value. One advantage of this approach is that it provides immediate financial protection for long-term care. A second advantage is that employees' ability to continue purchasing the plan after retirement becomes a surer prospect since the price would be substantially lower for long-time participants than if coverage were initially purchased at or near retirement.

The primary disadvantage to employees of an inside-funded long-term care insurance policy is the logistics of moving the value of one policy to another policy when an employee changes employers (see chapter VI). This could be an advantage for employers trying to encourage long employment tenures. However, by using graduated vesting schedules, it may be possible to allow terminated employees the option of buying into the plan or into a conversion policy from the same or another insurance carrier using most of the past policy value while still encouraging longer employment tenures.

---

[4]This classification scheme first appeared in Chollet and Friedland, 1988a.

An outside-funded long-term care insurance plan may be an employer-sponsored capital accumulation plan (for example, a defined contribution pension plan or a qualified cash or deferred arrangement) with guaranteed access to a group long-term care insurance policy at retirement. Assets and interest used to purchase long-term care in retirement would accumulate separately from the insurance plan, and the rate of asset accumulation could be independent of increases in the group plan cost. Employer and employee contributions to the cash accumulation plan, however, could be targeted to enable retirees to fully or substantially pay the projected premium. At retirement, the group insurance could be priced in at least two ways: on a "term" basis (increasing with retiree age and risk), or on an entry-age basis (reflecting the present value of the expected cost over the retiree's expected life). Purchasing a plan that is priced according to entry age is equivalent to an employee initiating an inside-funded plan at retirement.

An outside-funded plan would offer employers one significant advantage: they could avoid liability for increases in the cost of the long-term care benefit. The full indexation of retiree health liability associated with conventional retiree health plans that define benefits in terms of covered services has already posed a critical problem for employers. Presumably, they would want to avoid this situation in devising a long-term care insurance plan. Employers may, in fact, look to an outside funding approach like that described here to finance postretirement health insurance for future retirees in response to the new accounting requirements established by the Financial Accounting Standards Board. An outside-funded plan might also encourage employers to offer retirees coordinated or alternative plans to finance acute and long-term care. Even if an employer were liable for guaranteeing access to a group long-term care plan when participating workers retire, that obligation might be met in an expanding private insurance market for long-term care by negotiating an agreement with one or more insurance carriers.

An outside-funded plan would also offer employees some advantages, especially if such a plan were more acceptable to employers, since access to long-term care coverage would be more widespread. Most importantly, capital accumulation plans enable full portability and the most flexibility. Such plans, however, would place employees at risk for any shortfall between accumulated assets and the price of long-term care coverage at retirement. Although the concept of an outside-funded insurance plan borrows heavily from the concept of a defined contribution pension plan or a qualified cash or deferred arrangement, such as a 401(k) arrangement, it has little or no precedent in employee benefits. Furthermore, unless the tax code were explicitly amended to accommodate such an approach, there would be limitations inhibiting employers from trying to establish such a plan.

However, legislation directed at encouraging both retirement saving and the private market for long-term care could enable the establishment of such an account tied to the purchase or provision of long-term care insurance in the year contributions were made to the account. That is, long-term care coverage for the year could be added to the employer's acute health care plan in exchange for the establishment of a special-use 401(k)-type savings account or defined contribution pension fund for the explicit purpose of purchasing long-term care insurance, long-term care, or supplementing retirement income if all other sources of retirement income are considered to be too low.

Contributions to the account could be limited by age, with amounts targeted to sufficiently cover insurance premiums during retirement years. For workers under age 40, this amount should be around $250 a year and for older workers around $400 a year. Participation rates, however, would depend on whether the employer contributed to the account. In 1986, 61.7 percent of all eligible employees voluntarily participated in 401(k) arrangements (U.S. General Accounting Office, 1988a). Among employer plans that provide generous matches, however, participation has been known to exceed 90 percent.

Merrill Lynch (1988) proposed a variation of the outside-funded approach within the context of a single individual account, called a health care management account (HCMA). Contributions to the HCMA would be apportioned between a savings account and a long-term care insurance fund. A single financial intermediary would handle both the savings and insurance. Presumably, this intermediary might want to contract with an insurer to administer the insurance program. Employee and employer contributions to the HCMA would be on a pretax basis, and interest earned in either part of the account would be tax deferred. The insurance would pay a fixed dollar benefit for four years following a fairly long deductible period (one or more years). The deductible would be paid by the savings account portion of the HCMA with tax-free distributions. For example, if long-term care is needed for six years, the HCMA savings account would be used to finance the first two years. The insurance would contribute toward years three through five, and the balance in the savings account would be applied toward the sixth year. Any remaining balance in the savings portion of the account would belong to the estate. At all times, a portion of the savings account balance would be available for other purposes, but these distributions would be taxed as regular income.

Lewin/ICF analyzed two versions of the HCMA for Merrill Lynch using both their Brookings/ICF long-term care financing model and their macroeconomic demographic model (MDM). They simulated two scenarios, one voluntary and one mandatory. The voluntary scenario was based on the assumption that 80 percent of those who contributed to an IRA (prior to the Tax Reform Act of 1986) would contribute to an HCMA. The mandatory scenario required employee and employer contributions of 3 percent of the worker's earnings annually (6 percent total).[5] Under the voluntary scenario, the simulations suggest that by the year 2016, 37 percent of all elderly people would have an HCMA. Under the mandatory scenario, by the year 2016, 58 percent of the elderly would have an HCMA. Using the MDM, Lewin/ICF reported that with HCMAs, by the year 2020 the Gross National Product (GNP) would be 1.9 percent to 0.7 percent higher, depending on what is assumed about the impact of HCMA contributions on other savings. The more contributions to the HCMA tend to substitute for, and therefore reduce, individual savings, the lower the growth in GNP.[6]

## The Potential for Private Financing of Long-Term Care

### Affording Long-Term Care Insurance

The decision to purchase long-term care insurance depends in part on an individual's or family's income and assets. Using data that include income, assets, and disabilities of people aged 45 or older in 1984, a simple set of propositions was set forth to determine the potential for a broad cross-section of people to purchase long-term care insurance. The basic propositions used were as follows:

- Individuals with limitations that could be considered among either the standard limitations in activities of daily living (ADLs) or instrumental activities of daily living (IADLs) would not be eligible to purchase long-term care insurance.

---

[5]Unlike the Merrill Lynch proposal, which would have a three- or four-year deductible, Lewin/ICF (1988) assumed a three-month deductible.

[6]The supporting documentation does not indicate whether the health care medical account modeled in the macroeconomic demographic model was voluntary or mandatory.

- Individuals would not consider purchasing a long-term care insurance policy unless they had at least $10,000 in net wealth to protect.
- Married couples would not consider purchasing long-term care insurance policies unless their net wealth was at least $10,000.
- If the long-term care insurance policy was only affordable for one spouse, then neither spouse would purchase a policy.
- Individuals with employer-sponsored health insurance and their spouses would be eligible to purchase long-term care insurance for 25 percent less than policies purchased by individuals and couples who had no connection to an employment-based health insurance plan.

A hypothetical entry-age long-term care insurance policy was developed and priced according to the age of each individual eligible to purchase the insurance in 1984.[7] Prices were determined by averaging and interpolating prices from a small group of employment-based long-term care insurance policies that were available in the latter half of 1988 and the first half of 1989. In theory, the base price should reflect a three-year $100-a-day nursing home benefit and a $50-a-day home health benefit, available after a 60-day waiting period. Claims are not allowed until after the policy has been held for six months (i.e., preexisting conditions face a six-month deductible); the policy is guaranteed renewable for life; premiums are waived when benefits are received; prior hospitalization or prior nursing home confinement is not required; and all levels of care are covered. Benefits are triggered by a physician recommendation for care based on two ADL deficits, including cognitive capacity and personal care, such as dressing or bathing, moving about, using the toilet, and eating. Care for individuals with a degenerative brain disease like Alzheimer's disease would also be covered.

Premiums ranged from $254 a year for those who initially purchased the policy at age 45 with access to an employer-provided health insurance plan, to $6,520 a year for 80-year-olds with access to an employer-provided plan. Initial purchase at age 50 placed premiums at $356 a year. Although this simulation excluded people under age 45, initial purchase at age 30 would have placed premiums at around $120 a

---

[7]Entry-age price policies reflect the price at the time of initial purchase. The price does not go up each year with age unless the premiums for the age class must be adjusted. For example, if premiums are $100 a year for a person who initially purchases the policy at age 30, 10 years later that person should still be paying $100 a year, unless the premium charged all 30-year-olds (by the time that person is aged 40) has increased.

year; for those who enrolled in the plan at age 25, the yearly premium would have been closer to $100. For individuals who did not have access to a group long-term care insurance policy, the price was presumed to be 25 percent higher to account for the higher administrative and marketing costs of individual products.

The critical issue in simulating the potential for private insurance to be purchased by most people is determining what constitutes affordability.[8] The most straightforward approach would be to presume that anyone whose insurance premium is within a certain percentage of their income will purchase the insurance. Deciding what the specific percentage ought to be is more problematic. Without good household expenditure data, it is difficult to know how different people would value the insurance and, therefore, how much they would be willing to spend relative to their income. Therefore, this simulation arbitrarily assumed affordability based on the percentage of income premiums represented.

Clearly, while income is necessary to make premium payments, the decision to purchase insurance may be based on accumulated wealth and not on income. Income is not a good proxy for wealth (Cartwright and Friedland, 1985; Chollet and Friedland, 1987).[9] It has been suggested that the best way to measure the elderly's financial capacity is to subtract necessary expenditures (food, medical care, clothing, shelter, and taxes) from available resources (income and assets). The net result is discretionary resources.

Replicating the work of Cohen et al. (1987), discretionary resources were calculated by annuitizing all net wealth except the primary home, adding this to nonasset-produced income (mostly Social Security, earnings, pensions and other sources of retirement income), and using the budget estimates of Cohen et al. to subtract out necessary expenses (which were based on income levels).[10] To estimate who might be able to afford private long-term care insurance, discretionary resources instead of income were used. Discretionary resources are income and assets remaining after necessary expenses. Therefore, it is hypothesized, the percentages arbitrarily selected to determine affordability should be higher than those used for income alone.

---

[8]For other approaches to criteria concerning the decision to purchase long-term care insurance and the financial capacity of the elderly to meet the criteria, see Rivlin and Wiener (1988) and Cohen et al. (1987).

[9]See also chapter 5.

[10]The annuity factor used was based on life expectancy and an interest rate of 7 percent. Annuity factors are from Wade (1986).

280

Table VIII.1 shows the percentage of the 1984 U.S. population who could afford long-term care insurance, based on income, by benefit level and age. It includes those whose premiums are within 2.5 percent, 5 percent, and 10 percent of their income. Not surprisingly, there was a substantial difference between those under age 65, who were more likely to have access to an employment-based policy, and those over age 65, who were more likely to face individually priced premiums. More than 39 percent of all people aged 45 to 54 could afford a $100-a-day long-term care insurance policy if the criterion for affordability was that the premiums were within 2.5 percent of annual income. As this criterion moved toward premiums within 10 percent of annual income, the proportion of those who could afford the insurance exceeded one-half that age group.

Under the conditions established in this simulation, 41.1 percent of all people aged 45 to 64 could afford long-term care insurance premiums if affordability were measured as premiums within 5 percent of income. But if either the premiums were cut in half, or instead a $50-a-day nursing home benefit (and $25-a-day home health care benefit) was purchased, slightly more than one-half (53.7 percent) of those aged 45 to 64, and 7 percent of the elderly, could afford the premiums (table VIII.1).

Basing the concept of affordability on disposable wealth instead of income does not alter this basic differential in the proportions of the elderly and the nonelderly who would purchase long-term care insurance. If it is assumed that individuals would be willing to spend up to 20 percent of their discretionary resources on long-term care insurance, then the expected proportion of the population purchasing insurance would be substantially greater. Recall that discretionary resources are income plus the annuity value of nonhousing net wealth in excess of expected needs. It is presumed that somewhere between 74 percent and 97 percent of the value of nonhousing assets plus income is budgeted to food, clothing, housing, transportation, out-of-pocket medical expenses, and income taxes, depending on the level of income (the higher the level of income, the smaller the percentage for necessary expenses) and marital status (Cohen et al., 1987).

The distribution by age of those who could afford to purchase a $100-a-day policy is provided in table VIII.2. Slightly more than one-third (33.1 percent) of persons aged 45 to 64 and 71.2 percent of those aged 45 to 54 could afford long-term care insurance if the premiums were within 20 percent of their discretionary resources. However, less than 1 percent of the elderly would be able to afford the $100-a-day policy. If policy premiums were halved, or alternatively, if a $50-a-

TABLE VIII.1
# Percentage of People Who Could Afford Long-Term Care Insurance[a] Based on Income, by Benefit Level and Age

| | $100/Day Nursing Home Benefit[b] | | |
|---|---|---|---|
| Age Group | Annual premium within 2.5 percent of income | Annual premium within 5 percent of income | Annual premium within 10 percent of income |
| 45–54 | 39.1% | 55.1% | 61.3% |
| 55–64 | 8.6 | 27.0 | 46.0 |
| 65–74 | 0.2 | 2.3 | 11.0 |
| 75 or over | 0.0 | 0.1 | 0.5 |
| 45–64 | 23.8 | 41.1 | 53.7 |
| 65 or over | 0.1 | 1.4 | 7.0 |

| | $50/Day Nursing Home Benefit | | |
|---|---|---|---|
| Age Group | Annual premium within 2.5 percent of income | Annual premium within 5 percent of income | Annual premium within 10 percent of income |
| 45–54 | 55.1% | 61.3% | 63.5% |
| 55–64 | 27.0 | 46.0 | 58.8 |
| 65–74 | 2.3 | 11.0 | 31.1 |
| 75 or over | 0.1 | 0.5 | 3.3 |
| 45–64 | 41.1 | 53.7 | 61.2 |
| 65 or over | 1.4 | 7.0 | 20.5 |

Source: EBRI simulations using the 1984 Survey of Income and Program Participation, Bureau of the Census, U.S. Department of Commerce.

[a]Each cell represents the percentage of people for whom a hypothetical long-term care insurance premium would represent from 2.5 percent to 10 percent of family income. Calculated premiums vary by age, benefit level, and whether the insurance was purchased through an employment-based plan. Assignment of individuals to premium categories relies on the following assumptions:
- All workers with employer-provided health insurance and their dependents are assumed to be eligible for employer-sponsored group long-term care insurance.
- Married couples would not purchase the insurance unless they could afford to purchase policies for both spouses.
- Individuals with either an activity of daily living (ADL) or an instrumental activity of daily living (IADL) limitation are assumed to be ineligible for insurance.
- Family units would not purchase insurance unless their net wealth was in excess of $10,000.
- The $100/day benefit is assumed to cost twice the $50/day benefit and nongroup prices are assumed to be 25 percent higher than the group price.

[b]The group price per year for the $100/day benefit varies with age of initial purchase. At age 45 it is assumed to be $254; at age 50, $356; at age 60, $787; and at age 70, $1,680.

## TABLE VIII.2
# Percentage of People Who Could Afford Long-Term Care Insurance[a] Based on Discretionary Resources,[b] by Benefit Level and Age

| Age Group | $100/Day Nursing Home Benefit[c] | | |
|---|---|---|---|
| | Annual premium within 5 percent of resources | Annual premium within 10 percent of resources | Annual premium within 20 percent of resources |
| 45–54 | 22.6% | 52.0% | 71.2% |
| 55–64 | 3.2 | 14.2 | 36.7 |
| 65–74 | 0.3 | 1.2 | 6.0 |
| 75 or over | 0.0 | 0.1 | 0.5 |
| 45–64 | 2.6 | 12.9 | 33.1 |
| 65 or over | 0.0 | 0.2 | 0.8 |

| Age Group | $50/Day Nursing Home Benefit | | |
|---|---|---|---|
| | Annual premium within 5 percent of resources | Annual premium within 10 percent of resources | Annual premium within 20 percent of resources |
| 45–54 | 52.0% | 71.2% | 79.2% |
| 55–64 | 14.2 | 36.7 | 57.0 |
| 65–74 | 1.2 | 6.0 | 19.6 |
| 75 or over | 0.1 | 0.5 | 2.2 |
| 45–64 | 12.9 | 33.1 | 54.0 |
| 65 or over | 0.2 | 0.8 | 3.9 |

Source: EBRI simulations using the 1984 Survey of Income and Program Participation, Bureau of the Census, U.S. Department of Commerce.

[a]Each cell represents the percentage of people for whom a hypothetical long-term care insurance premium would represent from 5 percent to 20 percent of family income. Calculated premiums vary by age, benefit level, and whether the insurance was purchased through an employment-based plan. Assignment of individuals to premium categories relies on the following assumptions:
- All workers with employer-provided health insurance and their dependents are assumed to be eligible for employer-sponsored group long-term care insurance.
- Married couples would not purchase the insurance unless they could afford to purchase policies for both spouses.
- Individuals with either an activity of daily living (ADL) or an instrumental activity of daily living (IADL) limitation are assumed to be ineligible for insurance.
- Family units would not purchase insurance unless their net wealth was in excess of $10.000.
- The $100/day benefit is assumed to cost twice the $50/day benefit and nongroup prices are assumed to be 25 percent higher than the group price.

[b]Discretionary resources are measured by subtracting necessary expenditures (food, medical care, clothing, shelter, and taxes) from available resources (income and assets).

[c]The group price per year for the $100/day benefit varies with age of initial purchase. At age 45 it is assumed to be $254; at age 50, $356; at age 60, $787; and at age 70, $1,680.

day policy were purchased instead, and the same affordability criterion used, then 4 percent of the elderly would be able to afford a policy and, among those aged 45 to 54, more than 79 percent (table VIII.2). If this younger group continued purchasing the policy, the private financing of long-term care would be significantly increased.

The importance of age and access to an employer-sponsored insurance policy is illustrated in tables VIII.1 and VIII.2.[11] Table VIII.3 shows the elasticity or sensitivity of a 50 percent change in premiums on the affordability assumptions used in the simulations reported in tables VIII.1 and VIII.2. Numbers less than 1 in table VIII.3 reflect less sensitivity and numbers greater than 1 reflect more sensitivity. In nearly all cases, the simulations indicate that the elderly are more sensitive to a premium price change than are the nonelderly. Among the elderly, reductions in premiums by one-half increased the percentage of people who might purchase insurance by more than one-half. Using income as a proxy for affordability, a price reduction of 50 percent increased the number of potential purchases by far less than 50 percent. If the decision to purchase long-term care insurance, however, were based on discretionary resources, premium price changes would elicit a greater response. Among those aged 65 to 74, for example, the 50 percent reduction in price led to a nearly 80 percent increase in purchasers, using the 5-percent-of-income criterion (from table VIII.3). But among those aged 45 to 54, the cut in price added only 10 percent more policyholders.

There are also important differences by marital status. Table VIII.4 shows that married couples are most likely to be able to afford long-term care insurance. More than one-third of all married couples could afford a $100-a-day nursing home benefit policy (using 5 percent of income).[12] Not surprisingly, since widows are most likely to be older and poorer, they were the least likely to be able to afford any long-term care insurance. Fewer than 6 percent could afford a $100-a-day policy (using 5 percent of income), and slightly more than 10 percent could afford a $50-a-day policy. Using a resource-based approach to the decision (table VIII.5), at best 58 percent of all married couples

---

[11]About 24 percent of the population aged 45 or over had access to an employer-provided health insurance plan and, consequently, lower premiums for long-term care insurance.

[12]Although not included in these simulations, some insurance companies generally discount the premiums for married couples who both buy policies (Susan Van Gelder, Health Insurance Association of America, personal correspondence).

## TABLE VIII.3
## Sensitivity of Private Long-Term Care Insurance Affordability Simulations, by Affordability Criterion and Age[a]

| Age Group | Affordability Criterion | | | |
|---|---|---|---|---|
| | Annual premium within 2.5 percent of income | Annual premium within 5 percent of income | Annual premium within 10 percent of income | Annual premium within 20 percent of income |
| Based on Income | | | | |
| 45–54 | 0.58 | 0.20 | 0.07 | 0.03 |
| 55–64 | 1.37 | 0.82 | 0.44 | 0.14 |
| 65–74 | 1.79 | 1.59 | 1.29 | 0.77 |
| 75 or over | 2.00 | 1.81 | 1.71 | 1.40 |
| 45–64 | 0.84 | 0.47 | 0.25 | 0.08 |
| 65 or over | 1.79 | 1.60 | 1.32 | 0.84 |
| Based on Discretionary Resources[b] | | | | |
| 45–54 | 1.57 | 1.13 | 0.54 | 0.20 |
| 55–64 | 1.76 | 1.55 | 1.22 | 0.71 |
| 65–74 | 1.83 | 1.50 | 1.61 | 1.39 |
| 75 or over | 0.00 | 2.00 | 1.75 | 1.53 |
| 45–64 | 1.59 | 1.22 | 0.77 | 0.41 |
| 65 or over | 1.83 | 1.51 | 1.61 | 1.40 |

Source: EBRI simulations using the 1984 Survey of Income and Program Participation, Bureau of the Census, U.S. Department of Commerce (see tables VIII.1 and VIII.2).

[a]Each cell represents the percentage change in the number of people who could afford long-term care insurance (based on the different criterion for affordability) associated with a 50 percent decrease in the hypothetical premium. The greater the number, the larger the impact the price charge has.

[b]Discretionary resources are measured by subtracting necessary expenditures (food, medical care, clothing, shelter, and taxes) from available resources (income and assets).

## TABLE VIII.4
## Percentage of People Who Could Afford Long-Term Care Insurance[a] Based on Income, by Benefit Level and Marital Status

| | \$100/Day Nursing Home Benefit[b] | | | |
| --- | --- | --- | --- | --- |
| Marital Status | Annual premium within 2.5 percent of income | Annual premium within 5 percent of income | Annual premium within 10 percent of income | Annual premium within 20 percent of income |
| Married | 19.2% | 33.5% | 45.3% | 56.5% |
| Widowed | 1.9 | 5.1 | 10.9 | 19.0 |
| Divorced or Separated | 11.8 | 19.6 | 26.2 | 30.0 |
| Never Married | 11.0 | 17.7 | 23.6 | 29.9 |

| | \$50/Day Nursing Home Benefit | | | |
| --- | --- | --- | --- | --- |
| Marital Status | Annual premium within 2.5 percent of income | Annual premium within 5 percent of income | Annual premium within 10 percent of income | Annual premium within 20 percent of income |
| Married | 33.5% | 45.3% | 56.5% | 63.9% |
| Widowed | 5.1 | 10.9 | 19.0 | 27.5 |
| Divorced or Separated | 19.6 | 26.2 | 30.0 | 33.3 |
| Never Married | 17.7 | 23.6 | 29.9 | 36.7 |

Source: EBRI simulations using the 1984 Survey of Income and Program Participation, Bureau of the Census, U.S. Department of Commerce.

[a]Each cell represents the percentage of people for whom a hypothetical long-term care insurance premium would represent from 2.5 percent to 20 percent of family income. Calculated premiums vary by age, benefit level, and whether the insurance was purchased through an employment-based plan. Assignment of individuals to premium categories relies on the following assumptions:

- All workers with employer-provided health insurance and their dependents are assumed to be eligible for employer-sponsored group long-term care insurance.
- Married couples would not purchase the insurance unless they could afford to purchase policies for both spouses.
- Individuals with either an activity of daily living (ADL) or an instrumental activity of daily living (IADL) limitation are assumed to be ineligible for insurance.
- Family units would not purchase insurance unless their net wealth was in excess of $10,000.
- The $100/day benefit is assumed to cost twice the $50/day benefit and nongroup prices are assumed to be 25 percent higher than the group price.

[b]The group price per year for the $100/day benefit varies with age of initial purchase. At age 45 it is assumed to be $254; at age 50, $356; at age 60, $787; and at age 70, $1,680.

### TABLE VIII.5
## Percentage of People Who Could Afford Long-Term Care Insurance[a] Based on Discretionary Resources,[b] by Benefit Level and Marital Status

#### $100/Day Nursing Home Benefit[c]

| Marital Status | Annual premium within 2.5 percent of resources | Annual premium within 5 percent of resources | Annual premium within 10 percent of resources | Annual premium within 20 percent of resources |
|---|---|---|---|---|
| Married | 2.2% | 10.0% | 26.1% | 43.8% |
| Widowed | 0.1 | 1.0 | 3.6 | 8.5 |
| Divorced or Separated | 1.3 | 10.2 | 21.5 | 32.3 |
| Never Married | 1.0 | 7.5 | 16.1 | 24.2 |

#### $50/Day Nursing Home Benefit

| Marital Status | Annual premium within 2.5 percent of resources | Annual premium within 5 percent of resources | Annual premium within 10 percent of resources | Annual premium within 20 percent of resources |
|---|---|---|---|---|
| Married | 10.0% | 26.1% | 43.8% | 58.1% |
| Widowed | 1.0 | 3.6 | 8.5 | 14.6 |
| Divorced or Separated | 9.2 | 20.6 | 31.4 | 42.2 |
| Never Married | 7.5 | 16.1 | 24.2 | 31.5 |

Source: EBRI simulations using the 1984 Survey of Income and Program Participation, Bureau of the Census, U.S. Department of Commerce.

[a]Each cell represents the percentage of people for whom a hypothetical long-term care insurance premium would represent from 2.5 percent to 20 percent of family income. Calculated premiums vary by age, benefit level, and whether the insurance was purchased through an employment-based plan. Assignment of individuals to premium categories relies on the following assumptions:

- All workers with employer-provided health insurance and their dependents are assumed to be eligible for employer-sponsored group long-term care insurance.
- Married couples would not purchase the insurance unless they could afford to purchase policies for both spouses.
- Individuals with either an activity of daily living (ADL) or an instrumental activity of daily living (IADL) limitation are assumed to be ineligible for insurance.
- Family units would not purchase insurance unless their net wealth was in excess of $10,000.
- The $100/day benefit is assumed to cost twice the $50/day benefit and nongroup prices are assumed to be 25 percent higher than the group price.

[b]Discretionary resources are measured by subtracting necessary expenditures (food, medical care, clothing, shelter, and taxes) from available resources (income and assets).

[c]The group price per year for the $100/day benefit varies with age of initial purchase. At age 45 it is assumed to be $254; at age 50, $356; at age 60, $787; and at age 70, $1,680.

289

and nearly 15 percent of all widows would be able to afford a $50-a-day policy (using 20 percent of discretionary resources).

Microsimulation results presented by one study using the Brookings/ICF long-term care financing model indicated that relatively few individual policies would be purchased *during* retirement (Rivlin and Wiener, 1988). This modeling effort fails to include the potential of employment-based private long-term care insurance. However, two of the study's simulations offer some insights into this potential. The authors developed one scenario in which it was assumed that all people with an annual pension of $500 or more would purchase a policy, and another scenario in which it was assumed that all people aged 30 to 64 would purchase a policy if the premium were 1 percent or less of income and that all people aged 65 to 80 would purchase one if it were less than 3 percent of income and they had at least $10,000 in assets.

Under these two options, the model simulations suggest that for the period 2016 to 2020, 41.3 percent and 62.5 percent, respectively, of the elderly will have private long-term care insurance. Under both options, the model projects that total nursing home costs increase slightly under 2.5 percent, Medicaid expenditures fall by more than 12 percent, Medicare expenditures remain essentially the same, and private insurance expenditures increase by 15 percent to 18 percent.

## Affording Residency in a Life Care Community

Life care communities might be an important alternative to long-term care insurance for the elderly, but relatively few elderly could afford this option. As described in chapter III, life care communities integrate varying degrees of long-term care financial risk. For purposes of this simulation, the prices used reflected all-inclusive life care communities reported in the *National Continuing Care Directory, 1988* (Raper and Kalicki, 1988). The so-called modified and fee-for-service life care communities still offer a tremendous potential for financing long-term care, since they offer guaranteed access to care. But they do not completely share in the risk of incurring a catastrophic expense for long-term care. In theory, an insurance policy could be sold to supplement the risk that the life care community does not include. In that case, the cost of obtaining admission to the facility plus this supplemental insurance policy could offer the same amount of financial protection as an all-inclusive community.

To examine the potential of all-inclusive life care facilities to assist in the financing of long-term care, the income and assets of the elderly

290

were compared with the average entrance and monthly fees.[13] It was postulated that an individual or couple would be willing to consider moving into a life care community if, after paying the initial entrance fee and setting aside $10,000 in assets, the remaining income and annuitized value of the remaining assets (including their home) relative to the monthly fee were within a tolerable percentage. Those with ADL or IADL limitations, however, would not be allowed to seek admission.

In 1984, more than 85 percent of those aged 65 to 74 and more than 92 percent of those aged 75 or older would either not have had sufficient resources to seek admission or would have been ineligible for admission due to chronic disabilities. This left 12 percent of the elderly, or slightly more than 3 million people, in the position of deciding whether they could afford the monthly premium. Table VIII.6 shows this distribution by age.

## Obtaining Access to Home Equity

As shown in chapter IV, home equity is the most important asset held by most elderly people. More than 60 percent of the elderly own their homes, and 49 percent own them free of any debt. Overall, 52 percent of the elderly's net wealth is tied up in their homes. Nationwide, among elderly persons with no outstanding mortgage, 28 percent have between $30,000 and $75,000 in home equity. Another 10 percent of the elderly have more than $75,000 in home equity. It has been suggested that if there were a financially safe way for the elderly to obtain access to the equity in their homes when it was needed for medical emergencies, many people would be assisted. Although the Department of Housing and Urban Development has become very interested in supporting this concept, there has not, as yet, been much interest in sale-leaseback or reverse mortgage arrangements.[14]

Several states have looked into the feasibility of subsidizing and insuring lines of credit to low-income elderly homeowners. Under its Senior Home Equity Account, the State of Virginia, for example, will lend between 20 percent and 65 percent of a home's equity, depending on an individual's age. Assuming that a national program would lend

---

[13]The entrance fee was assumed to be $64,226 and the monthly fee was assumed to be $1,300 per person in 1988. For the analysis, these amounts were deflated to 1984 levels. These are the average entrance fees and monthly charges for the all-inclusive life care communities listed in the *National Continuing Care Directory* (Raper and Kalicki, 1988).

[14]See also chapter IV.

# TABLE VIII.6
## Percentage of People Who Could Afford to Live in Life Care Communities[a, b]

| Age Group | Would Not Purchase[c] | Monthly Fee as a Percentage of Remaining Income and Assets | | | |
|---|---|---|---|---|---|
| | | Less than 15 percent | 15–39 percent | 40–49 percent | 50 percent or over |
| 65–74 | 85.6% | 1.2% | 5.7% | 2.2% | 3.3% |
| 75 or over | 92.4 | 0.7 | 3.2 | 1.4 | 1.5 |

Source: EBRI simulations using the 1984 Survey of Income and Program Participation, Bureau of the Census, U.S. Department of Commerce.

[a]Prices used reflect all-inclusive life care communities reported in the *National Continuing Care Directory, 1988.* The entrance fee was assumed to be $64,226 and the monthly fee was assumed to be $1,300 per person in 1988. These amounts were deflated to 1984 levels.

[b]It is assumed that an individual or a couple would be willing to consider moving into a life care community if, after paying the initial entrance fee and setting aside $10,000 in assets, the remaining income and annuitized value of the remaining assets (including their home) relative to the monthly fee were within a tolerable percentage.

[c]Includes elderly with activity of daily living (ADL) or instrumental activity of daily living (IADL) limitations.

50 percent of the equity to those under age 75 and 60 percent to those aged 75 or older, and that the debt on these lines of credit would not have to be repaid until after the borrower died, data suggest that nearly one-half of the elderly in the United States would have been able to borrow $15,000 or more in 1984. However, only 10.1 percent of those aged 75 or older, and at most 14 percent of those aged 65 to 74, could borrow enough to stay two years or more in a nursing facility. The distribution of potential lines of credit under this assumption is provided in table VIII.7.

# Expanding and Restructuring Publicly Financed Programs

Generally, public programs are designed to finance long-term care, not to provide it. Historically, public financing of health care has relied on the private sector to provide the goods and services purchased by the public program. In theory, the sheer size of the government program could ensure competition among providers. Whether it could ensure competition and guarantee access to quality care depends in large part on the willingness of the program to meet provider costs.

### Creating a Welfare Program: Expanding Medicaid

The critical factor in most publicly financed programs is entitlement. Welfare programs do not confer entitlement unless an individual in need of assistance can prove that he or she does not have the means to be self-supporting at a legislatively determined level. Since Medicaid is already such an important component in financing long-term care, most welfare-based reform centers around incremental changes, such as liberalizing Medicaid eligibility rules and altering the range of covered benefits (such as mandatory coverage of home- and community-based services).

Most public policy discussion about Medicaid and long-term care has centered on containing current or anticipated expenditures. States have been aggressively trying to manage Medicaid expenditures, and since more than 40 percent of Medicaid payments go to nursing facilities, cost management activities have been primarily directed to that area (Buchanan, 1987). In 1986, Medicaid payments to providers for skilled nursing care, intermediate care, and home health care exceeded $10 billion, or $3,450 per Medicaid beneficiary aged 65 or older (Committee on Energy and Commerce, 1988). However, while states seek

## TABLE VIII.7
## Distribution of the Elderly Eligible for a Hypothetical Line of Credit, by Amount of Credit and Age, 1984

**Amount of Credit[a]**
**Percentage Eligible**

| Age Group | None | | | | | | | | |
|---|---|---|---|---|---|---|---|---|---|
| **65–74** | None | Under $5,000 | $5,000– $7,499 | $7,500– $9,999 | $10,000– $12,499 | $12,500– $14,999 | $15,000– $24,999 | $25,000– $37,499 | $37,500 and over |
| | 33.4% | 2.7% | 2.1% | 2.9% | 3.1% | 4.0% | 18.9% | 18.5% | 14.5% |
| **74 or over** | None | Under $6,000 | $6,000– $8,999 | $9,000– $11,999 | $12,000– $14,999 | $15,000– $17,999 | $18,000– $29,999 | $30,000– $44,999 | $45,000 and over |
| | 42.6% | 1.8% | 2.2% | 3.0% | 3.1% | 4.1% | 19.1% | 14.1% | 10.1% |
| **Total** | None | Under $5,000 | $5,000– $8,999 | $7,500– $11,999 | $10,000– $14,999 | $12,500– $18,000 | $15,000– $29,999 | $25,000– $44,999 | $37,500 and over |
| | 36.3% | 3.0% | 2.2% | 2.9% | 3.1% | 4.1% | 19.0% | 16.8% | 12.7% |

Source: EBRI tabulations of the 1984 Survey of Income and Program Participation, Bureau of the Census, U.S. Department of Commerce.

[a] Amount of credit available is based on 50 percent of the home equity for those under age 75, and 60 percent of home equity for those aged 75 or over.

ways to reduce expenditures, proposals have surfaced to liberalize Medicaid eligibility rules to enable more people to receive medical assistance.

Proposals to control the growth in program expenditures by changing Medicaid or replacing Medicaid with an alternative welfare program include instituting capitation payments for those eligible for long-term care services, and giving block grants to states to provide services to the needy elderly without federal requirements for cost-based reimbursement. By fixing the per capita payment or federal contribution at a given level, growth in federal program costs could be controlled by administrative fiat. States, conversely, could be given more flexibility in tailoring programs to fit the needs of their populations rather than being restricted to reimbursing the costs of a set of services defined by regulation. However, unless private providers receive a sufficient rate of return, they may be reluctant to serve program beneficiaries. Furthermore, as long as the financing is bifurcated (between private and public) and reimbursement rates differ, providers will be motivated to care for those who can pay the most and to shun those who pay the least.

It has been suggested that in terms of program efficiency and social equity, the Medicaid model ought to be highly rated. The program frugally directs public expenditures to those with the least amount of income and assets; therefore, assistance to the poor is well targeted and middle-income citizens are provided a safety net. The institutional bias ensures that public support is most likely to go to the most disabled and those without family support. Medicaid is financed in large part by progressive taxes and provides assistance to those with the least income and assets. In contrast, a social insurance program might assist relatively wealthier people, using tax revenues from low- and middle-income taxpayers. Furthermore, some contend, there is no public purpose to be served in protecting the assets of persons who are near the end of their lives (Rivlin and Wiener, 1988).

While it is difficult to criticize Medicaid's efficiency in directing assistance to the very poorest, it is difficult to defend the program in terms of efficient delivery of quality care.[15] Furthermore, fairness can be viewed in different ways. Some researchers discuss vertical equity (the treatment of individuals with different economic means) (Rivlin and Wiener, 1988); others look to horizontal equity (the treatment of people with the same economic means). Those who, on equity grounds,

---

[15]See also chapter III.

prefer a social insurance approach will stress the horizontal inequality of Medicaid. Since a small number of families need long-term care, there is a question of whether it is fair that two families of similar means face vastly different financial and physical burdens because one happens to need long-term care and the other does not (Lawlor and Pollak, 1985). This is a thorny question that many answer by rejecting means testing as inherently wrong and by focusing on the insurance nature of long-term care; that is, they ask why the need for long-term care should be treated differently from other potential financial catastrophes arising from a decline in health, such as a heart attack.

Furthermore, as shown in chapter III, the way in which long-term care is delivered is influenced by the way in which it is financed. Liberalizing Medicaid may not necessarily change the quantity, quality, or type of long-term care services delivered. Changing the services that Medicaid purchases and how these services are reimbursed would require substantially more changes than merely expanding Medicaid eligibility.

### Expanding Medicare

Social insurance for long-term care would entitle people who need assistance to receive services regardless of their financial circumstances. Participation in a social insurance plan could be either mandatory or voluntary, but no one could be excluded from eligibility by a means test. Financing for a social insurance scheme could be obtained from broad-based sources such as general revenues, a dedicated tax (like the Social Security payroll tax), or voluntary or mandatory premiums. Some proposals for coverage of long-term care benefits through Medicare include only home-based care or only nursing home care, but most include both.

Broad-based financing spreads the financial risks of a program over a larger pool. In a voluntary government program, the potential for adverse selection can be minimized by widespread public confidence in the program. In a mandatory program, adverse selection would be eliminated. Administrative costs per person are likely to be lower than those in a welfare program because there would be fewer costs for screening to determine eligibility. For both Medicaid and Medicare, the cost of administering claims for services rendered is about 5 percent of provider payments (*Annual Report*, 1988a; *Annual Report*, 1988c; Bureau of Data Management and Strategy, 1989). However, Medicaid administration costs do not include the cost of determining eligibility and the determination of recipients' contributions toward nursing home care. In any voluntary social insurance program, however, adverse selection is still likely to exist and could be exacerbated if the premiums necessary to finance the plan were perceived as high relative to the probability of receiving benefits.

A social insurance approach, especially if financed by payroll taxes, could create sufficient public identification with the program's benefits to make it less subject to cutbacks during tight fiscal periods. However, a program of universal coverage would give the government substantial influence over many of the resources devoted to long-term care. While this may raise concern about the responsiveness of a federally administered and regulated program to local and individual needs, it may enable the government to attract resources to areas without services and discourage the provision of additional services to areas already saturated, and to get providers to meet their price.

The American Association of Retired Persons (AARP), the Villers Foundation (Families USA), and the Older Women's League have proposed a program intended to cover all people with severe disabilities, perhaps beginning with coverage for people eligible for Medicare (Glasse, Pollack, and Rother, 1987; Rother, Gibson, and Varner, 1988). Under this program, people who need care at at least the intermediate care facility level would be eligible for services both at home and in institutions. An expanded array of community-based services would be made available, and beneficiaries would share costs in the form of copayments but not deductibles. Lower-income individuals would have their copayments paid by Medicaid. Eligible individuals would have an option of enrolling in a plan receiving capitated reimbursement, which would offer a richer variety of services than would be available if they retained their choice of fee-for-service providers. The future coverage of current workers would be financed by increasing payroll taxes. General revenues and dedicated taxes and premiums would finance those currently eligible.

The Harvard Medicare Project (1986) recommended changes in the Medicare program, including the addition of coverage for institutional and noninstitutional long-term care for chronic illness. However, the proposal would limit home health benefits strictly to health care related services and leave coverage of social services and custodial care to other payment sources. They recommended that Medicare cover nursing home stays following an initial one-month deductible period. After that month, Medicare would require residents to pay copayments equal to 80 percent of the resident's Social Security benefit, so that the copayment would be based on the beneficiaries' ability to pay the ordinary costs of room and board. The needs of eligible people who apply for benefits would be assessed by case managers who would authorize Medicare reimbursement for either institutional care or home health care services. Reimbursement to providers would be based on prospectively determined rates. Regional and national budgetary limits would be adjusted annually for inflation and anticipated increases in the number of potentially eligible people. Aggregate payments to providers could be exceeded only by borrowing from the following year's limit.

Current beneficiaries would be expected to pay 90 percent of the additional costs ($27.3 billion) through increased premiums and an income tax surcharge.[16] Payroll taxes would take effect in later years, and would finance an increasing share of the program. By the year 2000, 20 percent of the funds ($9.6 billion) would come from general revenues, 25 percent ($11.3 billion) from beneficiary premiums (both flat and income related), and the remaining 55 percent ($26.9 billion) from increases in the payroll tax. The Harvard Medicare Project projected that by the year 2000, total long-term care costs will be 32 percent, or $14.4 billion, more than they would be in the absence of such a program. Critical to this estimate is the assumption that current rates of institutionalization are too low and that they would increase, and that the supply of nursing home beds would expand to meet the increased need.[17]

It has also been proposed that long-term care coverage be made optional under Medicare. Services covered would include nursing home care, home health services, and day hospital services. The services would be subject to a 10 percent coinsurance but would limit out-of-pocket costs to $3,000 annually. People could enroll in this optional program any time between the ages of 60 and 70 but would not be eligible for covered services until they had been enrolled for at least five years. A premium would be set at 4 percent of income for those who enroll at age 60 (increasing for those who postpone enrollment), with a minimum annual premium of $200 (Davis and Rowland, 1986).

---

[16]The expanded Medicare benefits under the Medicare Catastrophic Coverage Act of 1988 were to be financed in this manner. The political fallout from this fundamental change in financing has, however, been significant.

[17]This assumes that: (1) all elderly needing assistance with personal care (eating, bathing, dressing, or using the toilet) who are living alone or are unmarried enter a nursing home; (2) one-half the elderly who have limitations in mobility and who live alone enter nursing homes; and (3) 20 percent of those now in nursing homes are able to live in the community due to improved home care. These assumptions represent a doubling in the rate of institutionalization of elderly persons with personal care needs and a sixfold increase in the institutionalization rate of elderly persons with impaired mobility (Harvard Medicare Project, 1986).

Another suggestion is that the Medicare long-term care benefit cover home health care immediately but that there be a two-year waiting period for Medicare-financed nursing home care. Home health care benefits would require a 10 percent coinsurance. In addition, beneficiaries would pay an income-related premium of approximately 2 percent of income, with a minimum premium of $200 and a maximum premium of $1,000 (Davis, 1989).

In a series of papers, commentaries, and discussions among a small group of nationally recognized health policy experts, which was published by the AARP, a consensus emerged concerning the financing of long-term care (Leader and Moon, 1989). Of particular note was the view that providers, while in the position to advocate the interests of any one individual, were not in a position to adequately protect the collective interests of all users and financers of health care. One author articulated the consensus quite pointedly when he wrote, ". . . it is inescapable that any long-term care system with any pretensions to adequacy must have some form of system gatekeeper" (Evans, 1989). It has been suggested that, in lieu of a universal and comprehensive health care system, some form of capitated long-term care delivery system with decentralized case management would be needed (Kane, 1989). Chapter VI discusses the possibility of using a case manager or care coordinator in this way and suggests this would also be an important component of any private long-term care insurance policy.

A recent study argued that public-sector spending for long-term care is already large and is likely to increase rapidly in the future, and that therefore it is now time to reexamine the role of public-sector financing (Rivlin and Wiener, 1988). Furthermore, based on that study's microsimulation of financing options sold at the point of retirement, the continued growth in private insurance will not have any appreciable impact on the growth of public expenditures. Consequently, the study argues, the public policy issue is how to structure these expenditures. The study sees the choice as either to continue with Medicaid as the major source of public financing or to move to a social insurance strategy, but it points out that the current system of public financing through a welfare program is the product of a series of historical accidents rather than a rational and deliberate public policy (Rivlin and Wiener, 1988).

The logical extension of the foregoing position is an argument for social insurance, which is reinforced by economic arguments (the broadest risk pool possible, no adverse selection, administrative efficiency) and psychosocial considerations—namely, that the need for long-term care should be viewed as a normal risk of getting old. If one accepts the assumption that the private market can only provide a limited amount of insurance at rates that almost everyone can afford, then, since the need for long-term care is a normal risk of growing old, government must play a role by providing social insurance. This line of reasoning could be used as an argument that individuals ought to be responsible for purchasing private long-term care insurance. However, the private insurance market, unlike a social insurance program, is not likely to cross-subsidize the disabled and low- or moderate-income people who do not—or cannot—purchase long-term care insurance.

The above study simulated four different publicly financed social insurance options. Under the most comprehensive scenario, Medicare benefits were expanded to provide unlimited coverage of skilled nursing and intermediate care facilities. Low-income beneficiaries would face only a 10 percent coinsurance rate that, for the very poorest, would be picked up by Medicaid. Relatively better-off beneficiaries would face an additional one-month deductible. Home health care benefits were also covered, but with a one-month deductible and a coinsurance rate that varied from zero to 20 percent, depending on income. Nursing homes and home health agencies would be paid 120 percent of the Medicaid rate. Medicaid would also be liberalized by increasing the personal needs allowance to $60, and protected assets would be raised to $1,800. Under this program, projections to the period 2016–2020 indicate that total long-term care expenses would increase 39 percent, private out-of-pocket expenses would decrease 34 percent, and public expenditures would be nearly double what they would have been without this program (Rivlin and Wiener, 1988).[18]

The least costly approach was a simulated catastrophic long-term care insurance program. Under this simulation, unlimited nursing home care would be provided after a two-year deductible. In addition,

---

[18]To assist in the determination of Medicaid expenditures, assets from the 1983 Survey of Consumer Finances, adjusted for inflation, were statistically matched to the individuals in the Brookings/ICF long-term care financing model. This process implies that the saving behavior of future elderly will be the same as that of those who were elderly in 1983. Furthermore, it assumed that, once retired, individuals would no longer continue to save. There is a substantial body of literature that has evolved concerning the question of why the elderly continue to save. It is important to recognize this limitation, since for most elderly Medicaid eligibility is contingent on the level of assets. If this statistical matching leads to asset levels that are lower than those that would actually occur, the model will overstate future Medicaid expenditures. The fact that the model imposes no supply constraints, however, ensures that it overstates long-term care utilization.

a 10 percent coinsurance rate would be imposed. Home health care benefits would not be expanded nor would Medicaid be liberalized. Nursing homes would be paid 115 percent of the Medicaid rate, and private insurance was assumed to be purchased at age 67, if among other conditions the premium was less than 5 percent of income. Under this scenario, total long-term care expenditures were projected to increase 20 percent, out-of-pocket expenses were projected to decrease 48 percent, and total public expenditures were projected to increase almost 44 percent more than they would otherwise.

Rivlin and Wiener (1988) simulated two other scenarios that differ in the treatment of Medicaid and the size of the coinsurance rate, but could be arrayed somewhere between comprehensive and strictly catastrophic coverage. In the less comprehensive scenario, Medicaid was not liberalized but there was a 25 percent coinsurance and 100-day deductible for nursing home care, regardless of income; home health care was limited to the most severely disabled (those with three or more ADL deficiencies) and was subject to a one-month deductible and a 20 percent coinsurance rate. Nursing homes and home health agencies would be paid 115 percent of the Medicaid rate. Under this scenario, total long-term care expenditures in the period 2016–2020 and total public expenditures were projected to be 87 percent higher than they would otherwise have been, and out-of-pocket expenditures were projected to be 34 percent lower (than they would have been if there were no program changes).

To finance the public insurance program, the authors estimate that the cost through the year 2050 would be about 3 percent of payroll. However, without any change in the financing of long-term care, the existing Medicaid program is expected to increase by one-half the cost anticipated with the establishment of a public insurance program (Rivlin and Wiener, 1988).

## Establishing a Public-Private Partnership

A public-private partnership already exists for organizing, delivering, and paying for long-term care. At issue is whether society wants to alter the current arrangement, and if so, in what way. Public expenditures through the Medicaid program already assist many of the poor and destitute who need long-term care in a nursing facility, and the preferential tax treatment of private long-term care insurance reserves is already subsidizing the development of this market. However, most long-term care is organized and delivered by the family and friends

301

of those needing assistance, and about one-half the cost of this care is paid by the dependents and their families.

This partnership could be altered in many ways, depending on the desired goals and on the financial commitment the public is willing to make. With limited public expenditures, it may be best to improve access to care by Medicaid recipients. This may include improving reimbursement rates and expanding the scope of services covered. With additional public expenditures, changes can be made to expand access to Medicaid and to facilitate the development of the private long-term care insurance market.

However, in the discussion of the potential for private long-term care financing it was demonstrated that while the market potential is tremendous—especially for the future elderly—there is little to justify substantial public expenditures to encourage the market for those currently elderly. Without direct subsidization of premiums, there are few public policy options that can ensure that a significant portion of the current elderly will have sufficient financial protection and guaranteed access to quality care, using financing mechanisms available in the private market. This raises the possibility of establishing or enhancing public programs to protect those who are currently at greatest risk of needing long-term care and of public intervention in the development and oversight of the private market to assist those who are now least likely to need long-term care. The challenge, however, is to create an entitlement that does not discourage the voluntary purchase of long-term care insurance or other forms of insurance such as life care communities.

Most states are grappling with how to deliver long-term care and control Medicaid expenditures. States are quite interested in encouraging a broad-based private insurance market to relieve Medicaid of some of its expenditures. In at least six states, task forces or commissions have been initiated to investigate the feasibility of waiving some of the Medicaid eligibility rules for those who purchase long-term care insurance. The Robert Wood Johnson Foundation has provided these states with planning grants.

Each of the states is approaching the issue from a slightly different perspective. Massachusetts, for example, is moving toward recommending guaranteed Medicaid coverage when qualified private long-term care insurance is purchased. This insurance could have a one-year deductible which, for low-income elderly, would be subsidized. The state would also consider subsidizing the cost of the insurance premiums, based on a sliding income scale, for low-income elderly persons. Connecticut is considering expanding its existing case management system as well as finding ways to waive Medicaid eligibility requirements for seniors who purchase insurance. Each dollar of insurance benefit paid would be subtracted from the assets Medicaid considers in determining eligibility. Legislation was passed in Indiana in April 1987 with the intent of establishing standards and guidelines so that the purchase of long-term care insurance would lead to a waiver of Medicaid eligibility rules. New Jersey and Wisconsin are investigating similar options. New York has proposed the development of a reinsurance fund that would assume insured persons' benefit payments when their private long-term care insurance benefits are exhausted. Funding for the reinsurance fund would come from a surcharge on long-term care insurance premiums, from the insurance premium directly when insurance benefits are exhausted, and from state revenues (Robert Wood Johnson Foundation, 1988).

In addition to finding ways to encourage and support consumer demand for long-term care insurance, all of these states are examining their delivery systems. It is anticipated that the case coordination infrastructure would be enhanced as part of the development of these programs. Although Medicaid does not have a provision that enables the waiver of Medicaid eligibility based on the purchase of long-term care insurance, it is possible, with six or more states pressing the Health Care Financing Administration and Congress, that either waivers will be granted or the law will be amended.

A commitment to universal access to long-term care in the very near term, however, will necessitate substantial public-sector expenditures. Social insurance could take many different forms, but would fundamentally provide "complete," "back-end," or "front-end" coverage. Back-end coverage would pay for covered services after a substantial waiting period; presumably, private insurance could be sold to cover this period. Such an approach could cover certain services, such as in-home care, without a waiting period, but could impose a waiting period for other care such as nursing home care. The very success of a back-end public program rests with how successfully private insurance fills the market niche.

Conversely, a front-end approach would pay for needed care from the start, but assistance would be limited in duration. Private insurance might be available after the public program assistance expires. Both the back-end and the front-end approaches suggest explicit partnerships between the government and the public and hold out a definite role for private insurance. The longer the front-end period of assistance, the more expensive the government commitment. Nearly 90 percent of those who return home from a nursing facility will do

303

so within six months. While 33 percent of those who leave a nursing facility after six months are alive, most (more than 90 percent) are discharged directly to a hospital (National Center for Health Statistics, 1989). Consequently, the front-end, rather than the back-end, approach to a public-private partnership offers the most potential for assisting more people when they are most likely to need assistance. It ensures that for those who are capable of leaving the nursing home, financial considerations will not be a barrier. On the other hand, needed financial assistance will end. This creates a very different niche for private insurance than the back-end public program does.

Regardless of the approach favored, serious questions remain concerning who would be eligible, how eligibility would be determined, what services would be covered, and how care would be controlled and coordinated so that services would be used effectively. The challenge for the design of any social insurance program will be to find ways to effect a delivery system that meets the needs of dependent people, their families, and the resources available in each community. Moreover, given that there is still more to know about how best to organize and deliver effective care, it is imperative that the system maintain flexibility to permit changes as lessons are learned. This suggests the need to include an assessment and case management team that has the flexibility to work with families and to arrange an array of services that will assist them in caregiving, or to substitute for the family when there is none.

## Conclusion

Part I of this book sets out to define long-term care and to isolate those factors most likely to affect the labor market, employers, and the financing of public programs designed to provide retirement income and security. It also identifies the problems of obtaining care for chronic disabling conditions and the population at risk for needing long-term care. Part II discusses how this care is financed and how fragmented, confusing, and institutionally biased the current financing system is. Relatively few people today or in the near future can be expected to afford very much long-term care for very long. This has resulted in a situation in which many people who depend on state assistance are likely to move to an institution, perhaps for the rest of their lives. Rarely are those who need state assistance offered a choice of facilities.

Concern over access to efficient care—i.e., the quantity and quality of care desired by society—during the last 25 years has slowly led to a persistent and growing call for reform of long-term care finance and delivery. The demographic changes that are upon us exacerbate the least desirable aspects of our delivery system. Consequently, more people will directly or indirectly confront the deficiencies in our system. But the window of opportunity, in terms of public policy options aimed at prefunding the cost of care for the next generation of elderly, diminishes with each passing year. After the year 2010, it will be too late for a very large number of future elderly to have prefunded their expected long-term care costs over their working years. When retirees in the year 2010 reach age 85, there will be more than twice as many 85-year-olds as there are today. Without some system of prefunding, transfer payments directly from either workers or taxpayers to beneficiaries are likely to be necessary for those who fall victim to disabling conditions that rob them of their ability to remain independent.

Private financing options are not likely to be broadly based for future generations unless employers are willing to take an aggressive lead in weaving long-term care insurance into the web of employee benefits. Part III of this book highlights the advantages of an employment-based group policy and discusses both the potential and the framework for establishing such a program. Employers, however, are preoccupied with controlling health care benefit costs, and are primarily concerned with health care cost management for active employees and retirees, new tax code rules, and accounting for the cost of postretirement medical benefits. Restructuring of employee compensation and benefits packages is feasible but is not likely to happen soon. Too few employees are affected by long-term care needs at any one time to constitute a critical mass agitating for change; demand is likely to evolve slowly. However, in general, the demographic changes in the work force are likely to work in favor of employees. Employees are likely to become even more valuable assets of production, with their increased value reflected in increases in real wages and salaries and ultimately in real retirement income. Concurrently, more people, including employees who are key members of a firm's management, are likely to learn firsthand about the frustrations and sometimes utter desperation involved in attempting to coordinate and provide long-term care for a loved one while continuing to fulfill their other responsibilities.

A lack of public policy response now will not change the explicit and implicit cost of long-term care, especially in the short run, but it could change the financing options, the quantity and quality of care, and the distribution of the cost of care. Any expansion in financing is likely to raise the cost of long-term care, since the demand for care exceeds the supply. Significant differences in ability to pay the cost of this care will lead to even more problems in obtaining access to assistance. The distribution of public and private dollars should be accounted for and treated with equal consideration. Too often, the argument that a public program costs too much is based solely on the public expenditures, without regard to the implications of the alternative—no public expenditures, but no services, either.

Financing long-term care is one of several challenges facing our society. But this challenge is also an opportunity to correct some of the problems in the current system. Insuring the cost of long-term care among a relatively large group is not an insurmountable problem. If we have the political and societal will to address this issue, financing options exist. Part of the answer lies in conducting a thorough examination of how to best organize and deliver long-term care. Regardless of how long-term care is financed, there will be a need for additional facilities and organizations to coordinate the system. The system must be able to marshal services to those who need assistance and be able to complement family caregiving.

As more people need long-term care, their claims on resources, regardless of how care is financed, will undoubtedly increase expenditures faster than many other health-related expenditures, but by how much is very speculative. An increasing number of frail and disabled people will have fewer children upon whom to depend, but their physical, emotional, and financial capacities, as well as their general life expectations, are not likely to be the same as those of the current elderly. At the very least, we can expect that the next generation of elderly will be even more diverse than the elderly today. However, if similar proportions of people are in need of assistance, public and private expenditures will increase. How we rationalize these expenditures and how we assist those who can no longer remain independent will be a measure of our civility and our humanity.

# Appendix A. Some Relevant Legislation Introduced during the 100th Congress

## Legislation to Increase Public Financing of Long-Term Care

At least 18 bills were introduced during the 100th Congress (1987–1988) that would directly increase public financing of long-term care. Three of the proposals would expand long-term care coverage under Medicaid, while the majority of bills would create an insurance or entitlement program along the lines of the Medicare program. Although none of the bills was enacted, they merit study because they may form the basis for future congressional proposals.

### Legislation to Expand or Alter Medicaid

A number of proposals were introduced to expand or alter Medicaid. Sen. Malcolm Wallop (R-WY) proposed a bill that would cap the federal contribution to Medicaid and index the cap for inflation but give states more flexibility in defining covered services and eligibility. Rep. Barbara Kennelly (D-CT) proposed legislation that would cover long-term care services under Medicaid for all individuals living below the poverty line. Her measure would also provide grants to states to subsidize the purchase of private long-term care insurance by low-income individuals. The bill would provide that beneficiaries' assets be protected to the extent they were protected by private insurance. Sen. Orrin Hatch (R-UT) proposed authorizing $100 million for home health services not already covered under Medicaid. None of these bills went beyond introduction and referral to the appropriate committees.

### Legislation to Expand Medicare

In the last six months of the 100th Congress, four bills were introduced to provide public financing of long-term care. These include Sen. George Mitchell's (D-ME) Long-Term Care Assistance Act of 1988 and the House companion bill, introduced by Rep. David Obey (D-WI); Sen. Edward Kennedy's (D-MA) Lifecare Long-Term Care Protection Act; Rep. Henry Waxman's (D-CA) Elder-Care Long-Term Care Assistance Act of 1988; and Rep. Pete Stark's (D-CA) Chronic Care

Medicare Long-Term Care Coverage Act of 1988. These bills represent three different approaches: comprehensive coverage, "back-end" coverage, and "front-end" coverage.

The proposals by Reps. Stark and Waxman would provide comprehensive coverage. In the proposal introduced by Sen. Mitchell, expenses for community-based care would be reimbursed once a level of functional dependency is attained but nursing home care would not be covered immediately. Sen. Mitchell's proposal would provide "back-end" coverage by excluding nursing home coverage for two years. However, this proposal includes a wide variety of incentives to encourage the private insurance market to sell products that would cover the two-year deductible. Under the Waxman and Stark proposals, nursing home care would not be covered for the first two months and three months, respectively. Sen. Kennedy's proposal, on the other hand, would provide "front-end" coverage by paying for nursing home care for the first six months without any waiting period or coinsurance payments.

The Stark, Waxman, and Mitchell proposals have coinsurance features varying from 20 percent to 35 percent of the cost. Rep. Stark has estimated that the cost of the coinsurance for each of these four proposals would range from $7,200 to $10,000 per year after the deductible. Of course, the deductible, which is the cost of nursing home care, could easily be $1,500 to $2,000 a month. Coinsurance for covered home- and community-based services would be 20 percent under the Stark, Waxman, and Mitchell proposals; under Sen. Kennedy's bill, it would be the lesser of 10 percent of the cost or 5 percent of the individual's monthly Social Security benefits. Sen. Mitchell's proposal also includes a $500 deductible for home- and community-based care.

All of the proposals would establish a program to assess an individual's physical or mental ability to perform activities deemed essential to living independently. Medicare beneficiaries would be eligible for participation under each of the proposals, and under Kennedy's proposal, children under age 19 would also be eligible. All would cover home health care services, including homemaker services, and adult day care, but only the bills introduced by Sens. Mitchell and Kennedy would pay for respite care, designed to enable primary caregivers to run errands or to take a break or vacation.

All of these proposals rely on Medicaid savings, especially premiums and copayments, to help defray a large part of the cost. Sen. Kennedy's proposal includes a provison for federally sponsored prefunded long-term care insurance that would cover nursing home expenses beyond the first six months provided in the bill and that would be offered to all people aged 45 or older. Eligibility would not begin until age 65, but the premiums paid during the preceding 20 years would be used to prefund the expected costs. Sen. Mitchell's proposal includes explicit incentives for private insurers to cover long-term care for people under age 65 and nursing home care for the first two years after they become Medicare eligible. The other proposals would not explicitly encourage insurers, and would restrict the potential insurance market to people under age 65 and include copayments and deductibles in policies for people aged 65 or older.

None of the proposals could be financed entirely by Medicaid savings, premiums, and copayments. Estimates of the additional cost of these programs to the federal government in 1993 range from $20 billion to $25 billion for the Kennedy and Mitchell bills to $40 billion to $46 billion for the Waxman and Stark types of proposals. Several sources have been considered for financing the additional expense. All of the proposals would either uncap or raise the amount of earnings subject to the Medicare Health Insurance portion of the payroll tax. Rep. Stark's proposal would also increase the Health Insurance tax imposed on employers and employees. Each of the proposals would increase Medicare premiums and raise estate taxes.

In addition to these bills, several pieces of legislation were introduced to expand long-term care coverage under a Medicare Part C program. Rep. Hal Daub (R-NE) introduced two bills to establish long-term nursing home and home health care benefits paid by Medicare after a beneficiary pays a substantial annual deductible based on income. Rep. Richard Gephardt (D-MO) and Sen. John Chafee (R-RI) each introduced measures to allow Medicare payments on a prepaid, capitated basis for people who enroll in an organization providing community nursing and ambulatory care services. The Secretary of Health and Human Services would be required to develop reimbursement rates for services not currently provided to Medicare beneficiaries. The late Rep. Claude Pepper (D-FL) and Sen. Jim Sasser (D-TN) introduced proposals cover long-term care services under Medicare by expanding the social health maintenance organization program.

Rep. Leon Panetta (D-CA) introduced a bill to cover 100 days of adult day care under Medicare for certified chronically impaired adults. He also introduced legislation to expand Medicare home health care coverage by removing the requirement that services be provided only to the homebound. His bill would also provide Medicare coverage of chore services and respite care for providers of care to dependent adults. Rep. Matthew Rinaldo (R-NJ) introduced legislation to authorize $50 million to provide funding for home health services under the Grants to States for Services portion of the Social Security Act (Title XX).

Rep. Pepper introduced an amendment to what became the Medicare Catastrophic Coverage Act of 1988. The amendment failed to pass and was subsequently introduced as a bill. However, the bill never came to a vote. Known as the Medicare Long-Term Home Care Catastrophic Protection Act of 1987, the bill would have amended Medicare to provide coverage of long-term home care services to chronically ill elderly, the disabled, and children who are functionally dependent in at least two activities of daily living. The elimination of the limit on wages subject to the Medicare Hospital Insurance tax would be the primary source of financing for the expansion of benefits.

## Legislation to Encourage Private Financing of Long-Term Care

More than 30 bills were introduced during the 100th Congress to encourage private financing of long-term care. At least four bills would encourage saving for long-term care or long-term care insurance by creating new savings accounts (usually referred to as health service accounts) that would resemble special-use individual retirement accounts (IRAs). Four other proposals would have allowed tax-free distributions from an IRA to be used to purchase long-term care insurance. At least one proposal would have allowed for an income tax deduction for the purchase of a qualified long-term care insurance policy to encourage individuals to purchase insurance. The deduction could be as large as the premium paid but would be capped at the lesser of $1,500 per beneficiary or the amount of taxable income.

Several bills were introduced to encourage employers to provide access to long-term care insurance. Proposals by Sen. Dave Durenberger (R-MN), Rep. Rod Chandler (R-WA), and Rep. Daub would create ways to finance long-term care on a tax-favored basis using existing pension plans or, as in one of the proposals, through an employer's 401(k) arrangement. The benefits paid would be exempt from income tax. In one version of this approach, long-term care or the purchase of long-term care insurance would only be provided to former employees or their dependents who are aged 70 or older. Many of the proposals can be found in the list of recommendations made by the Task Force on Long-Term Health Care Policies (1987). One of their primary proposals, which was also introduced in legislation, would enable individuals to withdraw funds from pension and retirement plans to purchase qualified long-term care insurance on a tax-free basis.

At least five bills would either clarify or amend the tax code so that qualified long-term care insurance would be treated as noncancelable accident or health insurance contracts. At least two other proposals would amend the definition of group health plans to include long-term care expenses so that long-term care could be provided by employers under the same terms that apply to group health plans. At least three bills would provide either a tax credit or a deduction for taxpayers who purchase long-term care outside of a nursing home or provide informal care to a functionally dependent family member. The family member would have to be aged 65 or older, under two of the bills, and at least aged 70 in another. One of the proposals had a prerequisite that the family member's annual family income be less than $15,000 and that the dependent have a Social Security-defined disability.

### Ensuring That Long-Term Care Insurance Receives the Same Tax Treatment as Accident or Health Insurance

During the 100th Congress many bills were introduced that sought to clarify the tax treatment of long-term care insurance. Rep. Michael Bilirakis (R-FL) proposed amending the Internal Revenue Code by adding the term "long-term care expenses" to the definition of group health plans. Reps. Rinaldo and John Hammerschmidt (R-AR) each introduced bills to allow qualified long-term care insurance contracts to receive the same tax treatment as noncancelable accident or health insurance contracts. Benefits received through qualified long-term care insurance would be treated in the same manner as benefits received for personal injury or sickness.

Rep. Ron Wyden (D-OR) introduced a bill to provide that qualified long-term care insurance contracts that are guaranteed renewable would be treated in the same manner for tax purposes as noncancelable accident or health insurance contracts. Qualified long-term health care is defined as necessary diagnostic, preventive, therapeutic, rehabilitative, and maintenance or personal care services required by an individual who is chronically ill or disabled or care provided in a qualified facility by a qualified provider. Home care could be a substitute for care in a qualified facility if the home care would cost less than institutional care, and if a medical practitioner certified that without home care the individual would have to be cared for in a nursing facility. The bill excludes family members as qualified providers.

311

Sen. Mitchell's bill, which would expand Medicare to include nursing home care two years after an individual is eligible for benefits, relies on the expansion of the private market to offer products covering the two-year deductible. His proposal would also treat qualified long-term care insurance as accident or health insurance in the tax code. Qualified polices would be guaranteed renewable and the benefits would be provided in a qualified facility, which could be an individual's home if a physician certifies that he or she would have to be institutionalized without the care. Furthermore, long-term care insurance reserves would be treated in the same manner as life insurance reserves. Long-term care insurance could be offered in an employer's cafeteria plan as long as the policy is not surrenderable for cash and is portable. Finally, employers would be able to deduct long-term care insurance premiums on the condition that any returns of premiums be applied to reduce the future costs of the plan or to increase benefits.

Reps. Judd Gregg (R-NH) and Kennelly each proposed legislation to provide that qualified long-term care insurance be treated as noncancelable accident and health insurance. Similarly, Rep. David Dreier (R-CA) proposed that contracts for the reserves of qualified long-term care insurance be treated in the same way as the reserves for noncancelable accident or health insurance. In all of these bills, qualified long-term care insurance would have to provide coverage for 12 months; be guaranteed renewable; and provide diagnostic, therapeutic, preventive, rehabilitative, and maintenance services in sites other than an acute care unit of a hospital. Benefits received would not be included as income, regardless of whether the plan is purchased by individuals or employers. Like the provisions in Sen. Mitchell's measures, these bills proposed to treat qualified long-term care expenses as medical care for purposes of personal deductions and to allow employers to deduct any premiums that they pay for long-term care. Sen. Kennelly's bill, like Sen. Mitchell's, would also permit long-term care insurance to be offered in an employer's cafeteria plan as long as the employee could not surrender it for cash and the policy is portable.

## Incentives for Individuals to Purchase Long-Term Care Insurance

Several proposals would have signaled to taxpayers the importance of long-term care insurance by offering a special tax preference to those who purchase it. Rep. Daub proposed a measure that would enable taxpayers to deduct the premiums of qualified long-term care insurance for themselves or for an eligible beneficiary (aged 50 or over) if the premiums were not in excess of unearned income and were no greater than $1,500. Legislation introduced by Rep. Duncan Hunter

(R-CA) would allow a deduction equal to one-half the amount paid for qualified long-term care insurance premiums.

Rep. Kennelly sponsored a measure that would amend the tax code to exclude from gross income the portion of distributions from qualified plans and tax-deferred annuities that are used to pay long-term care insurance premiums or qualified long-term care expenses. The same exclusion would apply to amounts received under an annuity, endowment, or life insurance contract.

### Long-Term Health Care Savings Accounts

During the 100th Congress several bills were introduced to encourage individuals to save for long-term care or long-term care insurance. Rep. Ralph Regula (R-OH) introduced a bill to enable individuals to deduct up to $2,000 for contributions to an account that could be used for long-term care or approved insurance, including catastrophic insurance. Earnings on the account would accrue with deferred taxation, and part of the distribution would be free from income taxes. In fact, the tax treatment of distributions would be designed to encourage the purchase of insurance over the direct purchase of care. Twenty percent of distributions for qualified health care expenses would be free from inclusion as taxable income; for the purchase of qualified insurance, 50 percent would be excluded.

Similar legislation was introduced by Rep. Gerald B. Solomon (R-NY) and by Sen. Barbara Mikulski (D-MD), except that in their versions all distributions would be tax free. Furthermore, their proposals would have enabled spouses and children acting as guardians to contribute to an individual's account without paying a gift tax. A different version of the individual savings account approach, introduced by Sen. Durenberger, would have enabled an individual to receive a tax credit of 10 percent of contributions for the taxable year, up to $200, if that person did not have long-term care insurance provided through an employer.

### Use of Retirement Savings to Purchase Long-Term Care Insurance

Rep. Roy Rowland (D-GA) introduced a bill to amend the Internal Revenue Code of 1986 relating to tax treatment of distributions for IRAs. The bill provided that taxation of IRA distributions would not apply to the applicable percentage of any amount paid to an individual from his or her IRA or annuity if the entire amount were used to purchase long-term care insurance within 90 days after the distribution and the individual had attained age 59 1/2 by the date of the distribution. If the taxpayer's adjusted gross income were less than

$45,000 (subject to inflation adjustments), all of the distribution would be nontaxable. If the taxpayer's income were between $45,000 and $100,000, only a portion of the distribution would be taxable, and if the income were greater than $100,000, the distribution would be fully taxable.

Similar proposals were included in two bills introduced by Rep. Daub and Sen. Durenberger. Rep. Daub's proposal would not adjust the percentage of the tax-deductible withdrawal by the beneficiary's adjusted gross income. Furthermore, it would specifically exclude certain kinds of care currently covered by Medicare. At least five bills (introduced by Reps. Rinaldo, Hammerschmidt, Bilirakis, Dreier, and Kennelly) would permit all distributions from IRAs for long-term care insurance to be fully deductible. In a similar vein, a bill introduced by Rep. Daub provided that the surrender or cancellation value of any life insurance policy used to pay long-term care insurance premiums would be excluded from gross income for individuals aged 65 or older.

Most of the proposals would establish standards for qualified long-term care insurance. At a minimum, most of the standards are similar to those established by the National Association of Insurance Commissioners when it developed a model act and model regulations to assist state legislatures in developing regulations pertaining to long-term care insurance. Most of the proposals call for certification by the Secretary of Health and Human Services.

Sen. Durenberger proposed adding to the tax code a "voluntary retiree health plan" trust to allow prefunding of retiree health and long-term care benefits in a manner similar to tax-qualified defined benefit pension plans. To qualify, the plan would have to meet non-discrimination rules, minimum and maximum funding standards, participation standards, minimum vesting standards, and distribution requirements, and would have to exclude self-direction of assets by participants or beneficiaries and place limitations on holdings of employer securities and employer real property. As proposed, voluntary retiree health plans would differ from other defined benefit plans in that both employer contributions and the receipt of any long-term care benefit under such a plan would not be included in an individual's gross income. A "qualified voluntary retiree health plan" would provide only postretirement long-term health care benefits through an acquired insurance plan, self-insurance by the employer, or reimbursement of expenses paid by a former employee or his or her spouse for long-term care insurance. The former employee or spouse would have to be aged 70 or over and be in need of necessary diagnostic, preventive, therapeutic, rehabilitative, maintenance, or personal care services provided in a qualified facility by a qualified provider.

Rep. Daub proposed two bills to allow group long-term care benefits to be provided through pension plans by allowing part of a pension plan to be put into a trust that would not be treated as a qualified pension trust.

### Providing Tax Credits or Deductions for Expenses Incurred in the Care of Dependents

Rep. Silvio Conte (R-MA) sponsored a bill to allow as a tax credit an amount equal to the applicable percentage of qualified expenses paid by the individual for the care of a qualifying family member. The applicable percentage would start at 30 percent of the amount of claimable expenses but would be reduced by one percentage point to a minimum of 20 percent for each $2,000 by which the taxpayer's adjusted gross income exceeds $25,000. The amount of credit would also be reduced by $1 for each dollar of adjusted income over $75,000, with maximum limits of $10,000 in total qualified expenses and no more than $5,000 per elderly family member. A qualifying family member would be any individual related to the taxpayer by blood or marriage who is at least aged 70, is diagnosed by a physician as having Alzheimer's disease or is disabled within the definition of section 216(i) of the Social Security Act, and has an annual income of less than $15,000.[1] Qualified elderly care expenses can include home health agency services, homemaker services, adult day care, respite care, health care equipment and supplies, and (for Alzheimer's victims only) nursing home payments. No credit would be permitted for payments for nursing home care for a sick elderly family member not institutionalized for Alzheimer's disease or related dementia.

Rep. Bilirakis introduced a bill to allow deduction of an amount equal to the amount by which qualified elder care expenses paid by the taxpayer during one year exceed 5 percent of the taxpayer's adjusted gross income. Qualified elder care expenses are defined as payments for in-home custodial care that does not require the continuing attention of trained medical or paramedical personnel. Qualifying elderly individuals are defined as the taxpayer's parents, grandparents, or dependents aged 65 or older. The bill provides that payment for med-

---

[1]Section 216(i) of the Social Security Act defines disabled as "inability to engage in any substantial gainful activity by reason of any medically determinable physical or mental impairment which can be expected to result in death, or has lasted, or can be expected to last, for a continuous period of not less than 12 months."

315

ical services or the provision of a medical good by a physician or registered professional nurse to an individual aged 65 or older would be treated, for tax purposes, as a charitable contribution. (The value of the contribution would be determined by its value under Medicare Part B.)

Rep. Panetta introduced a bill to establish an income tax credit for maintaining a household for dependents aged 65 or older. A $250 tax credit would be allowed for each qualified dependent whose principal place of residence is the same as that of the taxpayer or who is a dependent of the taxpayer and over age 65. In a different vein, Rep. Hunter introduced a measure to provide for a $10,000 deduction for those who care for a Medicare-eligible, chronically ill family member who is unable to perform at least two activities of daily living and who lives in the taxpayer's home.

### Creating a Federal Long-Term Care Reinsurance Corporation

Reps. Rinaldo, Hammerschmidt, and Robert Michel (R-IL) each introduced a measure during the 100th Congress to establish a private corporation to reinsure qualified insurance companies for their long-term care insurance. The proposals authorized that the Secretary of Health and Human Services provide the financial backing and seed money to establish a private corporation that would actively create a secondary market for long-term care insurance-backed securities. It would be similar to financial intermediaries in the student loan and housing markets. The corporation would provide reinsurance of insurance companies for extraordinary losses incurred in the issuance or payment of benefits for qualified long-term care insurance. It would issue common stock vested with full voting rights, one share being entitled to one vote. The full faith and credit of the U.S. government would *not* be pledged to the corporation's obligations and debts, but the corporation, including its capital reserves, surplus, security holdings, and income (everything except its property/real estate) would be exempt from all taxation by any state, county, district, or other local entity.

# Appendix B. Data Bases Used

## Introduction

Several data bases were used in this study. This appendix provides a brief overview of the four primary data bases used.[1]

## Survey of Income and Program Participation

The Census Bureau's Survey of Income and Program Participation (SIPP) was designed to measure household income and participation in private and public welfare programs. The survey interviews individuals every four months over a two and one-half year period. In 1984, SIPP interviewed a sample of about 21,000 households. The survey divides the sample into four rotation groups, returning to the same household every four months. When all four rotation groups have been interviewed, data are released as a single "wave." Because interviews of the four rotation groups occur in consecutive months, a wave spans seven months.

Each wave is processed independently. The Census Bureau calculates weights for each person interviewed so that the responses can be measured as national estimates. Responses to unanswered questions were imputed by the Census Bureau by matching the answers of nonresponding sample members with those of sample members of similar characteristics who did respond.

To capture responses from an individual over several interviews requires the examination of several waves of data. The Employee Benefit Research Institute (EBRI) created a 1984 calendar year research file by matching the records of individuals across waves. Certain questions, known as "core data," are asked every wave. Other sets of questions, known as "topical modules," are asked only during certain waves. Within the 1984 SIPP panel, the topical module dealing with questions of health and disability was conducted during the third wave of interviews, and the topical module on assets and liabilities was conducted during the fourth wave.

The EBRI calendar year file was based on data collected during waves 2 through 5 of the 1984 panel. Records from people who were interviewed in the first wave were linked with data from their records

---

[1]This appendix was prepared by Charles Betley of the Employee Benefit Research Institute.

317

in later waves. Individuals who entered the survey after the first wave were not included in EBRI's calendar year file because such individuals had a statistical probability that they would have been selected for the original sample during the first wave. Inclusion of the later entrants to the sample in the calendar year file would distort the sample's ability to represent the entire population.

Because the interviews in the survey design overlap, not all rotation groups include data for all of waves 2 through 5 in the calendar year file. Also, because individuals may leave the survey because of death, institutionalization, or emigration, data for some people are not available for all four waves and might be missing from one of the topical modules. Although marital status might change over the course of the year, individuals' marital status as of January 1984 was tabulated. The age the individual reported in December 1984 was tabulated, except if the individual left the sample before December 1984. Their age as of January 1984 was tabulated. The EBRI calendar year file includes people who left the survey. For some tabulations, only those individuals who had an entire year's data are included; where appropriate, partial year data were inflated to a full year.

Data from the topical modules of waves 3 and 4 were appended to each person's core data record. For purposes of this study, data from the wave 4 topical module on assets were used only when responses from individuals were given by the individuals themselves or by proxies residing in their households. People with asset data that had been imputed by the Census Bureau were deleted.

## Current Population Survey

The Current Population Survey (CPS) is a monthly sample survey of income, labor force participation, and receipt of public and private welfare benefits by households. The Census Bureau has conducted the CPS each month for nearly 35 years. Because the survey method has changed over time, tabulations of recent CPS data should be compared cautiously with earlier tabulations. However, no other source provides consistent data on income and labor force participation over as long a period for as large a sample.

Approximately 71,000 households are interviewed each month. Individuals are asked to describe their income sources, amounts, coverage under private and public welfare benefit programs and receipt of income from earnings, public transfer payments, interest and dividends, and other sources. EBRI performed its tabulations of the CPS using the public use data tape from the March 1987 CPS. For this

318

study, the CPS was used to estimate the rate of health care coverage among the elderly and nonelderly as well as to estimate income recipiency and poverty status.

## National Long-Term Care Survey

The National Long-Term Care Survey (NLTCS) began in 1982 under the auspices of the National Center for Health Statistics (NCHS) and the Health Care Financing Administration (HCFA) to determine the elderly's use of and need for functional assistance and how that assistance is financed. Administrative data from HCFA were used to select a random sample of Medicare beneficiaries, and those selected were telephoned and asked whether they had any functional impairments. Individuals who responded that they were functionally dependent were selected for face-to-face interviews.

NLTCS is not nationally representative of the entire elderly population. Rather, it represents the elderly who were eligible for Medicare and were functionally dependent yet living in the community in 1982. In 1984, the same individuals who had been interviewed in 1982 were contacted again. Respondents to the 1982 survey who were admitted to an institution in the intervening two years were included, along with information from surviving family members if the respondent had died before the 1984 survey. In addition to tracking people from the 1982 survey, the 1984 survey included new respondents, including those who had been 63 or 64 years old in 1982, making the total sample in 1984 approximately 30,000 persons.

NLTCS was used to examine various aspects of the elderly population with functional limitations. EBRI used the NLTCS public use data files produced by NCHS and HCFA.

## National Nursing Home Survey

To increase understanding of nursing home use, EBRI used published data from the National Nursing Home Survey (NNHS). NNHS is conducted irregularly by NCHS; EBRI used data collected in 1977 and in 1985.

NNHS is based on a representative sample of about 1,200 nursing homes in the 48 contiguous United States (excluding Alaska and Hawaii). Interviewers visited selected nursing homes and chose a sample of residents who had been living in the facilities on the evening before the interviewers' visits, a sample of discharge records from the 12 months preceding the visits, and a sample of registered nurses who were employed by the nursing homes or hired on a temporary or contract basis for the day of the visit.

# Bibliography

Aaron, Henry J. "When Is a Burden Not a Burden? The Elderly in America." *The Brookings Review* (Summer 1986): 17–24.

Aaron, Henry J., Barry P. Bosworth, and Gary Burtless. *Can America Afford to Grow Old? Paying for Social Security.* Washington, DC: Brookings Institution, 1989.

Abramowitz, Michael. "Long-Term Care Plans Aimed at the Elderly." *Washington Post*, 15 November 1987, Washington Business section, p. 28.

Advisory Committee on Long-Term Care. National Association of Insurance Commissioners. "Long Term Care: An Industry Perspective on Market Development and Consumer Protection." Exposure Draft (project begun March 1985), n.d.

————. "Long-Term Care Insurance Model Act." December 1988.

Altman, Lawrence K. "Alzheimer's: Progress in the Midst of Despair." *New York Times*, 18 November 1986, p. C1.

American Medical Association. Board of Trustees. "A Proposal for Financing Health Care of the Elderly." *Journal of the American Medical Association* (26 December 1986): 3379–3390.

Anderson, Kathryn H., and Richard V. Burkhauser. "The Retirement-Health Nexus: A New Measure of an Old Puzzle." *The Journal of Human Resources* (Summer 1985): 315–330.

Anderson, Kathryn H., Richard V. Burkhauser, and Joseph F. Quinn. "Do Retirement Dreams Come True? The Effect of Unanticipated Events on Retirement Plans." *Industrial and Labor Relations Review* (July 1986): 518–526.

Andolsek, Kathryn M., Nancy E. Clapp-Channing, Stephen H. Gehlbach, Irene Moore, Valerie S. Proffitt, Alverta Sigmon, and Gregg A. Warshaw. "Caregivers and Elderly Relatives: The Prevalence of Caregiving in a Family Practice." *Archive of Internal Medicine* (October 1988): 2177–2180.

Andrews, Emily S. *The Changing Profile of Pensions in America.* Washington, DC: Employee Benefit Research Institute, 1985.

————. Employee Benefit Research Institute. "Economic Incentives for Retirement in the Public and Private Sectors." *EBRI Issue Brief* no. 57 (August 1986).

————. "Expanding Opportunities for Older Workers." Employee Benefit Research Institute paper no. P–48, 15 February 1989.

Andrews, Emily S., and Deborah J. Chollet. "Future Sources of Retirement Income: Whither the Baby Boom?" In Susan M. Wachter, ed., *Social Security and Private Pensions: Providing for Retirement in the Twenty-First Century.* Lexington, MA: D.C. Heath and Company, 1988.

Andrews, Emily S., and Jennifer Davis. Employee Benefit Research Institute. "Earnings as an Employee Benefit: Growth and Distribution." *EBRI Issue Brief* no. 75 (February 1988).

Anlyan, William G., Jr., and Joseph Lipscomb. "The National Health Care Trust Plan: A Blueprint for Market and Long-Term Care Reform." *Health Affairs* (Fall 1985): 5–31.

321

*Annual Report of the Board of Trustees of the Federal Hospital Insurance Trust Fund.* Social Security Administration. U.S. Department of Health and Human Services. Baltimore, MD: Social Security Administration, 1988a.

*Annual Report of the Board of Trustees of the Federal Old-Age and Survivors Insurance and Disability Insurance (OASDI) Trust Funds.* Social Security Administration. U.S. Department of Health and Human Services. Baltimore, MD: Social Security Administration, 1987 and 1988b.

*Annual Report of the Board of Trustees of the Federal Supplementary Medical Insurance Trust Fund.* Social Security Administration. U.S. Department of Health and Human Services. Baltimore, MD: Social Security Administration, 1988c.

Applebaum, Robert A. "The Evaluation of the National Long Term Care Demonstration: 3. Recruitment and Characteristics of Channeling Clients." *HSR: Health Services Research* (April 1988): 51–66.

Applebaum, Robert A., Jon B. Christianson, Margaret Harrigan, and Jennifer Schore. "The Evaluation of the National Long Term Care Demonstration: 9. The Effect of Channeling on Mortality, Functioning, and Well-Being." *HSR: Health Services Research* (April 1988): 143–159.

Arrow, Kenneth J. "The Economics of Moral Hazard: Further Comment." *American Economic Review* (June 1968): 537–539.

———. "Uncertainty and the Welfare Economics of Medical Care." *American Economic Review* (December 1963): 941–973.

Bachman, Sara S., Ann F. Collard, Jay N. Greenberg, Edith Fountain, Thomas W. Huebner, Barbara Kimball, and Kathryn Melendy. "An Innovative Approach to Geriatric Acute Care Delivery: The Choate-Symmes Experience." *Hospital & Health Services Administration* (November 1987): 509–520.

Baldassare, Mark, Sarah Rosenfield, and Karen Rook. "The Types of Social Relations Predicting Elderly Well-Being." *Research on Aging* (December 1984): 549–559.

Baldwin, Carliss Y., and Christine E. Bishop. "Return to Nursing Home Investment: Issues for Public Policy." *Health Care Financing Review* (Summer 1984): 43–52.

Bazzoli, Gloria J. "The Early Retirement Decision: New Empirical Evidence on the Influence of Health." *The Journal of Human Resources* (Spring 1985): 214–234.

Bell, Nancy Sutton. "Financing the Long-Term Care Risk." *Journal of the American Society of CLU & ChFC* (September 1988): 72–78.

Benjamin, A.E. "Determinants of State Variations in Home Health Utilization and Expenditures Under Medicare." *Medical Care* (June 1986): 535–547.

Benjamin, A.E., Philip R. Lee, and Sharon N. Solkowitz. "Case Management of Persons with Acquired Immunodeficiency Syndrome in San Francisco." *Health Care Financing Review* (December 1988, annual supplement): 69–74.

Berk, Marc L., and Amy Bernstein. "Use of Home Health Services: Some Findings from the National Medical Care Expenditure Survey." *Home Health Care Services Quarterly* (Spring 1985): 13–23.

Berki, S.E. "A Look at Catastrophic Medical Expenses and the Poor." *Health Affairs* (Winter 1986): 138–145.

322

Bernstein, Aaron. "Help Wanted: America Faces an Era of Worker Scarcity that May Last to the Year 2000." *Business Week* (10 August 1987): 48–53.

"The Big Chill (Revisited). Or Whatever Happened to the Baby Boom?" *American Demographics* (September 1985): 22–29.

Bishop, Christine E. "A Compulsory National Long-Term-Care-Insurance Program." In James J. Callahan Jr. and Stanley S. Wallack, eds., *Reforming the Long-Term-Care System: Financial and Organizational Options.* Lexington, MA: D.C. Heath and Company, 1981.

————. "Use of Nursing Care in Continuing Care Retirement Communities." In Richard M. Scheffler and Louis F. Rossiter, eds., *Advances in Health Economics and Health Services Research: A Research Annual. Private-Sector Involvement in Health Care: Implications for Access, Cost, and Quality,* vol. 9. Greenwich, CT: JAI Press Inc., 1988.

Blank, Susan, and Thomas Brock. "Health, Health Care, and Economic Self-Sufficiency." In Jack A. Meyer and Marion Ein Lewin, eds., *Charting the Future of Health Care.* Washington, DC: American Enterprise Institute, 1987.

Blinder, Alan S. "Comment on Fuchs." *Journal of Labor Economics* (July 1986, part 2): S273–S277.

————. *Hard Heads, Soft Hearts.* New York, NY: Addison-Wesley Publishing Company, Inc., 1987.

Borden, Enid A., and Bruce D. Schobel. "Meeting the Future Needs of the Elderly." In Merrill Lynch & Co., Inc., *Financing Long-Term Care: A Tripartite Approach.* Selected papers from a conference in Washington, DC, December 6, 1988.

Boyd, Bruce. Teachers Insurance and Annuity Association and College Retirement Equities Fund. Memorandum, 1987.

Boyd, Bruce. Teachers Insurance and Annuity Association and College Retirement Equities Fund. Memorandum, 1987.

Branch, Laurence G. "Boston Elders: A Survey of Needs, 1978." Center for Survey Research. Report prepared for the City of Boston Commission on Affairs of the Elderly/Area Agency on Aging, Region VI, n.d.

————. "Continuing Care Retirement Communities: Self-Insuring for Long-Term Care." *The Gerontologist* (February 1987): 4–8.

————. "Home Care is the Answer: What is the Question?" *Home Health Care Services Quarterly* (Spring 1985): 3–11.

Branch, Laurence G., Daniel J. Friedman, Marc A. Cohen, Nancy Smith, and Elinor Socholitzky. "Impoverishing the Elderly: A Case Study of the Financial Risk of Spend-Down Among Massachusetts Elderly People." *The Gerontologist* (October 1988a): 648–652.

Branch, Laurence G., and Alan M. Jette. "A Prospective Study of Long-Term Care Institutionalization among the Aged." *American Journal of Public Health* (December 1982): 1373–1379.

Branch, Laurence G., Terrie T. Wetle, Paul A. Scherr, Nancy R. Cook, Denis A. Evans, Liesi E. Hebert, Eugenia Nesbitt Masland, Mary Ellen Keough, and James O. Taylor. "A Prospective Study of Incident Comprehensive Medical Home Care Use among the Elderly." *American Journal of Public Health* (March 1988b): 255–259.

Brody, Elaine M. "Parent Care as a Normative Family Stress." *The Gerontologist* (February 1985): 19–29.

Brody, Elaine M., Morton H. Kleban, Pauline T. Johnsen, Christine Hoffman, and Claire B. Schoonover. "Work Status and Parent Care: A Comparison of Four Groups of Women." *The Gerontologist* (April 1987): 201–208.

Brody, Elaine M., and Claire B. Schoonover. "Patterns of Parent-Care When Adult Daughters Work and When They Do Not." *The Gerontologist* (August 1986): 372–381.

Brody, Jacob A. "An Epidemiologist Views Senile Dementia—Facts and Fragments." *American Journal of Epidemiology* (1982, no. 2): 155–162.

———. "An Epidemiologist's View of the Senile Dementias—Pieces of the Puzzle." In *Senile Dementia: Outlook for the Future.* New York, NY: Allan R. Liss, Inc., 1984.

Brody, Jacob A., Dwight B. Brock, and T. Franklin Williams. "Trends in the Health of the Elderly Population." *Annual Review of Public Health* (1987): 211–234.

Brody, Jacob A., and Daniel J. Foley. "Epidemiologic Considerations." In Edward L. Schneider, ed., *The Teaching Nursing Home: A New Approach to Geriatric Research, Education, and Clinical Care.* New York, NY: Raven Press, 1985.

Brown, Randall S. "The Evaluation of the National Long Term Care Demonstration: 2. Estimation Methodology." *HSR: Health Services Research* (April 1988): 23–49.

Buchanan, Robert J. "Medicaid: Family Responsibility and Long-Term Care." *The Journal of Long-Term Care Administration* (Fall 1984): 19–25.

———. *Medicaid Cost Containment: Long-Term Care Reimbursement.* Cranbury, NJ: Associated University Presses, Inc., 1987.

Buck Consultants. "Long-Term Care Insurance—A Benefit in its Infancy." *For Your Benefit . . .* (February 1988).

Bureau of the Census. U.S. Department of Commerce. "Detailed Population Characteristics: Summary Section A." *1980 Census of Population.* Pub. no. PC80-1-D1-A. Washington, DC: U.S. Government Printing Office, 1984.

———. "Disability, Functional Limitation, and Health Insurance Coverage: 1984–1985." *Current Population Reports.* Household Economic Studies, Series P-70, no. 8. Washington, DC: U.S. Government Printing Office, 1986a.

———. *Historical Statistics of the United States: Colonial Times to 1970,* Bicentennial Edition, part 1. Washington, DC: U.S. Government Printing Office, 1975.

———. "Household After-Tax Income: 1986." *Current Population Reports.* Special Studies, Series P-23, no. 157. Washington, DC: U.S. Government Printing Office, 1988a.

———. "Household Wealth and Asset Ownership: 1984. Data from the Survey of Income and Program Participation." *Current Population Reports.* Household Economic Studies, Series P-70, no. 7. Washington, DC: U.S. Government Printing Office, 1986b.

———. "Marital Status and Living Arrangements, March 1988." *Current Population Reports.* Population Characteristics, Series P-20, no. 433. Washington, DC: U.S. Government Printing Office, 1989a.

———. "Money Income and Poverty Status of Families and Persons in the United States: 1984." *Current Population Reports.* Consumer Income, Series P-60, no. 189. Washington, DC: U.S. Government Printing Office, 1985.

————. "Pensions: Worker Coverage and Retirement Income, 1984." *Current Population Reports*. Household Economic Studies, Series P-70, no. 149. Washington, DC: U.S. Government Printing Office, 1987a.

————. "Poverty in the United States, 1986." *Current Population Reports*. Consumer Income, Series P-60, no. 160. Washington, DC: U.S. Government Printing Office, 1988b.

————. "Projections of the Population of the United States, by Age, Sex, and Race:1988 to 2080." *Current Population Reports*. Population Estimates and Projections, Series P-25, no. 1018. Washington, DC: U.S. Government Printing Office, 1989b.

————. "State Population and Household Estimates with Age, Sex, and Components of Change: 1981–1987." *Current Population Reports*. Population Estimates and Projections, Series P-25, no. 1024. Washington, DC: U.S. Government Printing Office, 1988c.

————. *Statistical Abstract of the United States: 1987*, 107th ed. Washington, DC: U.S. Government Printing Office, 1986c.

————. *Statistical Abstract of the United States: 1988*, 108th ed. Washington, DC: U.S. Government Printing Office, 1987b.

————. "United States Population Estimates by Age, Sex, and Race: 1980 to 1987." *Current Population Reports*. Population Estimates and Projections, Series P-25, no. 1022. Washington, DC: U.S. Government Printing Office, 1988d.

————. "Who's Helping Out? Support Networks Among American Families." *Current Population Reports*. Household Economics Studies, Series P-70, no. 13. Washington, DC: U.S. Government Printing Office, 1988e.

Bureau of Data Management and Strategy. Health Care Financing Administration. U.S. Department of Health and Human Services. Unpublished data, 1989.

Bureau of Labor Statistics. U.S. Department of Labor. *Employee Benefits in Medium and Large Firms, 1986*. Washington, DC: U.S. Government Printing Office, 1987a.

————. *Employee Benefits in Medium and Large Firms, 1988*. Washington, DC: U.S. Government Printing Office, 1989a.

————. "Employer-Sponsored Retiree Health Insurance." Unpublished paper, May 1986.

————. *Employment and Earnings* (July 1987 and Febuary 1989b).

————. *Handbook of Labor Statistics*. Washington, DC: U.S. Government Printing Office, 1985.

————. Unpublished data, 25 September 1987c.

Bureau of National Affairs. "Employers and Eldercare: A New Benefit Coming of Age." *The National Report on Work and Family*. Special Report no. 3. Washington, DC: Bureau of National Affairs, 1988.

Burke, Thomas R. "Long-Term Care: The Public Role and Private Initiatives." *Health Care Financing Review* (December 1988, annual supplement): 1–5.

Burkhauser, Richard V., Karen C. Holden, and Daniel Feaster. "Incidence, Timing, and Events Associated With Poverty: A Dynamic View of Poverty in Retirement." *Journal of Gerontology: Social Sciences* (March 1988): S46–S52.

Burkhauser, Richard V., and Joseph F. Quinn. "Is Mandatory Retirement Overrated? Evidence from the 1970s." *The Journal of Human Resources* (Summer 1983): 337–358.

Burtless, Gary. "Social Security, Unanticipated Benefit Increases, and the Timing of Retirement." *Review of Economic Studies* (October 1986): 781–805.

Burtless, Gary, ed. *Work, Health and Income among the Elderly.* Washington, DC: Brookings Institution, 1987.

Burwell, Brian, E. Kathleen Adams, and Mark [R.] Meiners. "Spend-Down of Assets Prior to Medicaid Eligibility Among Nursing Home Recipients in Michigan." Office of Research. Health Care Financing Administration. U.S. Department of Health and Human Services. HCFA contract no. 500-86-0016, February 1989.

Butler, John A., Judith D. Singer, Judith S. Palfrey, and Deborah K. Walker. "Health Insurance Coverage and Physician Use Among Children With Disabilities: Findings From Probability Samples in Five Metropolitan Areas." *Pediatrics* (January 1987): 89–98.

Butler, Robert N. *Why Survive? Being Old in America.* New York, NY: Harper & Row, 1975.

Butz, William P., Kevin F. McCarthy, Peter A. Morrison, and Mary E. Vaiana. *Demographic Changes in America's Future.* Santa Monica, CA: Rand Corporation, 1982.

Callahan, Daniel. *Setting Limits: Medical Goals in an Aging Society.* New York, NY: Simon and Schuster, 1987.

Callahan, James J., Jr., Lawrence [M.] Diamond, Janet Giele, and Robert Morris. "Responsibilities of Families for Their Severely Disabled Elderly." *Health Care Financing Review* (Winter 1980): 29–48.

Callahan, James J., Jr., and Stanley S. Wallack. "Major Reforms in Long-Term Care." In James J. Callahan Jr. and Stanley S. Wallack, eds., *Reforming the Long-Term-Care System: Financial and Organizational Options.* Lexington, MA: D.C. Heath and Company, 1981.

Cambridge Reports, Inc. *Trends and Forecasts* (October 1988).

Capitman, John A. "Case Management for Long-Term and Acute Medical Care." *Health Care Financing Review* (December 1988, annual supplement): 53–55.

Capitman, John A., Jeffrey [M.] Prottas, Margaret MacAdam, Walter [N.] Leutz, Don Westwater, and Donna L. Yee. "A Descriptive Framework for New Hospital Roles in Geriatric Care." *Health Care Financing Review* (December 1988, annual supplement): 17–25.

Carcagno, George J., and Peter Kemper. "The Evaluation of the National Long Term Care Demonstration: 1. An Overview of the Channeling Demonstration and its Evaluation." *HSR: Health Services Research* (April 1988): 1–22.

Carlsen, Melody A. "Census of Certified Employee Benefit Specialists, Results, May 1988: Growing Uncertainties—Mandated Benefits and Long Term Care." *Benefits Quarterly* (1988, third quarter): 108–113.

Cartwright, William S., and Robert B. Friedland. "The President's Commission on Pension Policy Household Survey 1980: Net Wealth Distributions by Type and Age." *Review of Income and Wealth* (September 1985): 285–308.

326

Cartwright, William S., Teh-wei Hu, and Lien-fu Huang. "Cost of Illness and the Elderly." Unpublished manuscript, March 1984, revised.

Chollet, Deborah J. "The Demographics of Health Care." *Journal of Compensation* (forthcoming, a).

_____. Employee Benefit Research Institute. "Issues and Trends in Retiree Health Benefits." *EBRI Issue Brief* no. 84 (November 1988a).

_____. Employee Benefit Research Institute. "A Profile of the Nonelderly Population without Health Insurance." *EBRI Issue Brief* no. 66 (May 1987a).

_____. *Financing the Elderly's Health Care: Public Policy and Private Options.* Washington, DC: Employee Benefit Research Institute, forthcoming, b.

_____. "Financing Retirement Today and Tomorrow: The Prospect for America's Workers." In Employee Benefit Research Institute. *America In Transition: Benefits for the Future.* Washington, DC: Employee Benefit Research Institute, 1987b.

_____. "Retiree Health Insurance Benefits: Trends and Issues." In Employee Benefit Research Institute. *Retiree Health Benefits: What Is the Promise?* Washington, DC: Employee Benefit Research Institute, 1989.

_____. *Uninsured in the United States: The Nonelderly Population without Health Insurance, 1986.* Washington, DC: Employee Benefit Research Institute, October 1988b.

Chollet, Deborah J., and Charles L. Betley. Employee Benefit Research Institute. "Financing Catastrophic Health Care Costs among the Nonelderly Population." *EBRI Issue Brief* no. 71 (October 1987).

Chollet, Deborah J., and Robert B. Friedland. "Assessing the Economic Status of the Elderly Using Income as a Proxy for Well-Being." Paper presented at the American Economic Association meetings in Chicago, IL, December 1987.

Chollet, Deborah J., and Robert B. Friedland. "Employer Financing of Long-Term Care." In Richard M. Scheffler and Louis F. Rossiter, eds., *Advances in Health Economics and Health Services Research: A Research Annual. Private-Sector Involvement in Health Care: Implications for Access, Cost, and Quality,* vol. 9. Greenwich, CT: JAI Press, Inc., 1988a.

Chollet, Deborah J., and Robert B. Friedland. "Employer-Paid Retiree Health Insurance: History and Prospects for Growth." In Robert D. Paul and Diane M. Disney, eds., *The Sourcebook on Postretirement Health Care Benefits.* Greenvale, NY: Panel Publishers, Inc., 1988b.

Chollet, Deborah J., and Robert B. Friedland. "Income as a Proxy for the Economic Status of the Elderly." Survey of Income and Program Participation Working Paper no. 8811. Washington, DC: Bureau of the Census, U.S. Department of Commerce, July 1988c.

Christianson, Jon B. "The Evaluation of the National Long Term Care Demonstration: 6. The Effect of Channeling on Informal Caregiving." *HSR: Health Services Research* (April 1988): 99–117.

Churchill, Larry R. *Rationing Health Care in America: Perceptions and Principles of Justice.* Notre Dame, IN: University of Notre Dame Press, 1987.

Clark, Robert L., and Joseph J. Spengler. *The Economics of Individual and Population Aging.* New York, NY: Cambridge University Press, 1980.

Clark, William F., Anabel O. Pelham, and Marleen L. Clark. *Old and Poor: A Critical Assessment of the Low-Income Elderly.* Lexington, MA: D.C. Heath and Company, 1988.

Cohen, Joel [W.], and John [F.] Holahan. "An Evaluation of Current Approaches to Nursing Home Capital Reimbursement." *Inquiry* (Spring 1986): 23–39.

Cohen, Marc A. "Life Care: New Options for Financing and Delivering Long-Term Care." *Health Care Financing Review* (December 1988, annual supplement): 139–143.

Cohen, Marc A., Eileen J. Tell, Helen L. Batten, and Mary Jo Larson. "Attitudes Toward Joining Continuing Care Retirement Communities." *The Gerontologist* (October 1988): 637–643.

Cohen, Marc A., Eileen J. Tell, Jay N. Greenberg, and Stanley S. Wallack. "The Financial Capacity of the Elderly to Insure for Long-Term Care." *The Gerontologist* (August 1987): 494–502.

Cohen, Marc A., Eileen J. Tell, and Stanley S. Wallack. "Client-Related Risk Factors of Nursing Home Entry Among Elderly Adults." *Journal of Gerontology* (November 1986a): 785–792.

Cohen, Marc A., Eileen J. Tell, and Stanley S. Wallack. "The Lifetime Risks and Costs of Nursing Home Use Among the Elderly." *Medical Care* (December 1986b): 1161–1172.

Cohen, Marc A., Eileen J. Tell, and Stanley S. Wallack. "The Risk Factors of Nursing Home Entry Among Residents of Six Continuing Care Retirement Communities." *Journal of Gerontology: Social Sciences* (January 1988): S15–S21.

Colerick, Elizabeth J., and Linda K. George. "Predictors of Institutionalization Among Caregivers of Patients with Alzheimer's Disease." *Journal of the American Geriatrics Society* (July 1986): 493–498.

Committee on Energy and Commerce. House. U.S. Congress. *Long-Term Care Services for the Elderly: Background Materials on Financing and Delivery of Long-Term Care Services for the Elderly.* Report prepared by the Congressional Research Service. 99th Cong., 2nd sess. Committee Print 99-EE. Washington, DC: U.S. Government Printing Office, 1986.

———. *Medicaid Source Book: Background Data and Analysis.* Report prepared by the Congressional Research Service. 100th Cong., 2nd sess. Committee Print 100-AA. Washington, DC: U.S. Government Printing Office, 1988.

Committee on Finance. Senate. U.S. Congress. *Quality of Long-Term Care.* 100th Cong., 1st sess. S. Hrg. 100-406. Washington, DC: U.S. Government Printing Office, 1987.

Committee on Nursing Home Regulation. Institute of Medicine. National Academy of Sciences. *Improving the Quality of Care in Nursing Homes.* Washington, DC: National Academy Press, 1986.

Committee on Ways and Means. House. U.S. Congress. *Background Material and Data on Programs Within the Jurisdiction of the Committee on Ways and Means,* 1988 ed. 100th Cong., 2nd sess. WCMP:100-29. Washington, DC: U.S. Government Printing Office, 1988.

———. *Retirement Income for an Aging Population.* 100th Cong., 1st sess. WMCP:100-22. Washington, DC: U.S. Government Printing Office, 1987.

Conference Board. News release, 12 January 1988.

Congressional Budget Office. U.S. Congress. *Changes in the Living Arrangements of the Elderly: 1960–2030.* Washington, DC: U.S. Government Printing Office, March 1988.

_____. Estimates of H.R. 3188. 13 October 1987.

Consumers Union. "Who Can Afford a Nursing Home?" *Consumer Reports* (May 1988): 300–311.

Cook-Deegan, Robert M. "Dealing with the Impact of Dementia." *Business and Health* (September 1986): 26–30.

Cornoni-Huntley, Joan C., Daniel J. Foley, Lon R. White, Richard Suzman, Lisa F. Berkman, Denis A. Evans, and Robert A. Wallace. "Epidemiology of Disability in the Oldest Old: Methodologic Issues and Preliminary Findings." *Milbank Memorial Fund Quarterly: Health and Society* (Spring 1985): 350–376.

Correia, Eddie W. "Options for Federal Financing of Long-Term Care." In Valerie LaPorte and Jeffrey Rubin, eds., *Reform and Regulation in Long-Term Care*. New York, NY: Praeger Publishers, 1979.

Corson, Walter, Thomas Grannemann, and Nancy Holden. "The Evaluation of the National Long Term Care Demonstration: 5. Formal Community Services under Channeling." *HSR: Health Services Research* (April 1988): 83–98.

Coughlin, Theresa A., and Korbin Liu. "Health Care Costs of Older Persons with Cognitive Impairments." *The Gerontologist* (April 1989): 173–182.

Council of Economic Advisers. *Economic Report of the President, 1988*. Transmitted to Congress February 1988. Washington, DC: U.S. Government Printing Office, 1988.

Cronin, Carol. *Health Benefits for an Aging Workforce: Issues and Strategies*. Washington, DC: Washington Business Group on Health and American Association of Retired Persons, 1988.

Curtis, Richard E., and Lawrence R. Bartlett. "High Cost of Long-Term Care Squeezes State Budgets." *Caring* (March 1985): 28–31.

Custer, William S. Employee Benefit Research Institute. "Managing Health Care Costs and Quality." *EBRI Issue Brief* no. 87 (February 1989).

Davis, Karen. "The U.S. Health Care System of the Future: A Long-Range Policy Proposal." In Shelah Leader and Marilyn Moon, eds., *Changing America's Health Care System: Proposals for Legislative Action*. American Association of Retired Persons. Glenview, IL: Scott, Foresman and Company, 1989.

Davis, Karen, and Diane Rowland. *Medicare Policy: New Directions for Health and Long Term Care*. Baltimore, MD: Johns Hopkins University Press, 1986.

DeFriese, Gordon H., ed. "Special Issue: The Evaluation of the National Long Term Care Demonstration." *HSR: Health Services Research* (April 1988).

Delaney, Meg. "Long-Term Care: Workable Options for Employers Now." *Health Cost Management* (July-August 1987): 21–27.

Densen, Paul M. "The Elderly and the Health Care System: Another Perspective." *The Milbank Quarterly* (1987, no. 4): 614–638.

Diamond, Peter, and Jerry Hausman. "The Retirement and Unemployment Behavior of Older Men." In H[enry J.] Aaron and G[ary] Burtless, eds., *Retirement and Economic Behavior*. Washington, DC: Brookings Institution, 1984.

Division of National Cost Estimates. Office of the Actuary. Health Care Financing Administration. U.S. Department of Health and Human Services. "National Health Expenditures, 1986–2000." *Health Care Financing Review* (Summer 1987): 1–36.

Doran, Phyllis A., Kenneth D. MacBain, and William A. Reimert. *Measuring and Funding Corporate Liabilities for Retiree Health Benefits.* Washington, DC: Employee Benefit Research Institute, 1987.

Doty, Pamela. "Family Care of the Elderly: The Role of Public Policy." *The Milbank Quarterly* (1986a, no. 1): 34–75.

―――――. "Long-Term Care for the Elderly Provided within the Framework of Health Care Schemes." Office of Legislation and Policy. Health Care Financing Administration. Report of the Permanent Committee on Medical Care and Sickness Insurance presented at the International Social Security Association's 22nd General Assembly in Montreal, September 2–12, 1986b.

―――――. "Long-Term Care in International Perspective." *Health Care Financing Review* (December 1988, annual supplement): 145–155.

Doty, Pamela, Korbin Liu, and Joshua [M.] Wiener. "An Overview of Long-Term Care." *Health Care Financing Review* (Spring 1985): 69–78.

Drèze, Jacques H. *Essays on Economic Decisions Under Uncertainty.* New York, NY: Cambridge University Press, 1987.

Duncan, G., M. Hill, and W. Rodgers. *The Changing Economic Status of the Young and Old.* Ann Arbor, MI: Survey Research Center, University of Michigan, 1985.

Edmondson, Brad. "Inside the Empty Nest." *American Demographics* (November 1987): 24–29.

Eggert, Gerald M., and Bruce Friedman. "The Need for Special Interventions for Multiple Hospital Admission Patients." *Health Care Financing Review* (December 1988, annual supplement): 57–67.

Employee Benefit Research Institute. *America in Transition: Benefits for the Future.* Washington, DC: Employee Benefit Research Institute, 1987.

―――――. *Business, Work, Benefits: Adjusting to Change.* Washington, DC: Employee Benefit Research Institute, 1989.

Estes, Carroll L., and Charlene Harrington. "Future Directions in Long Term Care." In Ida VSW Red, ed., *Long Term Care of the Elderly: Public Policy Issues.* Beverly Hills, CA: Sage Publications, Inc., 1985.

Estes, Carroll L., and Philip R. Lee. "Social, Political, and Economic Background of Long Term Care Policy." In Ida VSW Red, ed., *Long Term Care of the Elderly: Public Policy Issues.* Beverly Hills, CA: Sage Publications, Inc., 1985.

Estes, Carroll L., Philip [R.] Lee, Robert [J.] Newcomer, Charlene Harrington, James [H.] Swan, A.E. Benjamin, Lynn Paringer, and Wendy Max. "Correlates of Long Term Care Expenditures and Utilization in 50 States: Executive Summary." Report prepared for the National Center for Health Services Research and Health Care Technology Assessment, Rockville, MD. San Francisco, CA: California University, February 1985.

Evans, Robert G. "Notes of a Catskinner: Alternative Futures for American Health Care." In Shelah Leader and Marilyn Moon, eds., *Changing America's Health Care System: Proposals for Legislative Action.* American Association of Retired Persons. Glenview, IL: Scott, Foresman and Company, 1989.

Eve, Susan Brown. "A Longitudinal Study of Use of Health Care Services Among Older Women." *Journal of Gerontology: Medical Sciences* (March 1988): M31–M39.

Faber, Joseph F., and Alice H. Wade. *Life Tables for the United States: 1900–2050*. Office of the Actuary. Social Security Administration. U.S. Department of Health and Human Services. SSA pub. no. 11-11536. Washington, DC: U.S. Government Printing Office, 1983.

Farfel, Phillip. Author's personal communication, and unpublished results from the Robert Wood Johnson Hospital Based Long-Term Care Initiative at University Hospital, Baltimore, MD, 1988.

Feldblum, Chai R. "Home Health Care for the Elderly: Programs, Problems, and Potentials." *Harvard Journal on Legislation* (Winter 1985): 193–254.

Firman, James [P.]. "Reforming Community Care for the Elderly and Disabled." *Health Affairs* (Spring 1983): 66–82.

Firman, James P., William G. Weissert, and Catherine E. Wilson. *Private Long-Term Care Insurance: How Well Is It Meeting Consumer Needs and Public Policy Concerns?* Washington, DC: United Seniors Health Cooperative, 1988.

Fletcher, Susan, Leroy Stone, and William Tholl. "Cost and Financing of Long Term Care in Canada." In Mary Jo Gibson, ed., *Income Security and Long Term Care for Women in Midlife and Beyond: U.S. and Canadian Perspective*. Washington, DC: Women's Initiative of the American Association of Retired Persons, 1987.

Foundation for Hospice and Homecare. *Basic Home Care Statistics: The Industry, 1988*. Washington, DC: National Association for Home Care, 1988.

Friedland, Robert B. "Accumulation of Net Wealth: Effects of the United States Retirement System." Ph.D. diss., George Washington University, 1983.

——. "Assessing the Need For Catastrophic Health Care Cost Insurance." In Employee Benefit Research Institute, *Where Coverage Ends: Catastrophic Illness and Long-Term Health Care Costs*. Washington DC: Employee Benefit Research Institute, 1988a.

——. Employee Benefit Research Institute. "Issues Concerning the Financing and Delivery of Long-Term Care." *EBRI Issue Brief* no. 86 (January 1989).

——. Employee Benefit Research Institute. "Shifts in the Tide: The Impact of Changing Demographics on Employers, Employees, and Retirees." *EBRI Issue Brief* no. 77 (April 1988b).

——. "Financing Long-Term Care." In Frank B. McArdle, ed., *The Changing Health Care Market*. Washington, DC: Employee Benefit Research Institute, 1987a.

——. "A Foggy Tax Code Spells Out Uncertainties with Employer-Sponsored Long-Term Care Insurance." *Business and Health* (November 1988c): 30–33.

——. "Introduction and Background: Private Initiatives to Contain Health Care Expenditures." In Frank B. McArdle, ed., *The Changing Health Care Market*. Washington, DC: Employee Benefit Research Institute, 1987b.

Friedman, Bernard, and Larry M. Manheim. "Should Medicare Provide Increased Coverage for Long Term Care?" Center for Health Services and Policy Research Working Paper no. 144. Evanston, IL: Northwestern University, November 1986.

Fries, James F. "Aging, Natural Death, and the Compression of Morbidity." *New England Journal of Medicine* (17 July 1980): 130–135.

331

_____. "The Compression of Morbidity." *Milbank Memorial Fund Quarterly: Health and Society* (Fall 1983): 397–418.

Fuchs, Victor R. "His and Hers: Gender Differences in Work and Income, 1959–1979." *Journal of Labor Economics* (July 1986, part 2): S245–S272.

_____. *How We Live: An Economic Perspective on Americans from Birth to Death.* Cambridge, MA: Harvard University Press, 1983.

_____. " 'Though Much Is Taken': Reflections on Aging, Health, and Medical Care." *Milbank Memorial Fund Quarterly: Health and Society* (Spring 1984): 143–166.

Fullerton, Howard N., Jr. "Labor Force Projections: 1986 to 2000." *Monthly Labor Review* (September 1987): 19–29.

_____. "The 1995 Labor Force: BLS's Latest Projections." *Monthly Labor Review* (November 1985): 17–25.

Gabel, Jon [R.], Cynthia Jajich, Karen Williams, Kevin Haugh, Sarah Loughran, Susan Van Gelder, Deborah Ehrenworth, and Dianne Washington. "The State of Private Long Term Care Insurance: Results From a National Survey." Health Insurance Association of America. *Research and Statistical Bulletin* (25 November 1986).

Gabel, Jon R., Cindy Toth, and Karen Williams. "A Snapshot of the Private Market in Long-Term Care." *Business and Health* (May 1987): 34–39.

Gajda, Anthony J. "Long-Term Care: Who'll Pay the Bills?" *Personnel* (November 1988): 61–63.

Garber, Alan M. "Long-Term Care, Wealth, and Health of the Disabled Elderly Living in the Community." Working Paper no. 2328. Cambridge, MA: National Bureau of Economic Research, Inc., July 1987.

Gaumer, Gary L., Howard Birnbaum, Frederick Pratter, Robert Burke, Saul Franklin, and Kathy Ellingson-Otto. "Impact of the New York Long-Term Home Health Care Program." *Medical Care* (July 1986): 641–653.

George, Linda K., and Lisa P. Gwyther. "Caregiver Well-Being: A Multidimensional Examination of Family Caregivers of Demented Adults." *The Gerontologist* (June 1986): 253–259.

Getzen, Thomas E., and Charles P. Hall. "Achieving Financial Security Throughout Retirement: The Long Life Insurance Plan." *Benefits Quarterly* (1987, fourth quarter): 10–22.

Gibson, Mary Jo, ed. *Income Security and Long Term Care for Women in Midlife and Beyond: U.S. and Canadian Perspectives.* Washington, DC: Women's Initiative of the American Association of Retired Persons, 1987.

Gilford, Dorothy M., ed. *The Aging Population in the Twenty-First Century: Statistics for Health Policy.* Washington, DC: National Academy Press, 1988.

Ginzberg, Eli, Warren Balinsky, and Miriam Ostow. *Home Health Care: Its Role in the Changing Health Services Market.* Totowa, NJ: Rowman & Allanheld, 1984.

Glasse, Lou, Ron Pollack, and John Rother. "Review of Draft Outline for a Long Term Care Social Insurance Program Initiative." Preliminary draft, 16 July 1987.

Gornick, Marian, and Margaret Jean Hall. "Trends in Medicare Use of Post-Hospital Care." *Health Care Financing Review* (December 1988, annual supplement): 27–38.

Grad, Susan. *Income of the Population Age 55 or Older, 1986*. Office of Policy. Office of Research and Statistics. Social Security Administration. U.S. Department of Health and Human Services. SSA pub. no. 13-11871. Washington, DC: U.S. Government Printing Office, 1988.

Grad, Susan, and Karen Foster. "Income of the Population Age 55 and Older, 1976." *Social Security Bulletin* (July 1979): 16–32.

Graebner, William. *A History of Retirement*. New Haven, CT: Yale University Press, 1980.

Grana, John M., and David B. McCallum, eds. *The Impact of Technology on Long-Term Health Care*. Millwood, VA: Project HOPE Center for Health Affairs, 1986.

Greenberg, Jay N., and Walter N. Leutz. "A Basic Strategy For Financing Long Term Care." *Hospital Progress* (February 1984): 46.

Greenberg, Jay [N.], Walter [N.] Leutz, Merwyn Greenlick, Joelyn Malone, Sam Ervin, and Dennis Kodner. "The Social HMO Demonstration: Early Experience." *Health Affairs* (Summer 1988): 66–79.

Greene, Vernon L. "Nursing Home Admission Risk and the Cost-Effectiveness of Community-Based Long-Term Care: A Framework for Analysis." *HSR: Health Services Research* (December 1987): 655–669.

———. "Substitution Between Formally and Informally Provided Care for the Impaired Elderly in the Community." *Medical Care* (June 1983): 609–619.

Gruenberg, Ernest M. "The Failures of Success." *Milbank Memorial Fund Quarterly: Health and Society* (Winter 1977): 3–24.

Hadley, Jack. *More Medical Care, Better Health? An Economic Analysis of Mortality Rates*. Washington, DC: Urban Institute Press, 1982.

Hambor, John C. "Economic Policy, Intergenerational Equity, and the Social Security Trust Fund Buildup." *Social Security Bulletin* (October 1987): 13–18.

Hammond, J.D., and Arnold F. Shapiro. "AIDS and the Limits of Insurability." *The Milbank Quarterly* (1986, supplement 1): 143–167.

Harder, W. Paul, Janet C. Gornick, and Martha R. Burt. "Adult Day Care: Substitute or Supplement?" *The Milbank Quarterly* (1986, no. 3): 414–441.

Harney, Kenneth R. "Latest Reverse Mortgage Needs Scrutiny." *Washington Post*, 15 October 1988, p. E10.

Harrington, Charlene, Carroll L. Estes, Philip R. Lee, and Robert J. Newcomer. "Effects of State Medicaid Policies on the Aged." *The Gerontologist* (August 1986): 437–443.

Harrington, Charlene, and Leslie [A.] Grant. "Nursing Home Bed Supply, Access, and Quality of Care." Report prepared for the Committee to Study Nursing Home Regulation. Institute of Medicine. National Institutes of Health. San Francisco, CA: Aging Health Policy Center, University of California, January 1985.

Harrington, Charlene, and James H. Swan. "Medicaid Nursing Home Reimbursement Policies, Rates, and Expenditures." *Health Care Financing Review* (Fall 1984): 39–49.

Harrington, Charlene, and James H. Swan. "The Impact of State Medicaid Nursing Home Policies on Utilization and Expenditures." *Inquiry* (Summer 1987): 157–172.

Harrington, Charlene, James H. Swan, and Leslie A. Grant. "Nursing Home Bed Capacity in the States, 1978–1986." *Health Care Financing Review* (Summer 1988): 81–97.

Harris, Louis. "Results of a National Public Opinion Survey on Long-Term Care." Louis Harris and Associates, Inc. Testimony presented at a hearing of the Subcommittee on Health and Long Term Care. Select Committee on Aging. House. U.S. Congress. 29 March 1988.

Harris, Richard J. "Recent Trends in the Relative Economic Status of Older Adults." *Journal of Gerontology* (May 1986): 401–407.

Harvard Medicare Project. *Medicare: Coming of Age, A Proposal for Reform.* Cambridge, MA: Center for Health Policy and Management, John F. Kennedy School of Government, Harvard University, 1986.

Havens, Betty. "Assessment for Care: The Manitoba Model." *Provider* (January 1987): 26–29.

Hay, Joel W., and Richard L. Ernst. "The Economic Costs of Alzheimer's Disease." *American Journal of Public Health* (September 1987): 1169–1175.

Hayward, Mark D., William R. Grady, and Steven D. McLaughlin. "Recent Changes in Mortality and Labor Force Behavior Among Older Americans: Consequences for Nonworking Life Expectancy." *Journal of Gerontology: Social Sciences* (November 1988): S194–S199.

Health Care Financing Administration. U.S. Department of Health and Human Services. "Analysis of State Medicaid Program Characteristics, 1986." *Health Care Financing Program Statistics.* HCFA pub. no. 03249. Washington, DC: U.S. Government Printing Office, August 1987.

_____. "Long Term Care: Background and Future Directions." Discussion Paper no. HCFA 81-20047, 1981.

Henderson, Mary G., Barbara A. Souder, Andrew Bergman, and Ann F. Collard. "Private Sector Initiatives in Case Management." *Health Care Financing Review* (December 1988, annual supplement): 89–95.

Hendrickson, Michael C. "State Tax Incentives for Persons Giving Informal Care to the Elderly." *Health Care Financing Review* (December 1988, annual supplement): 123–128.

Hewitt Associates. *On Employee Benefits* (November-December 1987).

Hing, Esther. "Use of Nursing Homes by the Elderly: Preliminary Data from the 1985 National Nursing Home Survey." *Advancedata from Vital and Health Statistics* no. 135 (14 May 1987).

Hodgson, Thomas A., and Andrea N. Kopstein. "Health Care Expenditures for Major Diseases in 1980." *Health Care Financing Review* (Summer 1984): 1–12.

Holahan, John F., and Joel W. Cohen. *Medicaid: The Trade-off Between Cost Containment and Access to Care.* Washington, DC: Urban Institute, 1986.

Holahan, John [F.], and Joel [W.] Cohen. "Nursing Home Reimbursement: Implications for Cost Containment, Access and Quality." *The Milbank Quarterly* (1987, no. 1): 112–147.

Holahan, John [F.], and Lisa C. Dubay. "The Effects of Nursing Home Bed Supply on Hospital Discharge Delays." Working Paper no. 3710-01-01. Washington, DC: Urban Institute, December 1987.

Holahan, John [F.], and John L. Palmer. "Medicare's Fiscal Problems: An Imperative For Reform." Changing Domestic Priorities Discussion Paper. Washington, DC: Urban Institute, February 1987.

Holden, Karen C. "Poverty and Living Arrangements Among Older Women: Are Changes in Economic Well-being Underestimated?" *Journal of Gerontology: Social Sciences* (January 1988): S22–S27.

Holden, Karen C., Richard V. Burkhauser, and Daniel A. Myers. "Income Transitions at Older Stages of Life: The Dynamics of Poverty." *The Gerontologist* (June 1986): 292–297.

Horn, Jack. "Smaller is Better: Just Ask the Good-Times Generation." *Psychology Today* (June 1978): 24.

Howell, Embry [M.], Larry S. Corder, and Allen Dobson. "Out-of-Pocket Health Expenses for Medicaid Recipients and Other Low-Income Persons, 1980." *National Medical Care Utilization and Expenditure Survey.* Office of Research and Demonstrations. Health Care Financing Administration. U.S. Department of Health and Human Services. Series B, Descriptive Report no. 4, DHHS pub. no. 85-20204. Washington, DC: U.S. Government Printing Office, 1985.

Hu, Teh-wei, Lien-fu Huang, and William S. Cartwright. "Evaluation of the Costs of Caring for the Senile Demented Elderly: A Pilot Study." *The Gerontologist* (April 1986): 158–163.

Huang, Lien-Fu, William S. Cartwright, and Teh-Wei Hu. "The Economic Cost of Senile Dementia in the United States, 1985." *Public Health Reports* (January-February 1988): 3–7.

Hughes, Susan L. "Apples and Oranges? A Review of Evaluations of Community-Based Long-Term Care." *HSR: Health Services Research* (October 1985): 461–488.

————. *Long-Term Care: Options in an Expanding Market.* Homewood, IL: Dow Jones-Irwin, 1986.

Hughes, Susan L., Kendon J. Conrad, Larry M. Manheim, and Perry L. Edelman. "Impact of Long-Term Home Care on Mortality, Functional Status, and Unmet Needs." *HSR: Health Services Research* (June 1988): 269–294.

Hurd, Michael D. "Savings of the Elderly and Desired Bequests." *American Economic Review* (June 1987): 298–312.

Hurd, Michael D., and John B. Shoven. "Inflation Vulnerability, Income, and Wealth of the Elderly, 1969–1979." In T[imothy] M. Smeeding and M.H. David, eds., *Horizontal Equity, Uncertainty, and Economic Well-Being.* Chicago, IL: University of Chicago Press, 1985.

Hurd, Michael D., and David A. Wise. "The Wealth and Poverty of Widows: Assets Before and After the Husband's Death." Working Paper no. 2325. Washington, DC: National Bureau of Economic Research, July 1987.

ICF Incorporated. *Formulation of an Actuarial Cost Model for Federal Long-Term Care Programs.* Final Report. Washington, DC: ICF Incorporated, 1982.

————. *Health Care Coverage and Costs in Small and Large Businesses.* Prepared for the U.S. Small Business Administration. 15 April 1987a.

————. "Policy Options for Long Term Care." Final report submitted to the American Health Care Association. 15 May 1987b.

————. "Private Financing of Long Term Care: Current Methods and Resources, Phase I, Final Report." Report submitted to the Office of the Assistant Secretary for Planning and Evaluation, U.S. Department of Health and Human Services. Washington, DC: ICF Incorporated, January 1985a.

————. "Private Financing of Long Term Care: Current Methods and Resources, Phase II, Final Report." Report submitted to the Office of the Assistant Secretary for Planning and Evaluation, U.S. Department of Health and Human Services. Washington, DC: ICF Incorporated, January 1985b.

Ingram, D.K., and J.R. Barry. "National Statistics on Deaths in Nursing Homes: Interpretations and Implications." *The Gerontologist* (August 1977): 303–308.

Internal Revenue Service. U.S. Department of the Treasury. Revenue Ruling 89-43, 1989-15. *Internal Revenue Bulletin* no. 12, 10 April 1989.

Ippolito, Richard A. *Pensions, Economics and Public Policy.* Homewood, IL: Dow Jones-Irwin, 1986.

Isaacs, Joseph C., and Stephanie Tames. "Long-Term Care: In Search of National Policy." A Government Relations Monograph. New York, NY: National Health Council, Inc., December 1986.

Isaacs, Mareasa R., and Sybil K. Goldman. *State Initiatives in Long-Term Care: Report of a Survey of 32 States.* Submitted to Alpha Center for Health Planning. Office of Health Planning. Bureau of Health Maintenance Organizations and Resources Development. Public Health Service. U.S. Department of Health and Human Services. Pub. no. HRP-0905897. Springfield, VA: National Technical Information Service, U.S. Department of Commerce, August 1984.

Jacobs, Bruce, and William [G.] Weissert. "Home Equity Financing of Long-Term Care for the Elderly." In *Long-Term Care Financing and Delivery Systems: Exploring Some Alternatives.* Washington, DC: U.S. Government Printing Office, 1984.

Jacobs, Bruce, and William [G.] Weissert. "Using Home Equity To Finance Long-Term Care." *Journal of Health Politics, Policy and Law* (Spring 1987): 77–95.

Jazwiecki, Thomas. "Alternative Mechanisms for Financing the Care of Dementia." American Health Care Association. Paper prepared for the California Alzheimer's Disease Task Force symposium on Financing Dementia, February 20, 1986.

Johnston, William B., Arnold E. Packer, Matthew P. Jaffe, Marylin Chou, Philip Deluty, Maurice Ernst, Adrienne Kearney, Jane Newitt, David Reed, Ernest Schneider, and John Thomas. *Workforce 2000: Work and Workers for the Twenty-first Century.* Indianapolis, IN: Hudson Institute, 1987.

Joint Committee on Taxation. House. U.S. Congress. *Background on the Taxation of Life Insurance Companies and Their Products.* 98th Cong., 1st sess. Pub. no. JCS-11-83. Washington, DC: U.S. Government Printing Office, 1983.

Jones, Michael B., and Kenneth L. Sperling. "Designing a Long-Term Care Program." *Journal of Compensation and Benefits* (January-February 1989): 215–217.

Justice, Diane. *State Long Term Care Reform: Development of Community Care Systems in Six States.* Washington, DC: Health Policy Studies, Center for Policy Research, National Governors' Association, 1988.

Kamerman, Sheila B., and Alfred J. Kahn. *The Responsive Workplace: Employers and a Changing Labor Force.* New York, NY: Columbia University Press, 1987.

336

Kane, Robert L. "The U.S. Health Care System: Basic Goals." In Shelah Leader and Marilyn Moon, eds., *Changing America's Health Care System: Proposal for Legislative Action.* American Association of Retired Persons. Glenview, IL: Scott, Foresman and Company, 1989.

Kane, Robert L., and Rosalie A. Kane. "Alternatives to Institutional Care of the Elderly: Beyond the Dichotomy." *The Gerontologist* (June 1980, part 1): 249–259.

Kane, Robert L., and Rosalie A. Kane. "A Will and A Way: What Americans Can Learn About Long-Term Care from Canada." *A Rand Note.* Prepared for the Henry J. Kaiser Family Foundation (N-2154-HJK). Santa Monica, CA: Rand Corporation, August 1985a.

Kane, Robert L., and Rosalie A. Kane, eds. *Values and Long-Term Care.* Lexington, MA: D.C. Heath and Company, 1982.

Kane, Rosalie A. "The Noblest Experiment of Them All: Learning From the National Channeling Evaluation." *HSR: Health Services Research* (April 1988): 189–198.

Kane, Rosalie A., and Robert L. Kane. "The Feasibility of Universal Long-Term-Care Benefits: Ideas from Canada." *New England Journal of Medicine* (23 May 1985b): 1357–1364.

Kane, Rosalie A., and Robert L. Kane. *Long-Term Care: Principles, Programs, and Policies.* New York, NY: Springer Publishing Company, Inc., 1987.

Kastenbaum, R[obert], and S.E. Candy. "The 4% Fallacy: A Methodological and Empirical Critique of Extended Care Facility Population Statistics." *International Journal of Aging and Human Development* (1973, no. 4): 15–21.

Katz, Sidney, Thomas D. Downs, Helen R. Cash, and Robert C. Grotz. "Progress in Development of the Index of ADL." *The Gerontologist* (Spring 1970, part 1): 20–30.

Katz, Sidney, Amasa B. Ford, Roland W. Moskowitz, Beverly A. Jackson, and Marjorie W. Jaffe. "Studies of Illness in the Aged." *Journal of the American Medical Association* (21 September 1963): 914–919.

Katzman, Robert. "Alzheimer's Disease." *New England Journal of Medicine* (10 April 1986): 964–973.

Kemper, Peter. "The Evaluation of the National Long Term Care Demonstration: 10. Overview of the Findings." *HSR: Health Services Research* (April 1988): 161–174.

Kemper, Peter, Randall S. Brown, George J. Carcagno, Robert A. Applebaum, Jon B. Christianson, Walter Corson, Shari Miller Dunstan, Thomas Grannemann, Margaret Harrigan, Nancy Holden, Barbara [R.] Phillips, Jennifer Schore, Craig Thornton, Judith Wooldridge, and Felicity Skidmore. *National Long-Term Care Channeling Demonstration: The Evaluation of the National Long Term Care Demonstration: Final Report.* Mathematica Policy Research, Inc. Report prepared for the U.S. Department of Health and Human Services, HHS contract no. HHS-100-80-0157, revised May 1986.

Kenny, Kathleen, and Bronwyn Belling. "Home Equity Conversion: A Counseling Model." *The Gerontologist* (February 1987): 9–12.

Kerschner, Helen. "A Global Look at Long Term Care." *Provider* (January 1987): 6–8.

Kingson, Eric R., Barbara A. Hirshorn, and John M. Cornman. *Ties That Bind: The Interdependence of Generations.* Washington, DC: Seven Locks Press, 1986.

Knickman, James R. "Private Long-Term Care Insurance: Alleviating Market Failures With Public-Private Partnerships." In Richard M. Scheffler and Louis F. Rossiter, eds., *Advances in Health Economics and Health Services Research: A Research Annual. Private-Sector Involvement in Health Care: Implications for Access, Cost and Quality*, vol. 9. Greenwich, CT: JAI Press, 1988.

Knickman, James [R.], Nelda McCall, James Gollub, and Douglas Henton. *Increasing Private Financing of Long-Term Care: Opportunities for Collaborative Action*. Menlo Park, CA: SRI International, 1986.

Kolb, Deborah S., and Deborah J. Krueger. "Controlling Expansion of the Nursing Home Industry: Effects of Prospective Payment Systems on Capital Formation." *Topics in Health Care Financing* (Spring 1984): 77–87.

Korczyk, Sophie M. *Retirement Security and Tax Policy*. Washington, DC: Employee Benefit Research Institute, 1984.

Kosterlitz, Julie. "The Graying of America Spells Trouble for Long-Term Health Care for Elderly." *National Journal* (13 April 1985): 798–801.

Kovar, Mary Grace. "Expenditures for the Medical Care of Elderly People Living in the Community in 1980." *The Milbank Quarterly* (1986, no. 1): 100–132.

Kronenfeld, Jennie Jacobs, and Marcia Lynn Whicker. *U.S. National Health Policy: An Analysis of the Federal Role*. New York, NY: Praeger Publishers, 1984.

Kunreuther, Howard. "Even Noah Built an Ark: Would You Buy a Low-Priced Policy Against Natural Disaster? Do You Think Other People Would?" *The Wharton Magazine* (Summer 1978): 28–35.

Kusserow, Richard P. *Transfer of Assets in the Medicaid Program: A Case Study in Washington State*. Office of Analysis and Inspections. Office of Inspector General. U.S. Department of Health and Human Services. Pub. no. OAI-09-88-01340. May 1989.

Laitner, John. "Bequests, Gifts, and Social Security." *Review of Economic Studies* (April 1988): 275–299.

Lamberton, C.E., W.D. Ellingson, and K.R. Spear. "Factors Determining the Demand for Nursing Home Services." *Quarterly Review of Economics and Business* (Winter 1986): 74–90.

Lane, D., D. Uyeno, A. Stark, E. Kliewer, and G. Gutman. "Forecasting Demand for Long-Term Care Services." *HSR: Health Services Research* (October 1985): 435–460.

LaPorte, Valerie, and Jeffrey Rubin. "Introduction." In Valerie LaPorte and Jeffrey Rubin, eds., *Reform and Regulation in Long-Term Care*. New York, NY: Praeger Publishers, 1979.

Laudicina, Susan S., and Brian Burwell. "A Profile of Medicaid Home and Community-Based Care Waivers, 1985: Findings of a National Survey." *Journal of Health Politics, Policy and Law* (Fall 1988): 525–546.

Lave, Judith R. "Cost Containment Policies in Long-Term Care." *Inquiry* (Spring 1985): 7–23.

LaVor, Judith. "Long-Term Care: A Challenge to Service Systems." In Valerie LaPorte and Jeffrey Rubin, eds., *Reform and Regulation in Long-Term Care*. New York, NY: Praeger Publishers, 1979.

338

Lawlor, Edward F., and William Pollak. "Financing Long Term Care: Problems and Prospects." Paper presented at the Association for Public Policy Analysis and Management annual meetings, October 24–26, 1985.

Lawton, M. Powell. "Assessing the Competence of Older People." In Donald P. Kent, Robert Kastenbaum, and Sylvia Sherwood, eds., *Research Planning and Action for the Elderly: The Power and Potential of Social Science.* New York, NY: Behavioral Publications, Inc., 1972.

_____. "Competence, Environmental Press, and the Adaptation of Older People." In M. Powell Lawton, Paul J. Windley, and Thomas O. Byerts, eds., *Aging and the Environment: Theoretical Approaches.* New York, NY: Springer-Verlag, 1982.

Lawton, M. Powell, Miriam Moss, Mark Fulcomer, and Morton H. Kleban. "A Research and Service Oriented Multilevel Assessment Instrument." *Journal of Gerontology* (January 1982): 91–99.

Leader, Shelah, and Marilyn Moon, eds. *Changing America's Health Care System: Proposals for Legislative Action.* American Association of Retired Persons. Glenview, IL: Scott, Foresman and Company, 1989.

Lesnoff-Caravaglia, G. "The Five Percent Fallacy." *International Journal of Aging and Human Development* (1978-1979): 187–192.

Letsch, Suzanne W., Katharine R. Levit, and Daniel R. Waldo. "National Health Expenditures, 1987." *Health Care Financing Review* (Winter 1988): 109–122.

Leutz, Walter [N.]. "Long-Term Care for the Elderly: Public Dreams and Private Realities." *Inquiry* (Summer 1986): 134–140.

Leutz, Walter [N.], Ruby Abrahams, Merwyn Greenlick, Rosalie [A.] Kane, and Jeffrey [M.] Prottas. "Targeting Expanded Care to the Aged: Early SHMO Experience." *The Gerontologist* (February 1988): 4–17.

Leutz, Walter N., Jay N. Greenberg, Ruby Abrahams, Jeffrey [M.] Prottas, Larry M. Diamond, and Leonard Gruenberg. *Changing Health Care for an Aging Society: Planning for the Social Health Maintenance Organization.* Lexington, MA: D.C. Heath and Company, 1985.

Levin, Robert. "Employer Initiatives in Long-Term Care." *Business and Health* (June 1988): 6–9.

Levin, Robert, and Rebecca Frobom. *The Corporate Perspective on Long Term Care.* Survey Report. Washington, DC: Washington Business Group on Health, 1987.

Levine, Phillip B., and Olivia S. Mitchell. "The Baby Boom's Legacy: Relative Wages in the Twenty-First Century." *American Economic Review* (May 1988): 66–69.

Levit, Katharine R., Helen C. Lazenby, Daniel R. Waldo, and Lawrence M. Davidoff. "National Health Expenditures: 1984." *Health Care Financing Review* (Fall 1985): 1–35.

Lewin, Marion Ein, ed. *The Health Policy Agenda: Some Critical Questions.* Washington, DC: American Enterprise Institute for Public Policy Research, 1985.

Lewin/ICF. "Preliminary Estimates of the Impact of HCMAs." In Merrill Lynch & Co., Inc., *Financing Long-Term Care: A Tripartite Approach.* Selected papers from a conference in Washington, DC, December 6, 1988.

Lewis, Mary Ann, Shan Cretin, and Robert L. Kane. "The Natural History of Nursing Home Patients." *The Gerontologist* (August 1985): 382–388.

339

Liang, Jersey, and Edward Jow-Ching Tu. "Estimating Lifetime Risk of Nursing Home Residency: A Further Note." *The Gerontologist* (October 1986): 560–563.

Liu, Korbin, Pamela Doty, and Kenneth [G.] Manton. "Medicaid Spenddown in Nursing Homes and the Community." Unpublished manuscript, March 1989.

Liu, Korbin, and Kenneth G. Manton. "The Characteristics and Utilization Pattern of an Admission Cohort of Nursing Home Patients." *The Gerontologist* (February 1983): 92–98.

Liu, Korbin, and Kenneth G. Manton. "The Characteristics and Utilization Pattern of an Admission Cohort of Nursing Home Patients (II)." *The Gerontologist* (February 1984): 70–76.

Liu, Korbin, Kenneth G. Manton, and Barbara Marzetta Liu. "Home Care Expenses for the Disabled Elderly." *Health Care Financing Review* (Winter 1985): 51–58.

Liu, Korbin, Joshua [M.] Wiener, George Schieber, and Pamela Doty. "The Feasibility of Using Case Mix and Prospective Payment for Medicare Skilled Nursing Facilities." *Inquiry* (Winter 1986): 365–370.

Longman, Phillip. *Born to Pay: The New Politics of Aging in America.* Boston, MA: Houghton Mifflin Company, 1987.

Lubitz, James, and Ronald Prihoda. "The Use and Costs of Medicare Services in the Last 2 Years of Life." *Health Care Financing Review* (Spring 1984): 117–131.

Mace, Nancy [L.]. "Caregiving Aspects of Alzheimer's Disease." *Business and Health* (September 1986): 32–35.

Mace, Nancy L., and Peter V. Rabins. *The Thirty-Six Hour Day: A Family Guide to Caring for Persons With Alzheimer's Disease, Related Dementing Illnesses, and Memory Loss in Later Life.* Baltimore, MD: Johns Hopkins University Press, 1981.

Macken, Candace L. "A Profile of Functionally Impaired Elderly Persons Living in the Community." *Health Care Financing Review* (Summer 1986): 33–49.

Manheim, Larry M., and Susan L. Hughes. "Use of Nursing Homes by a High-Risk Long-Term Care Population." *HSR: Health Services Research* (June 1986, part 1): 161–176.

Manning, Willard G., Joseph P. Newhouse, Naihua Duan, Emmett B. Keeler, Arleen Leibowitz, and M. Susan Marquis. "Health Insurance and the Demand for Medical Care: Evidence from a Randomized Experiment." *American Economic Review* (June 1987): 251–277.

Manton, Kenneth G. "Cause Specific Mortality Patterns Among the Oldest Old: Multiple Cause of Death Trends 1968 to 1980." *Journal of Gerontology* (March 1986a): 282–289.

————. "Changing Concepts of Morbidity and Mortality in the Elderly Population." *Milbank Memorial Fund Quarterly: Health and Society* (Spring 1982): 183–244.

————. "A Longitudinal Study of Functional Change and Mortality in the United States." *Journal of Gerontology: Social Sciences* (September 1988): S153–S161.

_____. "Past and Future Life Expectancy Increases at Later Ages: Their Implications for the Linkage of Chronic Morbidity, Disability, and Mortality." *Journal of Gerontology* (September 1986b): 672–681.

Manton, Kenneth G., Dan G. Blazer, and Max A. Woodbury. "Suicide in Middle Age and Later Life: Sex and Race Specific Life Table and Cohort Analyses." *Journal of Gerontology* (March 1987): 219–227.

Manton, Kenneth G., and Korbin Liu. "The Future Growth of the Long-Term Care Population: Projections Based on the 1977 National Nursing Home Survey and the 1982 Long-Term Care Survey." Paper prepared for the Third National Leadership Conference on Long-Term Care Issues in Washington, DC, March 7–9, 1984a.

Manton, Kenneth G., and Korbin Liu. "Projecting Chronic Disease Prevalence." *Medical Care* (December 1984b): 511–526.

Manton, Kenneth G., Clifford H. Patrick, and Katrina W. Johnson. "Health Differentials between Blacks and Whites: Recent Trends in Mortality and Morbidity." *The Milbank Quarterly* (1987, supplement 1): 129–199.

Manton, Kenneth G., and Beth J. Soldo. "Dynamics of Health Changes in the Oldest Old: New Perspectives and Evidence." *Milbank Memorial Fund Quarterly: Health and Society* (Spring 1985): 206–285.

Marshall, Ray. "Reversing the Downtrend in Real Wages." *Challenge* (May-June 1986): 48–55.

Massachusetts Special Commission on Elderly Health Care. "Beyond Chaos and Catastrophic Costs: A Long Term Care Plan for Massachusetts Elderly." April 1987.

McArdle, Frank B., ed. *The Changing Health Care Market.* Washington, DC: Employee Benefit Research Institute, 1987.

McCaffree, Kenneth M., Suresh Malhotra, and John Wills. "Capital and the Reimbursement of the Costs of Nursing Home Services." In Valerie LaPorte and Jeffrey Rubin, eds., *Reform and Regulation in Long-Term Care.* New York, NY: Praeger Publishers, 1979.

McCall, Nelda. "Utilization and Costs of Medicare Services by Beneficiaries in Their Last Year of Life." *Medical Care* (April 1984): 329–342.

McConnel, Charles E. "A Note on the Lifetime Risk of Nursing Home Residence." *The Gerontologist* (April 1984): 193–198.

McDonnell, Nancy S., Teh-wei Hu, and Lon R. White. "A Review of Prevalence and Incidence of Senile Dementia Among the Elderly Population." Unpublished manuscript, n.d.

McKay, Niccie L. "An Econometric Analysis of Costs and Scale Economies in the Nursing Home Industry." *The Journal of Human Resources* (Winter 1988): 57–73.

McMillan, Alma, and Marian Gornick. "The Dually Entitled Elderly Medicare and Medicaid Population Living in the Community." *Health Care Financing Review* (Winter 1984): 73–85.

McMillan, Alma, Marian Gornick, Embry M. Howell, James Lubitz, Ronald Prihoda, Evelyne Rabey, and Delores Russell. "Nursing Home Costs for those Dually Entitled to Medicare and Medicaid." *Health Care Financing Review* (Winter 1987): 1–14.

McMillan, Alma, Penelope L. Pine, Marian Gornick, and Ronald Prihoda. "A Study of the 'Crossover Population': Aged Persons Entitled to Both Medicare and Medicaid." *Health Care Financing Review* (Summer 1983): 19–46.

341

Medicare Catastrophic Coverage Act of 1988 (P.L. 100-360, 1 July 1988), *U.S. Statutes at Large* 102, 683–817.

Meiners, Mark R. "The Case For Long-Term Care Insurance." *Health Affairs* (Summer 1983): 55–79.

_____. "Enhancing the Market for Private Long-Term Care Insurance." *Business and Health* (May 1988a): 19–22.

_____. "Long-Term Care Insurance." *Generations* (Summer 1985): 39–42.

_____. "Public Attitudes on Long-Term Care." Health Insurance Association of America. *Research Bulletin* (March 1989).

_____. "Reforming Long-Term Care Financing through Insurance." *Health Care Financing Review* (December 1988b, annual supplement): 109–112.

_____. "The State of the Art in Long-Term Care Insurance." National Center for Health Services Research. U.S. Department of Health and Human Services. Paper prepared for the Health Care Financing Administration conference on Long-Term Care Financing and Delivery Systems: Exploring Some Alternatives in Washington, DC, January 24, 1984.

Meiners, Mark R., and Arlene K. Tave. "Predicting the Determinants of Demand for Long-Term Care Insurance." National Center for Health Services Research. U.S. Department of Health and Human Services. Unpublished manuscript, preliminary draft, 7 December 1984.

Merrill Lynch & Co., Inc. *Financing Long-Term Care: A Tripartite Approach.* Selected papers from a conference in Washington, DC, December 6, 1988.

Miller, Dorothy A. "The Sandwich Generation: Adult Children of the Aging." *Social Work* (September 1981): 419–423.

Mitchell, Olivia [S.], and Gary Fields. "The Effects of Pensions and Earnings on Retirement: A Review Essay." In Ronald Ehrenberg, ed., *Research in Labor Economics*, vol. 5. Greenwich, CT: JAI Press, 1982.

Montgomery, Rhonda J.V. "Respite Care: Lessons from a Controlled Design Study." *Health Care Financing Review* (December 1988, annual supplement): 133–138.

Moody, H.R. "Ethical Dilemmas in Nursing Home Placement." *Generations* (Summer 1987): 16–23.

Moon, Marilyn. "Cost and Financing of Long Term Care in Canada: A U.S. Response." In Mary Jo Gibson, ed., *Income Security and Long Term Care for Women in Midlife and Beyond: U.S. and Canadian Perspectives.* Washington, DC: Women's Initiative of the American Association of Retired Persons, 1987.

Moon, Marilyn, and Timothy M. Smeeding. "Can the Elderly Really Afford Long Term Care?" Unpublished manuscript, 3 July 1986.

Mor, Vincent, Sylvia Sherwood, and Claire Gutkin. "A National Study of Residential Care for the Aged." *The Gerontologist* (August 1986): 405–417.

Moran, Donald W., and David Kennell. "Restructuring Long Term Care Financing." *Provider* (June 1987): 21–25.

Moran, Donald W., and Janet M. Weingart. "Long-Term Care Financing through Federal Tax Incentives." *Health Care Financing Review* (December 1988, annual supplement): 117–121.

Morford, Thomas G. "Nursing Home Regulation: History and Expectations." *Health Care Financing Review* (December 1988, annual supplement): 129–132.

Morris, Jonas. *Searching for a Cure: National Health Policy Considered.* New York, NY: Pica Press, 1984.

Morrison, Malcom H. "The Aging of the U.S. Population: Human Resource Implications." *Monthly Labor Review* (May 1983): 13–19.

Moscovice, Ira, Gestur Davidson, and David McCaffrey. "Substitution of Formal and Informal Care for the Community-Based Elderly." *Medical Care* (October 1988): 971–981.

Muse, Don, and Chuck Seagrave. Congressional Budget Office. U.S. Congress. Memorandum, 7 August 1989.

Muurinen, Jaana-Marja. "The Economics of Informal Care: Labor Market Effects in the National Hospice Study." *Medical Care* (November 1986): 1007–1017.

National Center for Health Statistics. Public Health Service. U.S. Department of Health and Human Services. "Advance Report of Final Natality Statistics, 1986." *Monthly Vital Statistics Report*, vol. 37, no. 3 supplement, DHHS pub. no. (PHS) 88-1120. Hyattsville, MD: Public Health Service, 12 July 1988a.

————. "Annual Summary of Births, Marriages, Divorces, and Deaths: United States, 1986." *Monthly Vital Statistics Report*, vol. 35, no. 13, DHHS pub. no. (PHS) 87-1120. Hyattsville, MD: Public Health Service, 24 August 1987a.

————. "Characteristics of Nursing Home Residents, Health Status and Care Received: National Nursing Home Survey, United States, May-December, 1977." *Vital and Health Statistics*, series 13, no. 51, DHHS pub. no. (PHS) 81-1712. Washington, DC: U.S. Government Printing Office, 1981.

————. "Current Estimates from the National Health Interview Survey: United States, 1986." *Vital and Health Statistics*, series 10, no. 164, DHHS pub. no. (PHS) 87-1592. Washington, DC: U.S. Government Printing Office, 1987b.

————. "Health Characteristics According to Family and Personal Income: United States." *Vital and Health Statistics*, series 10, no. 147, DHHS pub. no. (PHS) 85-1575. Washington, DC: U.S. Government Printing Office, 1985.

————. "Health Statistics on Older Persons: United States, 1986." *Vital and Health Statistics*. Analytical and Epidemiological Studies, series 3, no. 25. Washington, DC: U.S. Government Printing Office, 1987c.

————. *Health, United States, 1986.* DHHS pub. no. (PHS) 87-1232. Washington, DC: U.S. Government Printing Office, 1986.

————. *Health, United States, 1987.* DHHS pub. no. (PHS) 88-1232. Washington, DC: U.S. Government Printing Office, 1988b.

————. "Life Tables." *Vital Statistics of the United States, 1986*, vol. II, sect. 6, DHHS pub. no. 88-1147. Washington, DC: U.S. Government Printing Office, 1988c.

————. "The National Nursing Home Survey: 1977 Summary for the United States." *Vital and Health Statistics*, series 13, no. 43, DHEW pub. no. (PHS) 79-1794. Washington, DC: U.S. Government Printing Office, 1979.

————. "The National Nursing Home Survey: 1985 Summary for the United States." *Vital and Health Statistics*, series 13, no. 97, DHHS pub. no. (PHS) 89-1758. Washington, DC: U.S. Government Printing Office, 1989.

————. "1986 Summary: National Hospital Discharge Survey." *Advancedata from Vital and Health Statistics* no. 145 (30 September 1987d).

_____. *Vital Statistics of the United States, 1976,* Vol. 1–Natality. Washington, DC: U.S. Government Printing Office, 1980.

National Center for Home Equity Conversion and Health Policy Center of Brandeis University. "The Role of Home Equity in Financing Long Term Care: A Preliminary Exploration." Report submitted to the Minnesota Housing Finance Agency, 28 February 1986.

National Institute on Aging. National Institutes of Health. Public Health Service. U.S. Department of Health and Human Services. *Macroeconomic Demographic Model.* Washington, DC: U.S. Government Printing Office, 1984.

National Study Group on State Medicaid Strategies. "Restructuring Medicaid: An Agenda for Change." Washington, DC: Center for the Study of Social Policy, January 1983.

Neilson, George J., and Gerald L. Robinson. "The Economics of Dementia." Final report to the U.S. Office of Technology Assessment. Columbus, OH: Battelle Memorial Laboratories, December 1984.

Neuschler, Edward. *Medicaid Eligibility for the Elderly in Need of Long Term Care.* Health Policy Studies. Center for Policy Research. National Governors' Association. Washington, DC: National Governors' Association, September 1987.

Newcomer, Robert J., A.E. Benjamin Jr., and Carol E. Sattler. "Equity and Incentives in Medicaid Program Eligibility." In Ida VSW Red, ed., *Long Term Care of the Elderly: Public Policy Issues.* Beverly Hills, CA: Sage Publications, Inc., 1985.

Newhouse, Joseph P., William B. Schwartz, Albert P. Williams, and Christina Witsberger. "Are Fee-For-Service Costs Increasing Faster Than HMO Costs?" *Medical Care* (August 1985): 960–966.

Nocks, Barry C., Max Learner, Donald Blackman, and Thomas E. Brown. "The Effects of a Community-based Long Term Care Project on Nursing Home Utilization." *The Gerontologist* (April 1986): 150–157.

Nusberg, Charlotte. "Industrialized Countries Move Ahead." *Provider* (January 1987): 9–10.

Nyman, John A. "Excess Demand, the Percentage of Medicaid Patients, and the Quality of Nursing Home Care." *The Journal of Human Resources* (Winter 1988a): 76–92.

_____. "Improving the Quality of Nursing Home Outcomes: Are Adequacy- or Incentive-Oriented Policies More Effective?" *Medical Care* (December 1988b): 1158–1171.

_____. "Prospective and 'Cost-Plus' Medicaid Reimbursement, Excess Medicaid Demand, and the Quality of Nursing Home Care." *Journal of Health Economics* (1985, no. 4): 237–259.

O'Shaughnessy, Carol, Richard Price, and Jeanne Griffith. "Financing and Delivery of Long-Term Care Services for the Elderly." Report prepared for the Committee on Finance. Senate. U.S. Congress. Washington, DC: Congressional Research Service, 18 February 1987.

Office of the Assistant Secretary for Planning and Evaluation. U.S. Department of Health and Human Services. "Alzheimer's Disease." Report submitted to Congress, February 1985.

Office of Research and Statistics. Office of Policy. Social Security Administration. U.S. Department of Health and Human Services. "Monthly Tables." *Social Security Bulletin* (January 1989): 38–72.

Office of Technology Assessment. U.S. Congress. *Losing a Million Minds.* Washington, DC: U.S. Government Printing Office, April 1989.

————. *Losing a Million Minds: Confronting the Tragedy of Alzheimer's Disease and Other Dementias.* Pub. no. OTA-BA-323. Washington, DC: U.S. Government Printing Office, 1987.

————. *Technology and Aging in America.* Washington, DC: U.S. Government Printing Office, June 1985.

Olshansky, S.J., and A.B. Ault. "The Fourth Stage of the Epidemiologic Transition: The Age of Delayed Degenerative Diseases." *The Milbank Quarterly* (Summer 1986): 355–391.

Palmer, John L., Timothy [M.] Smeeding, and Christopher Jencks. "The Uses and Limits of Income Comparisons." In John L. Palmer, Timothy [M.] Smeeding, and Barbara Boyle Torrey, eds., *The Vulnerable.* Washington, DC: Urban Institute Press, 1988.

Palmer, John L., Timothy [M.] Smeeding, and Barbara Boyle Torrey, eds. *The Vulnerable.* Washington, DC: Urban Institute Press, 1988.

Palmore, Erdman [B.]. "Total Chance of Institutionalization Among the Aged." *The Gerontologist* (December 1976): 504–507.

Palmore, Erdman B., Bruce M. Burchett, Gerda G. Fillenbaum, Linda K. George, and Laurence M. Wallman. *Retirement: Causes and Consequences.* New York, NY: Springer Publishing Company, 1985.

Paringer, Lynn. "Forgotten Costs of Informal Long Term Care." *Generations* (Summer 1985): 55–58.

Pauly, Mark V. "The Economics of Moral Hazard: Comment." *American Economic Review* (June 1968): 531–537.

————. "Optimal Public Subsidies of Nursing Home Insurance in the United States." *Geneva Papers on Risk and Insurance* (January 1989).

Pear, Robert. "New Law Protects Rights of Patients in Nursing Homes." *New York Times,* 17 January 1988, p. 1.

Pearlman, Robert A., and Richard F. Uhlmann. "Quality of Life in Chronic Diseases: Perceptions of Elderly Patients." *Journal of Gerontology: Medical Sciences* (March 1988): M25–M30.

Peckman, David. Employee Benefit Research Institute. "Reverse Annuity Mortgages: A Viable Source of Retirement Income?" *EBRI Issue Brief* no. 12 (September 1982).

Pelham, Anabel O., and William F. Clark, eds. *Managing Home Care for the Elderly: Lessons from Community-based Agencies.* New York, NY: Springer Publishing Company, 1986.

Phillips, Barbara R., Peter Kemper, and Robert A. Applebaum. "The Evaluation of the National Long Term Care Demonstration: 4. Case Management Under Channeling." *HSR: Health Services Research* (April 1988): 67–81.

Piacentini, Joseph S. Employee Benefit Research Institute. "Pension Coverage and Benefit Entitlement: New Findings from 1988." *EBRI Issue Brief* no. 94 (September 1989).

Piacentini, Joseph S., and Timothy J. Cerino. *EBRI Databook on Employee Benefits.* Washington, DC: Employee Benefit Research Institute, forthcoming.

Pifer, Alan. "Our Aging Society, An Overview of the Challenge." In The Travelers Companies, *America's Aging Workforce*. Hartford, CT: The Travelers Companies, 1986.

Pillemer, Karl. "How Do We Know How Much We Need? Problems in Determining Need for Long-Term Care." *Journal of Health Politics, Policy, and Law* (Summer 1984): 281–290.

Pillemer, Karl, and David Finkelhor. "The Prevalence of Elder Abuse: A Random Sample Survey." *The Gerontologist* (February 1988): 51–57.

Polich, Cynthia L., Laura Himes Iversen, and Charles N. Oberg. *Who Will Pay? The Employer's Role in Financing Health Care for the Elderly*. Excelsior, MN: InterStudy Center for Aging and Long-Term Care, 1987.

Pollak, William. "The Financing of Long-Term Care: Practices and Principles." In John M. Grana and David B. McCallum, eds., *The Impact of Technology on Long-Term Health Care*. Millwood, VA: Project HOPE Center for Health Affairs, 1986.

Poterba, James M., and Lawrence H. Summers. "Public Policy Implications of Declining Old-Age Mortality." In Gary Burtless, ed., *Work, Health, and Income among the Elderly*. Washington, DC: Brookings Institution, 1987.

Prottas, Jeffrey M., and Eugenia Handler. "The Complexities of Managed Care: Operating a Voluntary System." *Journal of Health Politics, Policy and Law* (Summer 1987): 253–269.

Quinn, Jane Bryant. "Should Senior Citizens Foot the Bill for Long-Term Health Insurance?" *Washington Post*, 6 February 1989, Washington Business section, p. 71.

R L Associates. "The American Public Views Long Term Care." A survey conducted for the American Association of Retired Persons and the Villers Foundation. Princeton, NJ: R L Associates, October 1987.

Rabin, David L., and Patricia Stockton. *Long-Term Care for the Elderly: A Factbook*. New York, NY: Oxford University Press, 1987.

Radner, Daniel B. "Shifts in the Aged-Nonaged Income Relationship, 1979–85." ORS Working Papers 35. Washington, DC: Social Security Administration, January 1988.

————. "The Wealth of the Aged and Nonaged, 1984." ORS Working Papers 36. Washington, DC: Social Security Administration, January 1988.

Raper, Ann Trueblood, and Anne C. Kalicki, eds. *National Continuing Care Directory: Retirement Communities with Nursing Care*, 2nd ed. Glenview, IL: American Association of Retired Persons, 1988.

Ray, Wayne A., Charles F. Federspiel, David K. Baugh, and Suzanne Dodds. "Impact of Growing Numbers of the Very Old on Medicaid Expenditures for Nursing Homes: A Multi-State, Population-Based Analysis." *American Journal of Public Health* (June 1987a): 699–703.

Ray, Wayne A., Charles F. Federspiel, David K. Baugh, and Suzanne Dodds. "Interstate Variation in Elderly Medicaid Nursing Home Populations: Comparisons of Resident Characteristics and Medical Care Utilization." *Medical Care* (August 1987b): 738–752.

Reinhardt, Uwe E. Testimony presented at a hearing on Medicare catastrophic insurance of the Committee on the Budget. Senate. U.S. Congress. 25 February 1987.

Rice, Dorothy P. "Health Care Needs of the Elderly." In Ida VSW Red, ed., *Long Term Care of the Elderly: Public Policy Issues.* Beverly Hills, CA: Sage Publications, Inc., 1985.

Rice, Dorothy P., and Jacob J. Feldman. "Living Longer in the United States: Demographic Changes and Health Needs of the Elderly." *Milbank Memorial Fund Quarterly: Health and Society* (Summer 1983): 362–396.

Rice, Thomas. "An Economic Assessment of Health Care Coverage for the Elderly." *The Milbank Quarterly* (1987, no. 4): 488–520.

Rice, Thomas, Katherine Desmond, Jon [R.] Gabel, Steven DiCarlo, and Corinne Kyle. "Fear and Loathing in the Golden Years: The Elderly and Their Health Care Coverage." Unpublished paper, n.d.

Rice, Thomas, and Jon [R.] Gabel. "Protecting the Elderly Against High Health Care Costs." *Health Affairs* (Fall 1986): 5–21.

Rice, Thomas, and Nelda McCall. "The Extent of Ownership and the Characteristics of Medicare Supplemental Policies." *Inquiry* (Summer 1985): 188–200.

Riley, Gerald, James Lubitz, Ronald Prihoda, and Evelyne Rabey. "The Use and Costs of Medicare Services by Cause of Death." *Inquiry* (Fall 1987): 233–244.

Rivlin, Alice M., and Joshua M. Wiener. *Caring For the Disabled Elderly: Who Will Pay?* Washington, DC: Brookings Institution, 1988.

Robert Wood Johnson Foundation. "Program to Promote Long-Term Care Insurance for the Elderly." Program summary, 26 January 1989.

————. "Review of Robert Wood Johnson Foundation Grantee Activities." Unpublished manuscript, March 1988.

Robbins, Aldona, and Gary Robbins. "Encouraging Private Provision of Long-Term Care." *Compensation and Benefits Management* (Summer 1988): 301–305.

Rohrer, James E. "Access to Nursing Home Care: A Need-Based Approach." *Medical Care* (August 1987): 796–800.

Rosenwaike, Ira. "A Demographic Portrait of the Oldest Old." *Milbank Memorial Fund Quarterly: Health and Society* (Spring 1985): 187–205.

Ross, Christine M., Sheldon Danziger, and Eugene Smolensky. "Interpreting Changes in the Economic Status of the Elderly, 1949–1979." *Contemporary Policy Issues* (April 1987): 98–112.

Rother, John, Mary Jo Gibson, and Theresa Varner. "A Social Insurance Approach to Long-Term Care." In Employee Benefit Research Institute, *Where Coverage Ends: Catastrophic Illness and Long-Term Health Care Costs.* Washington, DC: Employee Benefit Research Institute, 1988.

Rubin, Robert J., Donald W. Moran, Katherine S. Jones, and Marie A. Hackbarth. *Critical Condition: America's Health Care in Jeopardy.* Washington, DC: National Committee for Quality Health Care, 1988.

Ruchlin, Hirsch S., and John N. Morris. "The Congregate Housing Services Program: An Analysis of Service Utilization and Cost." *The Gerontologist* (February 1987): 87–91.

Russell, Louise B. "An Aging Population and the Use of Medical Care." *Medical Care* (June 1981): 633–641.

————. *The Baby Boom Generation and the Economy.* Washington, DC: Brookings Institution, 1982.

Saltford, Nancy C. Employee Benefit Research Institute. "Dependent Care: Meeting the Needs of a Dynamic Work Force." *EBRI Issue Brief* no. 85 (December 1988).

Saltford, Nancy C., and Ramona K.Z. Heck. *An Overview of Employee Benefits Supportive of Working Families.* Paper prepared for Panel on Employer Policies and Working Families. Washington, DC: National Research Council, April 19, 1989.

Sandell, Steven H., ed. *The Problem Isn't Age: Work and Older Americans.* New York, NY: Praeger Publishers, 1987.

Scanlon, William J. "A Perspective on Long-Term Care for the Elderly." *Health Care Financing Review* (December 1988, annual supplement): 7–15.

————. "A Theory of the Nursing Home Market." *Inquiry* (Spring 1980): 25–41.

Scanlon, William [J.], Elaine Difederico, and Margaret Stassen. *Long-Term Care: Current Experience and A Framework For Analysis.* Health Policy and the Elderly Series, no. 1215-10. Washington, DC: Urban Institute, February 1979.

Schlesinger, Mark. "On the Limits of Expanding Health Care Reform: Chronic Care in Prepaid Settings." *The Milbank Quarterly* (1986, no. 2): 189–215.

Schmidt, K. Peter. "Retiree Health Benefits: An Illusory Promise?" In Employee Benefit Research Institute, *Retiree Health Benefits: What Is the Promise?* Washington, DC: Employee Benefit Research Institute, 1989.

Schneider, Don P., Brant E. Fries, William J. Foley, Marilyn Desmond, and William J. Gormley. "Case Mix for Nursing Home Payment: Resource Utilization Groups, Version II." *Health Care Financing Review* (December 1988, annual supplement): 39–52.

Schneider, E[dward] L., and J[acob] A. Brody. "Aging, Natural Death, and the Compression of Morbidity: Another View." *New England Journal of Medicine* (6 October 1983): 354–355.

Scholen, Ken. *Home-Made Money: Consumer's Guide to Home Equity Conversion.* Washington, DC: American Association of Retired Persons, 1987.

Schrimper, Ronald A., and Robert L. Clark. "Health Expenditures and Elderly Adults." *Journal of Gerontology* (March 1985): 235–243.

Schultze, Charles L. *The Public Use of Private Interest.* Washington, DC: Brookings Institution, 1977.

Schulz, James H. *The Economics of Aging,* 3rd ed. New York, NY: Van Nostrand Reinhold Company, 1985.

Schwartz, William B. "The Inevitable Failure of Current Cost-Containment Strategies." *Journal of the American Medical Association* (9 January 1987): 220–224.

Schwenger, Cope W. "Health Care for the Elderly in Canada." *Journal of Public Health Policy* (Summer 1987): 222–241.

Scott, Diana J., and Wayne S. Upton Jr. "Postretirement Benefits Other Than Pensions." In Financial Accounting Standards Board, *Highlights of Financial Reporting Issues* (December 1988): 1–4.

Seccombe, Karen. "Financial Assistance from Elderly Retirement-Age Sons to Their Aging Parents." *Research on Aging* (March 1988): 102–118.

Secretary's Commission on Nursing. Health Care Financing Administration. U.S. Department of Health and Human Services. *Interim Report.* Washington, DC: U.S. Government Printing Office, 1988.

Sekscenski, Edward S. "Discharges from Nursing Homes: Preliminary Data from the 1985 National Nursing Home Survey." *Advancedata from Vital and Health Statistics* no. 142 (30 September 1987).

Select Committee on Aging. House. U.S. Congress. *Abuses in Guardianship of the Elderly and Infirm: A National Disgrace.* 100th Cong., 1st sess. Comm. pub. no. 100-639. Washington, DC: U.S. Government Printing Office, 1987a.

————. *America's Elderly at Risk.* 99th Cong., 1st sess. Comm. pub. no. 99-508. Washington, DC: U.S. Government Printing Office, 1985a.

————. *The Attempted Dismantling of the Medicare Home Care Benefit.* 99th Cong., 2nd sess. Comm. pub. no. 99-552. Washington, DC: U.S. Government Printing Office, 1986a.

————. *Building a Long-Term Care Policy: Home Care Data and Implications.* 98th Cong., 2nd sess. Comm. pub. no. 98-484. Washington, DC: U.S. Government Printing Office, 1985b.

————. *Exploding the Myths: Caregiving in America.* 100th Cong., 1st sess. Comm. pub. no. 99-611. Washington, DC: U.S. Government Printing Office, 1987b.

————. *Financing Care for Patients with Alzheimer's Disease and Related Disorders.* 99th Cong., 2nd sess. Comm. pub. no. 99-596. Washington, DC: U.S. Government Printing Office, 1986b.

————. *Nursing Home Insurance: Exploiting Fear for Profit?* 100th Cong., 1st sess. Comm. pub. no. 100-647. Washington, DC: U.S. Government Printing Office, 1988.

————. *Nursing Home Insurance: Exploiting Fear for Profit? (An Examination of an Emerging Long-Term Care Insurance Market).* 100th Cong., 1st sess. Comm. pub. no. 100-634. Washington, DC: U.S. Government Printing Office, 1987c.

————. *Twentieth Anniversary of Medicare and Medicaid: Americans Still at Risk.* 99th Cong., 1st sess. Comm. pub. no. 99-538. Washington, DC: U.S. Government Printing Office, 1986c.

Shapiro, Evelyn, and Robert B. Tate. "Predictors of Long Term Care Facility Use among the Elderly." *Canadian Journal of Aging* (Spring 1985): 11–19.

Shapiro, Evelyn, and Robert B. Tate. "Who Is Really at Risk of Institutionalization?" *The Gerontologist* (April 1988): 237–245.

Shiley, Martha, and Robert Kalish. "Individual Income Tax Returns, Preliminary Data, 1986." *Statistics of Income: SOI Bulletin* (Winter 1987-1988): 39–52.

Short, Pamela Farley, Peter Cunningham, and Curt Mueller. "Standardizing Nursing Home Admission Dates for Short-Term Hospital Admissions." Paper presented at the American Statistical Association meetings in San Diego, CA, January 4–6, 1989.

Sickles, Robin C., and Paul Taubman. "An Analysis of the Health and Retirement Status of the Elderly." *Econometrica* (November 1986): 1339–1356.

Sirocco, Al. "Nursing and Related Care Homes as Reported from the 1986 Inventory of Long-Term Care Places." *Advancedata from Vital and Health Statistics* no. 147 (22 January 1988).

————. "An Overview of the 1982 National Master Facility Inventory Survey of Nursing and Related Care Homes." *Advancedata from Vital and Health Statistics* no. 111 (20 September 1985).

Slovic, Paul, Baruch Fischhoff, and Sarah Lichtenstein. "Cognitive Processes and Societal Risk Taking." In J.S. Carroll and J. Payne, eds., *Cognition and Social Behavior*. Hillsdale, NJ: Lawrence Erlbaum Associates, Inc., 1976.

Smallegan, Marian. "There Was Nothing Else to Do: Needs for Care before Nursing Home Admission." *The Gerontologist* (August 1985): 364–369.

Smeeding, Timothy M., and Lavonne Straub. "Health Care Financing Among the Elderly: Who Really Pays the Bills?" *Journal of Health Politics, Policy and Law* (Spring 1987): 35–52.

Smolensky, Eugene, Sheldon Danziger, and Peter Gottschalk. "The Declining Significance of Age in the United States: Trends in the Well-Being of Children and the Elderly Since 1939." In John L. Palmer, Timothy [M.] Smeeding, and Barbara Boyle Torry, eds., *The Vulnerable*. Washington, DC: Urban Institute Press, 1988.

Social Security Administration. U.S. Department of Health and Human Services. *Social Security Bulletin* (January 1989): 55.

_____. *Social Security Bulletin: Annual Statistical Supplement, 1987*. Washington, DC: U.S. Government Printing Office, 1987.

_____. *Supplemental Security Income for the Aged, Blind, and Disabled: Characteristics of State Assistance Programs for SSI Recipients*. SSA pub. no. 17-002. Washington, DC: U.S. Government Printing Office, 1985.

Soldo, Beth J., and Kenneth G. Manton. "Health Status and Service Needs of the Oldest Old: Current Patterns and Future Trends." *Milbank Memorial Fund Quarterly: Health and Society* (Spring 1985): 286–319.

Somers, Anne R. "Long Term Care for the Elderly and Disabled: An Urgent Challenge to New Federalism." In Burton D. Dunlop, ed., *New Federalism and Long-Term Health Care of the Elderly*. Millwood, VA: Project HOPE Center for Health Affairs, 1985.

Soule, Charles E. *Disability Income Insurance: The Unique Risk*. Homewood, IL: Dow Jones-Irwin, 1984.

Special Committee on Aging. Senate. U.S. Congress. *Aging America: Trends and Projections*. Washington, DC: U.S. Department of Health and Human Services, 1984.

_____. *Aging America: Trends and Projections*, 1987–88 ed. Washington, DC: U.S. Department of Health and Human Services, 1988.

_____. *The Cost of Caring for the Chronically Ill: The Case for Insurance*. 98th Cong., 2nd sess. S. Hrg. 98-1224. Washington, DC: U.S. Government Printing Office, 1985a.

_____. *How Older Americans Live: An Analysis of Census Data*. 99th Cong., 1st sess. S. Prt. 99-91. Washington, DC: U.S. Government Printing Office, 1985b.

_____. *Nursing Home Care: The Unfinished Agenda*. 99th Cong., 2nd sess. S. Prt. 99-160. Washington, DC: U.S. Government Printing Office, 1986.

Spence, Denise A., and Joshua M. Wiener. "Medicaid Spend-Down in Nursing Homes: Estimates from the 1985 National Nursing Home Survey." Brookings Institution. Draft, April 1989.

Steel, Knight. "Physician-Directed Long-Term Home Health Care for the Elderly—A Century-Long Experience." *Journal of the American Geriatrics Society* (March 1987): 264–268.

Strahan, Genevieve. "Nursing Home Characteristics: Preliminary Data from the 1985 National Nursing Home Survey." *Advancedata from Vital and Health Statistics* no. 131 (27 March 1987).

Strate, John M., and Steven J. Dubnoff. "How Much Income Is Enough? Measuring the Income Adequacy of Retired Persons Using a Survey Based Approach." *Journal of Gerontology* (May 1986): 393–400.

Strauss, Anslem, and Juliet M. Corbin. *Shaping a New Health Care System: The Explosion of Chronic Illness as a Catalyst for Change.* San Francisco, CA: Jossey-Bass Publishers, 1988.

"Survey Search: Consumers and Employers on Long-Term Care." *Health Cost Management* (July-August 1987): 28–33.

Sutton, Nancy A. "Long Term Health Care: A Comparison of Group and Individual Products." *Benefits Quarterly* (1987, fourth quarter): 23–30.

Swan, James H., and Charlene Harrington. "Estimating Undersupply of Nursing Home Beds in States." *HSR: Health Services Research* (April 1986): 57–83.

Swan, James H., and Charlene Harrington. "Medicaid Nursing Home Reimbursement Policies." In Ida VSW Red, ed., *Long Term Care of the Elderly: Public Policy Issues.* Beverly Hills, CA: Sage Publications, Inc., 1985.

Task Force on Long-Term Health Care Policies. Health Care Financing Administration. U.S. Department of Health and Human Services. *Report to Congress and the Secretary: Long-Term Health Care Policies.* Washington, DC: U.S. Government Printing Office, 21 September 1987.

Teachers' Insurance and Annuity Association and College Retirement Equities Fund Education Research Unit. "Long-Term Care—A Retirement Planning Issue." *Research Dialogues* (July 1986): 1–8.

Technical Work Group on Private Financing of Long-Term Care for the Elderly. U.S. Department of Health and Human Services. *Report to the Secretary on Private Financing of Long-Term Care for The Elderly.* Preliminary draft, November 1986.

Tell, Eileen J., Stanley S. Wallack, and Marc A. Cohen. "New Directions in Life Care: An Industry in Transition." *The Milbank Quarterly* (1987, no. 4): 551–574.

Thornton, Craig, Shari Miller Dunstan, and Peter Kemper. "The Evaluation of the National Long Term Care Demonstration: 8. The Effect of Channeling on Health and Long Term Care Costs." *HSR: Health Services Research* (April 1988): 129–142.

Thornton, Craig, Joanna Will, and Mark Davies. *National Long-Term Care Channeling Demonstration: Analysis of Channeling Project Costs.* Mathematica Policy Research, Inc. Report prepared for the U.S. Department of Health and Human Services, HHS contract no. HHS-100-80-0157, revised May 1986.

Tilly, Jane, and Debbie Brunner. *Medicaid Eligibility and Its Effect on the Elderly.* AARP Paper no. 8605. Washington, DC: American Association of Retired Persons, January 1987.

Toff, Gail E. *Alternatives to Institutional Care for the Elderly: An Analysis of State Initiatives.* Washington, DC: Intergovernmental Health Policy Project, George Washington University, September 1981.

Tompkins, Arnold R., Margaret E. Porter, and Mary F. Harahan. "Financing Services for Developmentally Disabled People: Directions for Reform." *Health Care Financing Review* (December 1988, annual supplement): 103–107.

Torrey, Barbara Boyle. "Sharing Increasing Costs on Declining Income: The Visible Dilemma of the Invisible Aged." *Milbank Memorial Fund Quarterly: Health and Society* (Spring 1985): 377–394.

The Travelers Companies. *America's Aging Workforce.* Hartford, CT: The Travelers Companies, 1986.

_____. "Employee Caregiver Survey: A Survey on Caregiving Responsibilities of Travelers Employees for Older Americans." Unpublished survey results, June 1985.

U.S. Department of Health and Human Services. "Catastrophic Illness Expenses." Report to the President. Washington, DC: U.S. Department of Health and Human Services, November 1986.

_____. *HHS News* (18 November 1988).

_____. *National Invitational Conference on Long-Term Care Data Bases,* May 21–22, 1987. Washington, DC: U.S. Department of Health and Human Services, 1987.

U.S. General Accounting Office. *An Aging Society: Meeting the Needs of the Elderly While Responding to Rising Federal Costs.* Pub. no. GAO/HRD-86-135. Washington, DC: U.S. Government Printing Office, 1986a.

_____. *The Elderly Should Benefit From Expanded Home Health Care But Increasing These Services Will Not Insure Cost Reductions.* Pub. no. GAO/IPE-83-1. Washington, DC: U.S. Government Printing Office, 1982.

_____. *Entering a Nursing Home—Costly Implications for Medicaid and the Elderly.* Pub. no. PAD-80-12. Washington, DC: U.S. Government Printing Office, 1979.

_____. *401(k) Plans: Incidence, Provisions, and Benefits.* Pub. no. GAO/PEMD-88-15BR. Washington, DC: U.S. Government Printing Office, 1988a.

_____. *Long-Term Care for the Elderly: Issues of Need, Access, and Cost.* Pub. no. GAO/HRD-89-4. Washington, DC: U.S. Government Printing Office, 1988b.

_____. *Long-Term Care Insurance: Coverage Varies Widely in a Developing Market.* Pub. no. GAO/HRD-87-80. Washington, DC: U.S. Government Printing Office, 1987a.

_____. *Long-Term Care Insurance: State Regulatory Requirements Provide Inconsistent Consumer Protection.* Pub. no. GAO/HRD-89-67. Washington, DC: U.S. Government Printing Office, 1989.

_____. *Medicaid: Determining Cost-Effectiveness of Home and Community-Based Services.* Pub. no. GAO/HRD-87-61. Washington, DC: U.S. Government Printing Office, 1987b.

_____. *Medicaid: Improvements Needed in Programs to Prevent Abuse.* Pub. no. GAO/HRD-87-75. Washington, DC: U.S. Government Printing Office, 1987c.

_____. *Medicaid and Nursing Home Care: Cost Increases and the Need for Services are Creating Problems for States and the Elderly.* Pub. no. GAO/IPE-84-1. Washington, DC: U.S. Government Printing Office, 1983.

_____. *Medicare: Comparison of Catastrophic Health Insurance Proposals—An Update.* Pub. no. GAO/HRD-88-19BR. Washington, DC: U.S. Government Printing Office, 1987d.

_____. *Retirement Before Age 65*. Pub. no. GAO/HRD-86-86. Washington, DC: U.S. Government Printing Office, 1986b.

Ullmann, Steven G. "Ownership, Regulation, Quality Assessment, and Performance in the Long-Term Health Care Industry." *The Gerontologist* (April 1987): 233–239.

Utz, John L. "Employers and Long Term Health Insurance: What to Buy, Where to Get It and How to Fund It." *Employee Benefits Journal* (March 1988): 13–20.

Van Gelder, Susan, and Diane Johnson. "Long-Term Care Insurance: Market Trends." Health Insurance Association of America. *Research Bulletin* (March 1989).

Varner, Theresa. "Catastrophic Health Care Costs for Older Americans: The Issue and Its Implications for Policy Development." Working Paper no. 8702. Washington, DC: American Association of Retired Persons, 1987.

Venti, Steven F., and David A. Wise. "Aging, Moving, and Housing Wealth." Working Paper no. 2324. Cambridge, MA: National Bureau of Economic Research, Inc., July 1987.

Verbrugge, Lois M. "Longer Life But Worsening Health? Trends in Health and Mortality of Middle-Aged and Older Persons." *Milbank Memorial Fund Quarterly: Health and Society* (Summer 1984): 475–519.

_____. "Sex Differentials in Health." *Public Health Reports* (September-October 1982): 417–437.

Verbrugge, Lois M., and Jennifer H. Madans. "Social Roles and Health Trends of American Women." *Milbank Memorial Fund Quarterly: Health and Society* (Fall 1985): 691–735.

Vertrees, James, and Kenneth G. Manton. "The Complexity of Chronic Disease at Later Ages: Practical Implications for Prospective Payment and Data Collection." *Inquiry* (Summer 1986): 154–165.

Vicente, Leticia, James A. Wiley, and R. Allen Carrington. "The Risk of Institutionalization before Death." *The Gerontologist* (August 1979): 361–367.

Vignola, Margo L. "At the Threshold Of Major Change." *Provider* (May 1987): 4–6.

Villers Foundation. *On the Other Side of Easy Street*. Washington, DC: Villers Foundation, 1987.

Virginia Housing Development Authority and Virginia Department for the Aging. "Virginia Senior Home Equity Account: Program Summary." Richmond, VA: Virginia Housing Development Authority, 1988.

Vladeck, Bruce C. "The Dilemma Between Competition and Community Service." *Inquiry* (Summer 1985a): 115–121.

_____. "The Static Dynamics of Long-Term Care Policy." In Marion Ein Lewin, ed., *The Health Policy Agenda*. Washington, DC: American Enterprise Institute for Public Policy Research, 1985b.

_____. *Unloving Care: The Nursing Home Tragedy*. New York, NY: Basic Books Inc., 1980.

Wade, Alice [H.]. *Actuarial Tables Based on the U.S. Life Tables: 1979–1981*. Office of the Actuary. Social Security Administration. U.S. Department of Health and Human Services. Actuarial Study no. 96, SSA pub. no. 11-11543. Washington, DC: U.S. Government Printing Office, 1986.

Waldo, Daniel R., and Helen C. Lazenby. "Demographic Characteristics and Health Care Use and Expenditures by the Aged in the United States: 1977–1984." *Health Care Financing Review* (Fall 1984): 1–29.

Waldo, Daniel R., Katharine R. Levit, and Helen [C.] Lazenby. "National Health Expenditures, 1985." *Health Care Financing Review* (Fall 1986): 1–20.

Walker, Clare. "Long Term Care of the Elderly." Paper presented at the American Enterprise Institute conference on Health Policy Reform in the Broader Policy Debate, October 4–5, 1983.

Wallack, Stanley S. "Recent Trends in Financing Long-Term Care." *Health Care Financing Review* (December 1988, annual supplement): 97–102.

Wallack, Stanley S., and Marc A. Cohen. "Trends in Financing and Delivery of Care." *Provider* (May 1987): 10–14.

Wan, Thomas T.H. "Health Consequences of Major Role Losses in Later Life." *Research on Aging* (December 1984): 469–489.

Washington Business Group on Health. *The Corporate Perspective on Long Term Care.* Survey Report, December 1987.

Wattenberg, Ben J. *The Birth Dearth.* New York, NY: Pharos Books, Inc., 1987.

Weinrobe, Maurice D. *Home Equity Conversion for the Elderly: An Analysis for Lenders.* Washington, DC: American Association of Retired Persons, 1986.

————. "Home Equity Conversion and the Financing of Long-Term Care." *Health Care Financing Review* (December 1988, annual supplement): 113–115.

Weissert, William G. "Estimating the Long-Term Care Population: Prevalence Rates and Selected Characteristics." *Health Care Financing Review* (Summer 1985): 83–91.

————. "The National Channeling Demonstration: What We Knew, Know Now, and Still Need to Know." *HSR: Health Services Research* (April 1988): 175–187.

White, Lon [R.], William S. Cartwright, Joan [C.] Cornoni-Huntley, and Dwight B. Brock. "Geriatric Epidemiology." *Annual Review of Gerontology and Geriatrics* (July 1986).

Wiener, Joshua M. "Financing and Organizational Options for Long-Term-Care Reform: Background and Issues." *Bulletin of the New York Academy of Medicine* (January-February 1986): 75–86.

Wiener, Joshua M., Ray Hanley, Denise [A.] Spence, and Diana Coupard. "Money, Money, Who's Got The Money? Financing Options For Long-Term Care." Paper presented at a conference on Health in Aging: Sociological Issues and Policy Directions at the State University of New York in Albany, NY, April 18–19, 1986.

William M. Mercer Meidinger Hansen, Inc. *Long-term Care: The Newest Employee Benefit.* New York, NY: William M. Mercer Meidinger Hansen, Inc., 1988.

Williams, T. Franklin, John G. Hill, Matthew E. Fairbank, and Kenneth G. Knox. "Appropriate Placement of the Chronically Ill and Aged: A Successful Approach by Evaluation." *Journal of the American Medical Association* (10 December 1973): 1332–1335.

Winfield, Fairlee E. "Workplace Solutions for Women Under Eldercare Pressure." *Personnel* (July 1987): 31–39.

Wingard, Deborah L., Denise Williams Jones, and Robert M. Kaplan. "Institutional Care Utilization by the Elderly: A Critical Review." *The Gerontologist* (April 1987): 156–163.

Winklevoss, Howard E., and Alwyn V. Powell. *Continuing Care Retirement Communities: An Empirical, Financial, and Legal Analysis.* Homewood, IL: Richard D. Irwin, Inc., 1984.

Wisensale, Steven K., and Michael D. Allison. "An Analysis of 1987 State Family Leave Legislation: Implications for Caregivers of the Elderly." *The Gerontologist* (December 1988): 779–785.

Wooldridge, Judith, and Jennifer Schore. "The Evaluation of the National Long Term Care Demonstration: 7. The Effect of Channeling on the Use of Nursing Homes, Hospitals, and Other Medial Services." *HSR: Health Services Research* (April 1988): 119–127.

Wyszewianski, Leon. "Financially Catastrophic and High-Cost Cases: Definitions, Distinctions, and Their Implications of Policy Formulation." *Inquiry* (Winter 1986): 382–394.

Yaggy, Duncan, ed. *Health Care for the Poor and Elderly: Meeting the Challenge.* Durham, NC: Duke University Press, 1984.

Ycas, Martynas A., and Susan Grad. "Income of Retirement-Aged Persons in the United States." *Social Security Bulletin* (July 1987): 5–14.

Yordi, Cathleen L. "Case Management in the Social Health Maintenance Organization Demonstrations." *Health Care Financing Review* (December 1988, annual supplement): 83–88.

Zawadski, Rick T., and Catherine Eng. "Case Management in Capitated Long-Term Care." *Health Care Financing Review* (December 1988, annual supplement): 75–81.

Zopf, Paul E., Jr. *America's Older Population.* Houston, TX: Cap and Gown Press, Inc., 1986.

# Index

## M

361

construction of, 78, 85
discharges from, 48, 49
employer-provided plans and,
130
expenditures for, 4, 35, 37, 45–
46, 137, 150, 159, 197, 198,
266, 290
—SDAT and, 34
"heavy care" patients, 85, 87
ICF/SNF distinctions, 75–76,
89–91
impact of Medicaid policies
on, 84–86
lengths of stay, 45–46, 48
Medicare/Medicaid standards,
83–84
number of facilities and beds,
76
—distribution of, 78, 86–87
ownership of, 76
payment sources, 52, 137
—private insurance, 4, 45, 137,
197
quality of care, 87–91
staffing of, 78, 84
utilization of, 46–49, 61, 71,
93–97, 213
welfare system and, 78

## O

Omnibus Budget Reconciliation
Act of 1981 (OBRA '81), 151
Omnibus Budget Reconciliation
Act of 1987 (OBRA '87)
ICF/SNF distinctions, 89–91
Medicaid waivers, 146
Older Americans Act, 150, 151–152
Older Women's League, 297
Out-of-pocket expenditures, 38–42
employer-provided plans and,
130–133
nursing home care and, 45, 46,
137

## P

Pension and retirement income
simulation model (PRISM), 184–
190
Pension coverage, 240, 241
Pension recipiency, 19
Personal care homes, 92
Physician services
expenditures, 35–37, 150
—out-of-pocket, 38
Portability
long-term care insurance and,
236–237, 275, 276
Postretirement health benefits see
Retiree health benefits
Poverty
catastrophic health expenditures and, 126
disability and, 190
health insurance coverage and,
135
rates, 167–172
widowhood and, 175–176
Preferred provider organizations
(PPOs), 216–217
PRISM see Pension and retirement
income simulation model
Productivity, 16, 28, 189, 249, 257
Public employees, 241
Public policy
aging population and, 16
long-term care and, 205–206,
239, 251, 265, 166–168, 271–
278
Medicaid long-term care
financing and, 293–295

## Q

Quality of care, 267
home health care and, 98
nursing homes and, 87–91

## R

Race
nursing home utilization and,
46, 49, 61

363

nursing home investigation,
88–89
U.S. Veterans Administration pro-
grams, 150, 153
Uninsured, 135–137, 254
University of Maryland Center on
Aging, 251–252

## V

Vesting
long-term care insurance and,
236–237
Veterans, 153
Villers Foundation, 252, 297
Virginia home equity program,
156, 291
Voluntary employee beneficiary
association (VEBA), 234

## W

Wages, 188–189, 250
Washington Business Group on
Health, 236
Wealth, 176–183
disability and, 190–191
Widowhood poverty, 175–176
Women
as informal caregivers, 257–258
labor force participation of,
17–19, 243, 246–248
Medicaid eligibility and, 159–
164
nursing home utilization and,
46, 61
poverty rates and, 167–168,
170–172
PRISM simulations and, 187,
189
wages and, 250